·四川大学精品立项教材·

公共卫生口译教程

Interpreting for Public Health: A Course Book

主　编　秦　丹
副主编　杨　敏　何　琳

四川大学出版社

责任编辑:余　芳
责任校对:周　洁
封面设计:墨创文化
责任印制:王　炜

图书在版编目(CIP)数据

公共卫生口译教程 / 秦丹主编. —成都：四川大学出版社，2017.1
四川大学精品立项教材
ISBN 978-7-5690-0347-5

Ⅰ.①公… Ⅱ.①秦… Ⅲ.①公共卫生-英语-口译-高等学校-教材 Ⅳ.①R126.4

中国版本图书馆 CIP 数据核字（2017）第 012229 号

书名　**公共卫生口译教程**
Gonggong Weisheng Kouyi Jiaocheng

主　　编　秦　丹
出　　版　四川大学出版社
地　　址　成都市一环路南一段 24 号 (610065)
发　　行　四川大学出版社
书　　号　ISBN 978-7-5690-0347-5
印　　刷　郫县犀浦印刷厂
成品尺寸　185 mm×260 mm
印　　张　34.75
字　　数　826 千字
版　　次　2017 年 10 月第 1 版
印　　次　2017 年 10 月第 1 次印刷
定　　价　110.00 元

◆读者邮购本书,请与本社发行科联系。
电话:(028)85408408/(028)85401670/
(028)85408023　邮政编码:610065
◆本社图书如有印装质量问题,请
寄回出版社调换。
◆网址:http://www.scupress.net

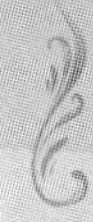

编写说明

公共卫生领域是各国交流的活跃领域之一，与商务活动一样，有专业性。无疑，国际公共卫生活动中的口译行为专业性较强。

翻译硕士专业学位（MTI）的目标是培养应用型翻译人才。翻译硕士专业学位教育指导委员会颁布的指导性教学大纲规定了必修课之外的选修课程。根据这一要求，本教材设计在培训双语知识的过程中，凸显口译训练的专业化与应用性。本教材编撰者认为，课堂上专业针对性的训练可为学生在一个特定领域打下基础，引导学生分流到专业性强的口译领域。考虑到与现有MTI方面其他口译类教材之间的衔接以及在专业方面的区别，本教材侧重公共卫生领域的专业针对性。

本教材适用于选修课或口译工作坊，教材使用对象为修过基础口译的口译方向研究生及高年级本科生。由于在基础口译阶段，各种基础教材对口译原理都有较为详尽的介绍，并且以口译技巧为主的口译专题练习也是教学的重点，因此在口译选修课这一阶段，教学应配合基础课程，在继续强化口译的准确度、流畅度的同时，增加练习量，均衡翻译速度，提高学生在口译过程中的综合掌控能力。因此，本教材针对不少学生抓不住文章讲话重点的弱点，将一些文章用于复述或详细的摘要练习，而在篇章安排上尽量编排相近的内容，以使学生对所学内容更加熟悉。为了提供背景知识，每单元以主题相关知识介绍开始，然后将两篇英语文章作为总结性的复述练习。为了让学生学会更完整地掌握篇章内容，练习后附有复述要点提示。接着是词汇准备，以及供英译汉、汉译英翻译练习用各两篇文章。为了便于教师教学和学生自练，每一单元后都有参考答案。考虑到教材可能也会用于医学英语专业以及医学生的口译练习，本教材仍然编排一般性的口译理论与口译技巧。

需要说明的是，本书不是一本公共卫生专业的书，而是一本为英语专业口译方向学生编写的涉及公共卫生领域的书。在选材上，教材注意收集真实的语料，包括出自诸如新闻发布会、会议讲话的语料等，尽量反映口译真实场景。材料内容尽量涵盖公共卫生领域有代表性的专题。在不同专题之下，兼顾英译汉、汉译英训练。

需要说明的另一点是，笔译的“信、达、雅”原则虽是文字翻译的基本原则，但本书的参考答案在遵循“信”这一原则的同时根据“达”的原则带有实际口译场景之中的“概括”或“解释”之痕迹。

本书主编秦丹为四川大学外国语学院副教授、硕士生导师，加拿大多伦多大学访问学者，四川大学国家级精品课程“英汉口译”主讲教师；所编教材《综合大学英语》第六册（外研社）曾获四川大学优秀教材奖；曾参加MTI教材《交替传译》（外研社）的编写。副主编杨敏为四川大学外国语学院讲师，主讲专业英语写作和综合英语，多次参与文学作品笔译和卫生系统口译工作，曾发表数篇美国文学研究性文章。副主编何琳为四川大学外国语学院讲师，长期在四川省公共卫生领域担任口译译员，参译了三本医学教育、公共卫生教材。另外三位参编人员，王艳妮、胡益鑫、魏梦颖，系四川大学外国语学院口译硕士专业研究生。

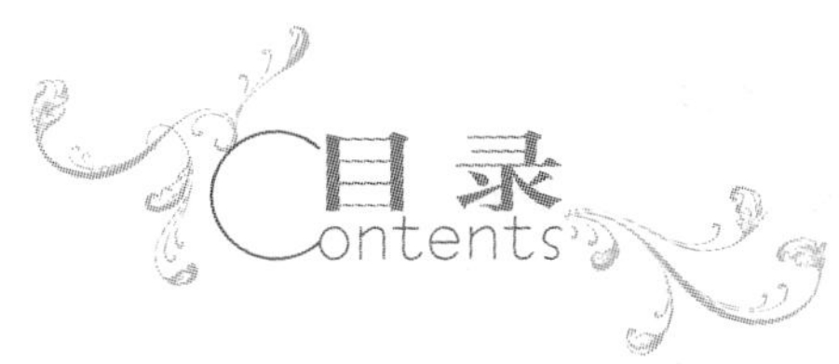
目录
Contents

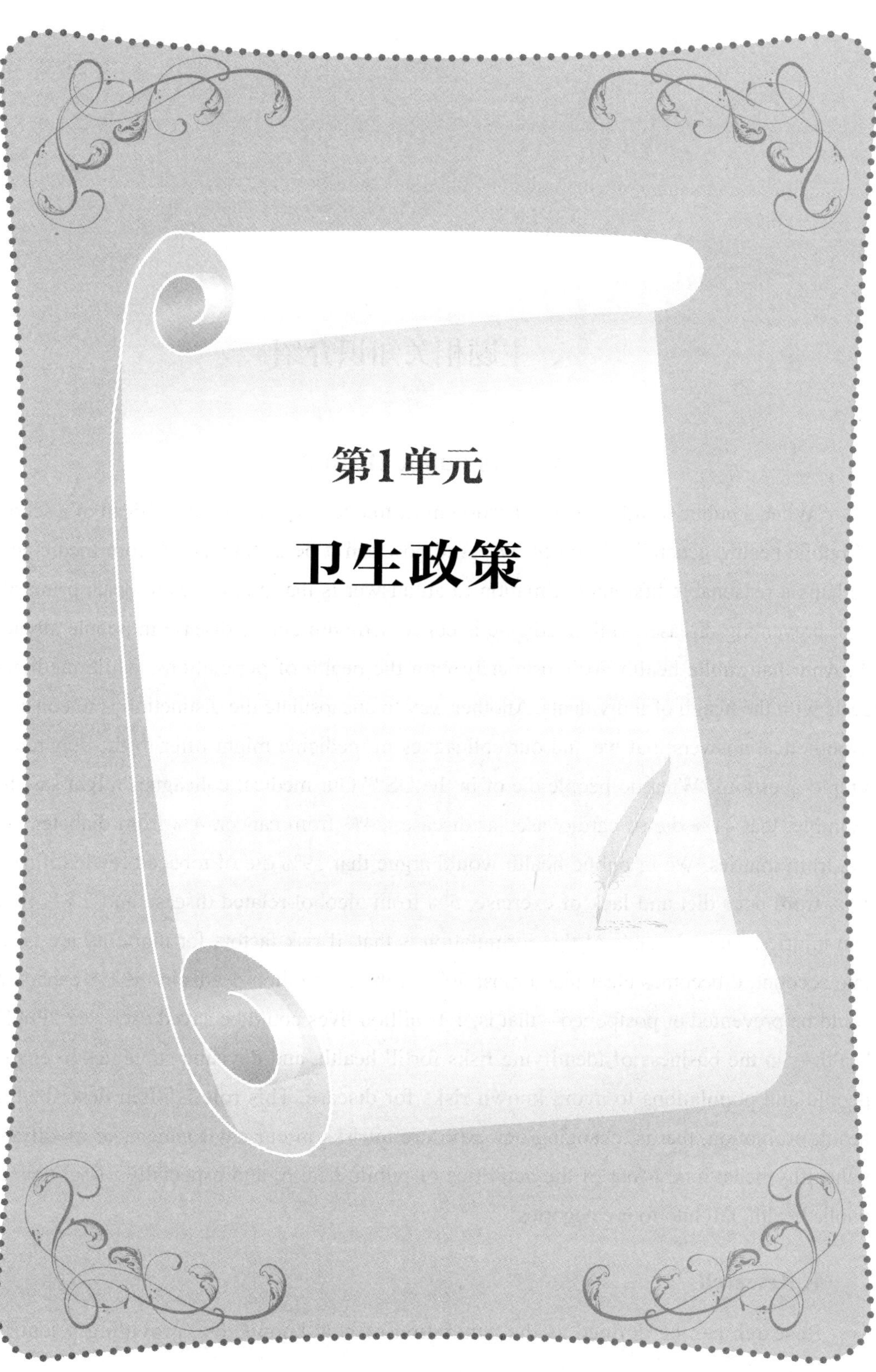

第1单元

卫生政策

一、主题相关知识介绍

What Is Public Health?

"What is public health?" is the question most frequently asked of every dean of a school of public health, generally followed by, "And how can it be distinguished from medicine?" Perhaps a reasonable first approximation to an answer is that public health deals primarily with preventing disease, while medicine is concerned with curing disease in people already ill. And that public health deals primarily with the health of populations, while medicine deals with the health of individuals. Another way to encapsulate the distinction is to consider hypothetical answers that we and our colleagues in medicine might offer to the apparently simple question, "What do people die of in the US?" Our medical colleagues might say, for example, that 41% die of cardiovascular disease, 24% from cancer, 4% from diabetes and 8% from injuries. We in public health would argue that 19% die of tobacco-related illness, 14% from poor diet and lack of exercise, 5% from alcohol-related disease and 2.5% from gun injuries. The relevance of this formulation is that, if risk factors for mortality are taken into account, it becomes clear that almost 50% of the 2.3 million deaths in the US each year could be prevented or postponed—that is, 1.1 million lives could be saved each year. Public health is in the business of identifying risks for ill health, and devising strategies to enable people and populations to avoid known risks for disease. This role is often described as health promotion, that is, changing our exposure to risks in our environment, or modifying unhealthy behaviors. Most of the activities of public health, and especially of schools of public health, fall into four categories.

1. Research

Research can be defined as the generation of new knowledge, providing scientific evidence for decision-making at the individual or societal level. The discipline of public health embraces a wide variety of approaches to knowledge of the public's health and risk factors for disease. These include epidemiological and statistical sciences to look for disease associations and to design and analyze clinical trials and interventions; laboratory science to elucidate mechanisms of disease and risk; social science to uncover social determinants of illness and behavioral and societal changes that result in better health; and finally policy sciences, particularly to analyze the economic costs of illness, the costs and cost effectiveness of interventions, and the quality of health systems. As Julio Frank says, "A health system is a population's organized social response to its health problems... It represents the common vehicle through which all interventions we talk about are actually delivered to actual populations."

2. Training

If half of the deaths in the US and perhaps a greater fraction globally can be prevented or postponed, there is a huge mission for training in public health. Public health training is essential not only for degree students in public health and medicine but also for police, firefighters, social workers, teachers, national leaders, and most importantly, the public. It is a sad fact that fewer than half of the workforce in state, county and municipal public health departments in the US have any formal training in public health. Yet they bear responsibility for decisions that affect the health of millions. The public health workforce has become far more diverse in recent years. In the case of graduates of the Harvard School of Public Health, about one-third serve the public through federal, state, county and municipal health departments; one-third work for the private sector in HMOs, hospitals, consulting companies, and the pharmaceutical industry; and the remaining one-third become motivated to go into research and academic public health.

3. Communication

If public health is to fulfill its responsibility to prevent death and illness and promote health, it will have to do a great deal better in communicating risks in ways that inform and motivate, rather than scaring people. It is crucial for our leaders and the public to have access to accurate information to tell the truth in ways that are empowering, not terrifying. And with only 2% or less of health care dollars spent on public health, we must do a better job of explaining what we do and why it counts.

4. Practice

All the knowledge from the laboratory and from populations will be squandered if it is not put into practice in ways to improve the health of the public. There is a greatly underappreciated but enormously dedicated group of people doing the work of public health. They can, of course, only be effective if our elected officials and policy makers understand their importance and support their work. What have been the achievements of public health in the last century? Life expectancy is perhaps the crudest, least sensitive index of health (one is scored as either dead or alive); nevertheless, life expectancy has risen in the US from 47 years in 1900 to 77 in 1999. How can we account for that? The Centers for Disease Control and Prevention (CDC) summarized the major achievements of public health in the US during the last century as follows:

10 Major Achievements of Public Health

- Vaccination and childhood immunization
- Motor vehicle safety
- Safer workplaces
- Control of infectious diseases
- Decline in deaths from coronary heart disease and stroke
- Safer and healthier foods
- Healthier mothers and babies
- Family planning
- Fluoridation of drinking water
- Recognition of tobacco as a health hazard

Source: Adapted from Barry R. Bloom, School of Public Health, Harvard University

二、技巧指导：口译的质量概念

在开始本课程的学习之前，我们需要首先明确口译质量有哪些必要的评价根据，以使自己心中有数。本教材聚焦于连续传译技能（Consecutive Interpreting Skills），因此这里只聚焦连续传译质量概念。

从听众的角度看，普通人有以下几种需求：（1）译员能够在听完原文之后迅速开始翻译，不拖沓。从听完不太明白甚至完全不知所云的原文到翻译开始之间，观众的心理等待时间大约只有2～3秒，总是超过这个时间，观众就会感到翻译拖沓、冗长，甚至为译员着急或怀疑译员是否能够胜任翻译工作。（2）译文准确、流畅。由于口译的现场性与即时性，观众听到明白无误的内容是一个基本的需求，这就要求译员将原文主题、精神和论点忠实地表达出来。（3）用词准确，干净利落，没有多余的辅助词。“嗯”“啊”“就是”“他说”等词都很累赘，让人感到厌烦，译员要避免。（4）语速适中，不快也不慢，让人轻松听明白。（5）声音干净清晰，吐词清楚，音量适中。声音沙哑、过于低沉都会影响吐词的清晰度，使人听得吃力；音量过大或过小都会使人感到疲惫或费力。（6）译员面部表情自然放松，或面带微笑；无论是站还是坐，体态自然。这样听众心里便不会紧张，能够轻松地聆听讲话。

从专业角度看，口译的质量取决于即时、准确、流畅。即时的意义即迅速启动翻译，前文已讲。准确的概念涵盖以下几个方面：主题准确、精神准确、论点准确、风格准确、词语准确、数字准确、表达准确、语速准确以及口吻准确。关于流畅的概念，除了与听众要求契合的起译迅速、译文准确、用词利落、吐词清楚、语速适中、音量适中外，还要风格近似，语音语调正确。以全国口译大赛要求为例，大赛考察的要点是：（1）完整、准确地译出原语信息，无错译、漏译；（2）熟练运用口译技巧，如笔记、信息重组、逻辑处理、语言转换等；（3）语言表达规范，语流顺畅，语速适中；（4）语体符合原语的基本特点，无明显偏移；（5）语音语调正确，吐字清晰。

从比赛的具体评分标准，可以看到细化的要求：

表1-1　口译评分标准

评分参考标准	90～100分	80～89分	70～79分	60～69分	59分及以下
信息传达（50%）	完整传达源语的信息，语气和风格与源语一致，逻辑清晰，术语、数字准确。	除个别次要信息有遗漏外，源语的全部重要信息都得到传达。语气和风格与源语基本一致，逻辑清晰，术语、数字准确。	有少量漏译但无严重错译，准确度一般，但能够基本传达源语信息。	有个别重大漏译或错译现象。部分信息含混，但总体上基本可以达意。	漏译、错译非常严重。目标语译文不能达意，曲解或歪曲原文要点和精神。

续表1-1

评分参考标准	90~100分	80~89分	70~79分	60~69分	59分及以下
技巧运用（30%）	目标语表达流畅，能够综合运用口译技巧，选词贴切，表达符合目的语习惯，语法无误，语音语调准确、清晰、地道。	目标语表达流畅，能够使用口译技巧，语言规范，基本无语法错误，语音语调准确。	较少使用灵活口译技巧，目标语表达比较死板。有不流畅或不地道的情况，语音语调比较准确。	目标语几乎没有灵活运用口译技巧，译文僵硬，不符合目标语表达习惯，语音语调不太准确。	大量语法和用词错误。句子生搬硬套，表达十分不地道，语音语调不准确。
职业素养（20%）	状态稳健，充分展示职业口译工作者的心理素质和整体风貌，非言语交流能力强。	状态大方得体，心理素质比较稳定，具备从事职业口译工作的潜力。	不怯场，能够较好地完成比赛，能积极主动地进行非言语交流。	能够完成比赛，没有重大的临场失误，有一定的非言语交流。	心理素质差，紧张怯场，基本上没有目光交流和身体语言。

三、词汇准备

Text 1

universal health care 全民医疗保健
National Health Service （英国）国民医疗服务制度
social solidarity 社会团结
commitment 承诺
preventable and treatable 可预防的，可治疗的
impoverish 使……陷于贫困
Bill and Melinda Gates Foundation 比尔和梅林达·盖茨基金会
United Nations Population Fund 联合国人口基金
make... accountable 使……承担起责任
hospitalization 住院治疗

Text 2

legal entity 法人实体

the Public Health Agency of Canada (PHAC) 加拿大公共卫生局

advantaged and disadvantaged 优势的和弱势的

the Human Pathogens and Toxins Act (HPTA) 人类病原体和毒素法案

all levels of government (provincial, territorial and municipal) 各级政府（省级、地区级、市级）

World Health Organization (WHO) 世界卫生组织

Assistant Deputy Minister (ADM) 副部长助理

Infectious Disease Prevention and Control (IDPC) 传染病预防和控制

Health Promotion and Chronic Disease Prevention (HPCDP) 健康促进与慢性病预防

Emergency Management and Corporate Affairs (EMCA) 应急管理和企业事务

Text 3

inextricably 密不可分地

WHO's Constitution 世界卫生组织章程

attainable standard 可达标准

aspirations 愿望

macro-economic stability 宏观经济的稳定

health financing 卫生筹资，健康筹资

cost-effectiveness 成本效益

resource allocation 资源分配

confidentiality 保密

equity 平等性

social exclusion 社会排斥

vulnerable population 弱势群体

benchmarks and indicators 基准和指标

enshrine 铭记

Text 4

the Affordable Care Act 平价医疗法案

health legislation 卫生立法

the National Prevention Council 国家预防委员会

National Prevention Strategy 国家预防策略

drug abuse 滥用药物

vaccinations 接种疫苗

prevention 预防
predictor 预测
empower 授权
disparity 差异
the Strategic Directions 战略方向
evidence-based (medicine) 循证（医学）

Text 5

新农合制度 the new rural cooperative medical system
健康风险保护 health risk protection
住院费用支付 payment for hospital expense
重特大疾病保障机制 security mechanism for serious diseases
医疗救助 medical assistance
异地即时结算 offsite immediate settlement
强筋健骨 strengthening the muscles and bones
基本药物 essential drugs
综合评价体系 comprehensive evaluation system
多渠道补偿机制 multi-channel compensation mechanism
定编定岗不定人，全员按岗竞聘 fixed number of personnel, fixed number of posts, and all staff obtain posts through competition
改善群众就医感受 improve patients' experience of hospital visits
我们要进一步凝心聚力，攻坚克难，奋力拼搏 we must further concentrate our thoughts and strength, tackle tough problems, and work hard

Text 6

人均期望寿命 the average life expectancy
孕产妇 pregnant and lying-in women
死亡率 the mortality rate
基本医疗保障覆盖面 the coverage of basic medical insurance
消费结构的转变升级 the change and upgrading of consumption structure
后顾之忧 worries
扩大内需 expand domestic demand
公益性质 commonweal nature
保基本，强基层，建机制 insuring essentials, strengthening services for the grass-

roots, and establishing mechanism

优化资源配置和利用 optimizing resource allocation and utilization

高血压 hypertension

糖尿病 diabetes mellitus

心脑血管疾病 cardiovascular and cerebrovascular diseases

恶性肿瘤 malignant tumor

慢性非传染性疾病 chronic non-communicable diseases

乙肝疫苗接种 hepatitis B vaccination

宫颈癌 cervical cancer

乳腺癌 breast cancer

育龄妇女 women of childbearing age

叶酸 folic acid

四、摘要练习

请听下面英语语篇，第一篇用源语言复述此段主要信息逻辑点及层次，第二篇用译入语复述此段主要信息逻辑点及层次。注意信息点之间的逻辑联系。

Text 1

Universal Health Care

Andrew Lansley, World Health Association[1]

21 May 2012

I am delighted to be here today to talk on the vital topic of universal health care.

Universal healthcare has been at the heart of the National Health Service in the United Kingdom for over 60 years. And it will remain so. Universal access to a comprehensive health service—free, based on need, is part of our social solidarity and an essential basis for improving the population's health.

When we came into government two years ago we made two very clear commitments.

1 本书选用的演讲、讲话、文件材料的作者，其职务近年来有些变动，因部分作者的单位、职务变动情况无法明确，为全书统一，均标注的是发表演讲、讲话，发布文件时所在单位及职务。

Firstly that we would increase the budget of our National Health Service in real terms, and secondly that we would increase our spending on development to meet our historic 0.7% commitment. I am proud of our performance on both of those commitments.

Across the globe, each year, tens of millions of poor people fall ill and die due to diseases and conditions that are preventable and treatable. Out-of-pocket costs stop many of these people getting the help they need. The solution is efficient and effective healthcare that does not exclude or impoverish the poor. Governments have a duty to manage this.

In July, the UK government and the Bill and Melinda Gates Foundation, with the United Nations Population Fund, and others, will host an international family planning summit in London. The aim is to launch a global movement to give 120 million extra women in the world's poorest countries access to contraceptive information, services and supplies by 2020. I am sure many of your governments will wish to participate. And I am extremely pleased that our Director General will be playing a key role in the event.

Back home our investment in the National Health Service is strengthening our universal primary care infrastructure. We are focused on developing preventative services, on early interventions and minimizing unnecessary hospitalization. We are reforming the National Health Service to empower clinical leaders to deliver outcomes for patients which are amongst the best in the world. We are giving more autonomy to healthcare providers; but we are making them increasingly accountable for the results they achieve.

We are reforming our public health system, to ensure we are able to tackle the social determinants of health. Nationally and locally, improving the health of the population is a government-wide responsibility. We are recognizing and acting on the effects which employment, education, housing and the environment have on health outcomes.

Our approach to tackling public health issues is to maximize our impact at key moments in people's lives, for example, through support in maternity and the early years of children. We are also focused on the major risk factors such as obesity, tobacco, drugs, alcohol and sexual health. We will be strong and effective in tobacco control. With food, drink and retail industries we are forming a partnership, based on a shared understanding that public health is everyone's business and that by co-operation we can achieve more progress, more quickly, towards an environment which enables consumers to lead a healthier lifestyle.

We have a busy week ahead of us. Our agenda here underlines the importance of the WHO being the best it can be. We need the WHO to facilitate the sharing of ideas and strategies for member states to build strong universal healthcare systems. We need continued action to tackle emerging and continuing public health threats. When these things happen, we must be ready to act collectively.

The reform of WHO, supporting these objectives, will enable us to make more progress in improving the health of all our peoples. A strong WHO, ready to face these challenges in the 21st Century is vital. It is in all our interests to ensure the reforms of WHO are advanced this week.

复述要点提示（主要信息逻辑点及层次）

Universal healthcare enables universal access to a free comprehensive health service. It is part of social solidarity and an essential basis for improving the population's health.

In the world, tens of millions of poor people fall ill and die of preventable and treatable diseases, because they cannot access help they need. The solution is efficient healthcare that covers all.

In July, the UK government and the Bill and Melinda Gates Foundation, with the United Nations Population Fund, etc., will host an international family planning summit in London. The aim is to launch a global movement to give 120 million women in the world's poorest countries access to contraceptive information, services and supplies by 2020.

Two years ago we made two clear commitments: to increase the budget of National Health Service, and increase spending on development to meet our historic 0.7% commitment. Our investment in the National Health Service is now strengthening our universal primary care infrastructure. We are developing preventative services, on early interventions and minimizing unnecessary hospitalization.

We are reforming the National Health Service. We give more autonomy to healthcare providers, but making them more accountable for the results they achieve. We are reforming our public health system, by recognizing and acting on the effects which employment, education, housing and the environment have on health outcomes.

We are maximizing our impact on various issues, such as on supporting maternity, the early years of children, obesity, tobacco, drugs,. alcohol and sexual health. We are strengthening tobacco control. We are forming partnership with food, drink and retail industries.

Our agenda here underlines the importance of the WHO. We need the WHO to facilitate the sharing of ideas and strategies for member states to build strong universal healthcare systems to collectively tackle public health threats. The reform of WHO support all these objectives. Let's ensure the reforms of WHO are advanced this week.

Text 2

Canadian Public Health Agency and Its Mission

Confirmed as a legal entity in December 2006 by the Public Health Agency of Canada Act and established in September 2004 in part as a response to the SARS outbreak in 2003, the Public Health Agency of Canada (PHAC) is the main Government of Canada agency responsible for public health in Canada. PHAC's primary goal is to strengthen Canada's capacity to protect and improve the health of Canadians and to help reduce pressures on the health-care system. To do this, the Agency is working to build an effective public health system that enables Canadians to achieve better health and well-being in their daily lives by promoting good health, helping prevent and control chronic diseases and injury, and protecting Canadians from infectious diseases and other threats to their health. PHAC is also committed to reducing health disparities between the most advantaged and disadvantaged Canadians.

To address concerns about human pathogens and toxins, Parliament passed the Human Pathogens and Toxins Act (HPTA) in 2009. PHAC is charged with enforcing the Act and developing a program and regulatory framework. Because public health is a shared responsibility, PHAC works in close collaboration with all levels of government (provincial, territorial and municipal) to build on each other's skills and strengths. The Agency also works closely with non-government organizations, including civil society and business, and other countries and international organizations like the World Health Organization (WHO) to share knowledge, expertise and experiences.

PHAC is one of the six departments and agencies that make up the federal government's Health Portfolio and reports to Parliament through the Minister of Health. PHAC is managed by the Chief Public Health Officer of Canada, currently Dr. David Butler-Jones, who plays a dual role:

● Deputy Minister in the federal public service, heading the Agency and advising the Minister of Health on matters of public health and the function of the Agency; and

● Lead federal public health professional tasked with communicating directly with Canadians and governments on important public health matters.

PHAC consists of three main branches, each led by an Assistant Deputy Minister (ADM):

● Infectious Disease Prevention and Control (IDPC)

● Health Promotion and Chronic Disease Prevention (HPCDP)

- Emergency Management and Corporate Affairs (EMCA)

Together with these ADMs, key advisors and offices report directly to the CPHO and Associate Deputy Minister. To maintain the knowledge and skills needed to develop and deliver the public health advice and tools required by Canadians, the Agency relies on the efforts of its dedicated staff. PHAC's approximately 2,700 employees work across Canada in a wide range of operational, scientific, technical and administrative positions.

The PHAC mission is to promote and protect the health of Canadians through leadership, partnership, innovation and action in public health. Its vision is "Healthy Canadians and communities in a healthier world".

We have the following values:

Leadership: We value, at the organization level, leaders who foster long-term planning, strategic thinking, open communication and who create an atmosphere of enthusiasm and team collaboration. At the individual level, we take ownership and exercise accountability in everyday responsibilities.

Healthy Work Environment: We value an organization that openly acknowledges and recognizes the contributions of its employees, that is supportive of equity, diversity and inclusiveness, and encourages a balance between work life and personal/family life.

Ethical Behaviour: We value a workplace that fosters respect, fairness and equality and where people, at all levels, demonstrate integrity, honesty and trust in fulfilling their roles and responsibilities and their internal and external relationships.

Commitment to Excellence: We value excellence in achieving the mandate of PHAC through professional behaviour, continuous learning, career development activities, creativity and innovation and a continued commitment to the principles and the science of public health.

Dedication to Service: We value respectful and high quality service to all those with whom we interact on a daily basis; we care about and take pride in our work and in the contribution the organization makes to society in reducing health disparities in Canada and the world.

We value commitment to Excellence and dedication to Service.

The role of PHAC is to:

Promote health; prevent and control chronic diseases and injuries; prevent and control infectious diseases; prepare for and respond to public health emergencies; serve as a central point for sharing Canada's expertise with the rest of the world; apply international research and development to Canada's public health programs; and strengthen intergovernmental collaboration on public health and facilitate national approaches to public health policy and planning.

Public health focuses on the entire population at both the individual and the community level. It encompasses a range of activities performed by all three levels of government (federal, provincial/territorial, and municipal) in collaboration with a wide variety of stakeholders and communities across the country.

Through our research, programs and services, our goals are to bring about healthier Canadians, reduced health disparities, and a stronger capacity to deliver on and support public health activities.

As part of PHAC's program activities, the Agency uses Grants and Contributions to fund community, voluntary and not-for-profit agencies to support government policies and priorities. PHAC currently has 25 Grants and Contributions programs which fund approximately 1,200 projects across the country and account for almost 33 percent of PHAC's annual budget.

复述要点提示（主要信息逻辑点及层次）

成立于2004年的加拿大公共卫生署（PHAC）是一个法律实体，是加拿大政府机构，主要负责加拿大的公共卫生事宜。该机构的宗旨是强化加拿大在保护和改善加拿大人的健康方面的能力，帮助减轻卫生保健系统的压力，建立一个有效的公共卫生体系，以促进身体健康，协助预防控制慢性疾病和损伤，减少传染病和其他威胁。它致力于减小加拿大的优势和弱势群体之间的健康差距。

PHAC负责执行人类病原体和毒素法（HPTA）并建立监管框架。它与省政府、区域政府、市政府、非政府组织、民间团体、企业、其他国家和国际组织密切合作。PHAC是联邦政府健康机构的六个部门之一，通过卫生部长向议会报告，由加拿大首席公共卫生长官管理。该卫生长官既是联邦公共服务部副部长，主管卫生公署并在公共卫生事宜和机构功能方面向卫生部长提供建议，同时领导担责的联邦公共卫生专业人士，就重大公共健康问题与市民和政府进行沟通。

PHAC有三个主要分支，有三名副部长助理（ADM）。三个分支分别为传染病预防和控制部（IDPC）、健康促进和慢性病预防部（HPCDP）、应急管理及部门事务部（EMCA）。其主要办事处直接向CPHO和副部长助理汇报。

我们的价值观如下：1. 看重那些有长远规划、战略思维、开放性的沟通方式，认同能够创造热情氛围并能够引领团队协作的领导。在个体方面，我们在日常工作中履行自己的职责。2. 看重健康的工作环境，在此环境中员工的贡献得到公开的承认，机构公正待人，宽以待人，支持多样性，鼓励员工平衡工作与个人以及家庭生活之间的关系。3. 看重道德行为，在工作场所培养尊重他人、公平待人与平等待人的意识。所有员工都表现出正直、诚实和值得信赖的品质。4. 看重通过职业行为表现出精益求精的工作，看重不断学习、职业发展活动、创造力以及持续的贡献精神。5. 重视服务奉献，为我们的工作感到骄傲，为机构对社会的贡献而感到骄傲。

公共卫生为全体居民服务，包括由联邦、省和市政府组织的活动，以及与利益相关者和社区活动一起举行的活动。卫生署利用拨款和捐款资助社区、志愿者机构和非营利机构，以支持政府的政策和优先事项。

五、英译汉练习

Text 3

Health, Dignity and Human Rights

Director-General, Keynote Address at the 7th Conference of European Health Ministers

Oslo, Norway

12 June 2003

Secretary-General, distinguished ministers, friends and colleagues,

You have chosen a critically important theme for your meeting: health, dignity and human rights. Three sets of ideas that are inextricably linked, and that are central to the development of health systems and services, both in Europe and throughout the rest of the world.

Fifty-five years ago, the creators of WHO's Constitution stated that the enjoyment of the highest attainable standard of health is a fundamental right of every human being. In our daily work—and in yours as health ministers—we are all striving to make this right a reality, and turn aspirations and policies into practice.

Rarely is this easy. The pressures we all are facing are intense. Ageing populations, rapid technological developments, increasing public expectations, all these factors generate pressure to increase health spending.

But convincing colleagues in treasuries and ministries of finance—whose prime concern is macro-economic stability—can be hard.

We have to be able to deliver results. Better health outcomes are what matters in the end. But, how they are achieved, and who benefits, are equally important. This is where human rights and the right to health can help. We are all engaged in debates about the future of health financing. How do we increase cost-effectiveness in resource allocation and promote efficiency in spending whilst, at the same time, maintaining solidarity in the way we are funding the services?

The key point here is that, while securing adequate financing is critical, ensuring that the burden of costs is shared fairly is equally important.

Similarly, we are not just concerned with access to health care, but with how people are treated when they need services.

We regard responsiveness of health systems—which includes ensuring confidentiality, reducing waiting times, involvement in decision making—as a proper and legitimate goal in its own right.

Here, there is a direct link with human rights. For, at the root of the concern for equality and freedom from discrimination in human rights thinking and practice, lies the notion of human dignity: the equal and inherent value of every human being.

In recent years, we have become clearer as to what the right to health should actually mean. First and foremost, it is an inclusive right: it is not just about health care services—it is also about the underlying determinants of ill health.

These are much broader and include access to safe drinking water, adequate sanitation, a supply of safe and nutritious food, healthy occupational and environmental conditions and access to information, including information about sexual and reproductive health.

Chair,

At the heart of the primary health care and Health for All movement, which has been so influential in shaping health policies in Europe, lies a concern for equity.

But, we all know that, in every country represented here today, there are groups of people that are missing out on what our health systems have to offer. The human rights framework can help us address the needs of these groups.

The causes of social exclusion are many and varied. Some groups, such as ethnic minorities and the economically disadvantaged get overlooked when we work with national averages. But, there are also those whose needs are obvious, but whose cause is politically unpopular—I think here of irregular migrants, for example.

Paying attention to vulnerable population groups constitutes an essential element in a human rights approach because the right to health demands giving priority attention to those most in need. This is important in itself, but the fact that these rights are part of an internationally recognized legal framework also places an obligation on governments.

The right to health is a goal for which all governments, rich and poor, should strive. Of course, this cannot be achieved overnight. All nations face constraints, in many cases posed by limited resources. This is why the principle of progressive realization is central to the achievement of all human rights.

But, this principle is not an excuse for inaction. The right to health also contains immediate obligations to take concrete, deliberate and targeted steps towards full realization. This is why we need good benchmarks and indicators.

When WHO reviewed national constitutions globally, we found that over half of the countries in the Council of Europe had enshrined health as a human right.

This commitment is expressed in various ways—some constitutions commit the government to providing the best health care that is available and practicable; most recognize health as a right expressed variously in terms such as the right to protection of health, the right to a healthy environment, or the right to social security, medical insurance and medical services.

Within the European Union, the debate on the Convention on the future of Europe and the publication of a draft constitutional treaty, has similarly raised to the forefront the debate on the level of priority afforded to health in the context of Community policies and activities. We welcome the move to include an explicit reference to the fundamental human right to health in the draft constitutional treaty outlining the Union's basic values. Let me end these remarks by looking beyond Europe.

The reality is that public health, as never before, is a priority on the global agenda. This is for the simple reason that so many of the challenges we now face have a global impact, requiring solutions and a global response. We are living in an interconnected and interdependent world.

SARS has been a wake-up call. It has shown us the potential gains from international collaboration, as well as some of the pitfalls when collaboration fails.

But, there are many other issues which should claim our attention. The right of those in developing countries to enjoy better health depends on the actions of all governments, in the north as well as the south. Meeting obligations to provide development finance; building trust in trade negotiations; advancing human development and institution building—which may mean looking hard at our own health service recruitment policies; financing the public goods such as surveillance systems—from which all can benefit, but none can individually afford.

Let me end with a simple message. There can be no real growth without healthy populations.

No sustainable development without tackling disease and malnutrition.

No international security without assisting crisis-ridden countries.

And no hope for the spread of freedom, democracy and human dignity unless we treat health as a basic human right.

Thank you.

Text 4

2011 National Prevention Strategy of the United States (Excerpt)

National Prevention, Health Promotion and Public Health Council

The Affordable Care Act, landmark health legislation passed in 2010, created the National Prevention Council and called for the development of the National Prevention Strategy to realize the benefits of prevention for all Americans' health. The National Prevention Strategy is critical to the prevention focus of the Affordable Care Act and builds on the law's efforts to lower health care costs, improve the quality of care, and provide coverage options for the uninsured.

Preventing disease and injuries is key to improving the American's health. When we invest in prevention, the benefits are broadly shared. Children grow up in communities, homes, and families that nurture their healthy development, and people are productive and healthy, both inside and outside the workplace.

1. Most of our nation's pressing health problems can be prevented. Eating healthfully and engaging in regular physical activity, avoiding tobacco, excessive alcohol use, and other drug abuse, using seat belts, and receiving preventive services and vaccinations are just a few of the ways people can stay healthy. Health is more than merely the absence of disease; it is physical, mental, and social well-being.

2. Investments in prevention complement and support treatment and care. Prevention policies and programs can be cost-effective, reduce health care costs, and improve productivity (Appendix 1).

The National Prevention Strategy's core value is that Americans can live longer and healthier through prevention. Many of the strongest predictors of health and well-being fall outside of the health care setting. Social, economic, and environmental factors all influence health.

3. People with a quality education, stable employment, safe homes and neighborhoods, and access to high quality preventive services tend to be healthier throughout their lives and live longer. When organizations, whether they are governmental, private, or nonprofit, succeed in meeting these basic needs, people are more likely to exercise, eat healthy foods, and seek preventive health services. Meeting basic needs and providing information about personal health and health care can empower people to make healthy choices, laying a foundation for lifelong wellness. Preventing disease requires more than providing people with information to make healthy choices. While knowledge is critical, communities must reinforce and support health, for example, by making healthy choices easy and affordable. When all sectors (e.g., housing, transportation, labor, education, and defense) promote prevention-oriented environments and policies, they all contribute to health.

The National Prevention Strategy builds on the fact that lifelong health starts at birth and continues throughout all stages of life. Prevention begins with planning and having a healthy pregnancy, develops into good eating and fitness habits in childhood, is supported by preventive services at all stages of life, and promotes the ability to remain active, independent, and involved in one's community as we age. Students who are healthy and fit come to school ready to learn; employees who are free from mental and physical conditions take fewer sick days, are more productive, and help strengthen the economy; and older adults who remain physically and mentally active are more likely to live independently.

4. To ensure that all Americans share in the benefits of prevention, the National Prevention Strategy includes an important focus on those who are disproportionately burdened by poor health.

In the United States, significant health disparities exist and these disparities are closely linked with social, economic, and environmental disadvantage (e.g., lack of access to quality affordable health care, healthy food, safe opportunities for physical activity, and educational and employment opportunities).

The National Prevention Strategy aims to guide our nation in the most effective and achievable means for improving health and well-being. The Strategy prioritizes prevention by integrating recommendations and actions across multiple settings to improve health and save lives. This Strategy envisions a prevention-oriented society where all sectors recognize the value of health for individuals, families, and society and work together to achieve better health for all Americans.

This Strategy focuses on both increasing the length of people's lives and ensuring that people's lives are healthy and productive. Currently Americans can expect to live 78 years, but only 69 of these years would be spent in good health.

5. Implementing the National Prevention Strategy can increase both the length and quality of life. To monitor progress on this goal, the Council will track and report measures of the length and quality of life at key life stages (Appendix 2 for baselines and targets). To realize this vision and achieve this goal, the Strategy identifies four Strategic Directions and seven targeted Priorities. The Strategic Directions provide a strong foundation for all of our nation's prevention efforts and include core recommendations necessary to build a prevention-oriented society. The Strategic Directions are

● Healthy and Safe Community Environments: Create, sustain, and recognize communities that promote health and wellness through prevention.

● Clinical and Community Preventive Services: Ensure that prevention-focused health care and community prevention efforts are available, integrated, and mutually reinforcing.

● Empowered People: Support people in making healthy choices.

● Elimination of Health Disparities: Eliminate disparities, improving the quality of life for all Americans. Within this framework, the Priorities provide evidence-based recommendations that are most likely to reduce the burden of the leading causes of preventable death and major illness.

The seven Priorities are

● Tobacco Free Living

● Preventing Drug Abuse and Excessive Alcohol Use

● Healthy Eating

● Active Living

● Injury and Violence Free Living

● Reproductive and Sexual Health

● Mental and Emotional Well-Being

六、汉译英练习

Text 5

突出重点强化责任　深入推进医药卫生体制改革
——在全国深化医药卫生体制改革工作会议上的发言

中华人民共和国卫生部部长　陈竺

2012年4月17日

过去的三年，是新中国成立以来卫生事业发展史上极为不平凡的三年。三年来，深化医改这一事关13亿人民健康福祉的重大民生工程取得了明显成效。站在新的起点上，卫生系统要进一步统一思想，明确任务，充分发挥行业组织优势和专业优势，认真贯彻李克强副总理重要讲话和本次会议精神，全面落实"十二五"医改规划和2012年医改主要工作安排确定的各项任务，坚定不移地将医改推向深入。

一、抓重点，解难题，加快推进"十二五"时期医改工作

（一）加快推进新农合制度，实现从扩大范围向提升质量转变

随着新农合筹资水平的不断提高，卫生部门要把增强农民健康风险保护作为巩固完善新农合制度的突出重点。一要巩固覆盖面和提高保障水平。2012年新农合政策范围内住院费用支付比例要达到75%左右，继续降低农村居民的个人医药费用负担。二要推动支付方式改革。发挥新的支付方式对于规范医疗服务行为、控制医药费用、推动医疗机构综合改革的作用。三要探索建立重特大疾病保障机制。不断扩大保障范围，并与医疗救助和购买商业大病保险衔接，尽力减轻患者个人负担。四要提高管理服务水平。依托信息化加快推进异地即时结算，同时要推进商业保险机构参与经办新农合服务。

（二）巩固完善基本药物制度和基层运行新机制，实现基层医疗卫生机构由"强筋健骨"向全面发展转变

要从四个方面继续巩固完善基本药物制度。一是有序推进基本药物制度向村卫生室和非政府办基层医疗卫生机构扩展，推动其他医疗机构优先使用基本药物。二是调整国家基本药物目录，规范地方增补非目录药品。三是继续规范基本药物采购机制，推动建立完善符合行业发展规律的药品质量综合评价体系。四是加强政府宏观调控和指导，建立基本药物生产供应新机制。

巩固完善基层医疗卫生机构综合改革要抓住以下关键环节：一是落实政府举办基层医疗卫生机构的责任，保障基层医疗卫生机构发展建设支出。二是建立稳定

长效的多渠道补偿机制。协调财政部门建立基本药物制度经常性补助渠道并纳入预算。三是建立竞争性用人制度。实行定编定岗不定人，全员按岗竞聘，合同管理。四是推进分配制度改革。建立多劳多得、优绩优酬的分配制度。五是加大基层卫生人才培养力度。开展全科医生规范化培训，把落实全科医生制度作为“强基层”的关键举措。

（三）大力推进县级公立医院改革，实现公立医院改革由局部试点向全面推进转变

公立医院改革是医改的重点和难点之一。今年将选择300个左右的县（市）开展县级医院改革试点，采取调整医疗服务价格、改革医保支付方式、落实政府投入责任等综合措施，破除以药补医机制。同时，继续深化城市公立医院改革试点，推进便民惠民服务，改善群众就医感受。

要建立符合医疗卫生行业特点的薪酬制度，进一步落实“多劳多得，优劳优得”的分配原则，促进改革后医务人员收入合理增加。加快推进形成多元化办医格局，落实鼓励社会资本办医的相关政策措施。

在完成重点医改任务的同时，要统筹推进提高基本公共卫生服务均等化水平、加快卫生信息化建设和创新卫生人才培养使用等相关卫生工作。

二、强化责任抓落实，确保全面完成医改各项任务

一是严格落实责任。各级卫生部门要把医改作为中心工作，强化责任落实和追究，切实加大推进医改工作的力度。

二是注重开拓创新。卫生部门要继续大胆探索，积极创新，不断破解医改难题，把工作抓细抓实，扎实推进各项工作。

三是加强宣传引导。卫生系统要主动宣传医改中好的做法、经验和成效，坚持正确的舆论导向，积极引导社会预期，使医改在宽松、有利的环境中稳步推进。

卫生领域是医改的主战场，广大医务人员是医改的主力军，做好医改工作是我们的应尽之责。下一步，我们要进一步凝心聚力，攻坚克难，奋力拼搏，全面完成医改各项工作任务，推进卫生事业又好又快发展。

Text 6

深化医药卫生体制改革　促进卫生事业科学发展（节选）

中华人民共和国卫生部党组书记　张茅

2012年8月1日

党的十六大以来，在科学发展观指导下，我国医药卫生事业取得了显著成就。2010年我国人均期望寿命达到73.5岁，2011年我国孕产妇死亡率和婴儿死亡率分别下降到26.1/10万和12.1‰，接近中等发达国家水平。特别是2009年4月党中央、国务院全面深化医药卫生体制改革启动实施以来，我国基本医疗保障覆盖面从2008年的87%提高到2011年的95%以上，全民医保框架基本建立，为近13亿居民构建了抵御疾病经济风险的安全屏障。2011年，全国医疗卫生机构诊疗62.71亿人次，入院人数1.5亿，达到历史最高水平。总结卫生事业发展取得的成绩，关键在于深入贯彻落实科学发展观，坚持走中国特色卫生发展道路，正确处理卫生事业与经济社会事业协调发展的关系，正确处理影响卫生事业科学发展的若干重要关系，努力探索出医改这一世界性难题的中国式解决办法。

一、坚持科学发展理念，统筹推进卫生事业与经济社会事业协调发展

卫生事业是社会公益性事业，体现着人民群众最关心、最直接、最现实的利益诉求，承担着维护和促进人民健康的光荣使命。党和政府历来高度重视卫生工作，努力维护人民群众身心健康。实践证明，经济社会事业的持续发展、消费结构的转变升级和广大居民健康需求的不断增长，为卫生事业发展提供了前进动力和不竭源泉，也为深化医改奠定了坚实的物质基础；虽然区域间、城乡间经济发展差距难以在短期内大幅度缩小，但通过实施包括卫生在内的公共服务均等化措施，能较快缩小区域和城乡之间社会事业的发展差距，有效维护社会公平公正；卫生事业的科学发展，居民健康水平的大幅提高，既为经济社会发展提供了大量高素质的劳动力，又缓解了群众看病就医的后顾之忧，增强了居民消费信心，从而为扩大内需、转变经济发展方式、实现经济社会又好又快发展起到重要的支撑作用。

二、坚持公共医疗卫生的公益性质，统筹发挥政府主导与市场机制作用

如何发挥好政府主导和市场机制的作用，是我们多年来努力探索的重大问题。新医改提出“保基本，强基层，建机制”的基本原则，明确了医疗卫生事业的公益性质，突出了政府在医疗卫生事业中的主导作用，有效弥补了医疗卫生领域“市场失灵”的问题，切实维护了基本医疗卫生的公益性，促进了社会公平公正。

新医改三年来，公共财政前所未有地加大卫生投入，全国财政医疗卫生累计支出15 166亿元。政府在优化资源配置和利用、加强对贫困地区及薄弱领域和环节的支

持力度等方面充分发挥了主导作用，“保基本”的职责得到进一步加强。经过多年努力，世界上最大的基本医疗保障安全网得以建立，基本药物制度在政府办基层医疗卫生机构全面实施，城乡基层医疗卫生服务体系更加健全，服务能力大幅提高，公立医院改革试点有序推进。

三、坚持以农村为重点，统筹城乡和区域卫生事业协调发展

在卫生资源配置、卫生服务利用、居民健康水平等方面，我国城乡、区域和群体之间存在着明显差异，大部分卫生资源集中在大城市，高新技术、优秀卫生人才基本上集中在城市的大医院，农村和城市基层卫生服务能力较为薄弱，城乡居民在享有卫生服务及主要健康指标方面均存在较大差距，实现公共卫生和医疗服务均等化面临诸多挑战。

新医改通过改善和优化卫生资源配置结构，着力缩小城乡、区域和群体间的差距，以卫生事业的均衡发展促进城乡之间经济社会的均衡发展。一是明显加大了对中西部地区和欠发达地区的财政支持力度，逐步完善了医疗卫生资源区域、城乡间优化调整的政策措施。二是加强对欠发达地区人才、技术、政策、管理、资金等方面的扶持力度。三年来，中央财政投入470多亿元，用于支持2 233个县级医院、6 213个乡镇卫生院和2.5万个村卫生室的基础设施建设。三是加大城市优质资源对农村地区和基层的支持力度，推动建立公立医院与基层医疗卫生机构分工协作机制。通过建立医院间的远程会诊、组建医疗集团和医疗联合体等多种形式，促进优质医疗资源下到基层，并充分发挥其辐射带动作用和倍增效应。

四、坚持发挥中医药特色优势，统筹中西医协调发展

中医药是中华民族的瑰宝。实践证明，中医与西医优势互补、相互促进，共同维护和增进人民健康，已经成为中国特色医疗卫生事业的显著特征和独特优势。但是，目前中医也面临着扶持力度不够、服务领域缩小、优势特色淡化等困难和问题。

作为深化医改的重要配套文件，国务院2009年出台了《关于扶持和促进中医药事业发展的若干意见》，系统提出了中医药事业发展的指导思想、基本原则和主要任务。各级党委政府对扶持促进中医药事业发展的认识明显提高，对中医药工作的支持力度进一步加大，中医药服务越来越受到广大群众的欢迎和认可，中医药在防治疾病、促进健康方面的作用明显增强。

五、坚持预防为主，统筹公共卫生和医疗服务体系发展

坚持预防为主，是我们一贯的卫生工作方针，也是最经济、最有效的健康策略。但是，受多种因素影响，长期以来预防为主的卫生工作方针没有得到很好落实，不同程度地存在重治疗、轻预防的问题。

当前，我国经济社会发展进入新阶段，人民群众生活方式发生很大变化，健康

问题变得更为复杂。尤其值得关注的是，我国现有2亿多高血压病人、9 000多万糖尿病病人，每年有200万人死于心脑血管疾病，190万人死于恶性肿瘤，慢性非传染性疾病已经成为我国居民的主要死因。在新医改中，我们坚持把加强公共卫生服务体系建设放在首位，用制度建设落实预防为主的方针。在防治策略上，坚持传染病与慢性非传染性疾病防治并重；在防治机构上，坚持依靠专业公共卫生机构和医疗服务机构及医学科研机构并重；在防治方式上，坚持社会动员和全员参与；在防治重心上，坚持以基层医疗卫生机构为基础，主要发挥全科医生的作用，实现城乡居民的全面健康管理。针对新时期人民群众健康状况的新特征，国家启动实施包括建立健康档案、高血压、糖尿病管理等10大类41项国家基本公共卫生服务项目，基本公共卫生服务补助经费逐步提高到2011年的人均25元。此外，针对重点人群和重点区域的重大公共卫生服务项目顺利实施，累计完成乙肝疫苗补种6 700万人，分别对1 169万、146万名农村适龄妇女免费进行了宫颈癌、乳腺癌检查，对2 356万名育龄妇女免费补服了叶酸等。

虽然我国卫生事业和医改工作取得了巨大成就，但我国医疗资源总体供给短缺，特别是优质资源难以满足群众需求的状况没有改变，医疗卫生资源配置不合理、城乡和区域不平衡的矛盾依然存在。我们要继续深入贯彻落实科学发展观，按照中央确定的深化医改的基本理念、基本原则和基本路径，加快健全全民医保体系，进一步完善基本药物制度和基层医疗卫生机构运行新机制建设，积极推进公立医院改革，统筹开展深化医改各项工作，以优异的成绩迎接党的十八大胜利召开！

资料来源：

Text 1 http://mediacentre.dh.gov.uk/2012/06/08/21-may-2012-andrew-lansley-world-health-association/

Text 2 http://www.phac-aspc.gc.ca/about_apropos/index-eng.php

Text 3 http://www.who.int/dg/brundtland/speeches/2003/conference_european_healthministers/en

Text 4 http://www.healthcare.gov/prevention/nphpphc/strategy/report.pdf

Text 5 http://www.moh.gov.cn/publicfiles/business/htmlfiles/mohzcfgs/s7857/201205/54643.htm

Text 6 http://www.moh.gov.cn/publicfiles/business/htmlfiles/mohbgt/s6717/201208/55537.htm

参考答案

四、摘要练习

Text 1

全民医疗保健制度

世界卫生协会　安德鲁·兰斯利

2012年5月21日

发表于2012年6月8日

今天我很高兴来到这里谈全民保健这一重要问题。

在英国，全民医疗保健一直是国家医疗服务制度的重点，已有60年历史。普及综合、免费、以需求为基础的卫生服务是社会团结和改善人民健康这一重要基础的一个组成部分。

两年前，我们做出两项承诺：一是提高我们国家医疗服务的预算，二是增加我们曾做出的0.7%的承诺方面的开支。关于上述两项承诺我们做得还不错。

今天，每年世界数以百万计的贫困人口生病或死于可预防和可治疗的疾病，因为自付费用使许多人得不到所需要的帮助。解决方案只能是不排除穷人也不令其致贫的既高效又有效的医疗保健制度。

今年7月，英国政府、比尔与梅林达·盖茨基金会、联合国人口基金，以及其他机构将在伦敦举办国际计划生育峰会。目标是推出一个全球性的运动，到2020年给世界上最贫穷国家的1.2亿妇女提供避孕信息、服务和用品。我相信很多人都希望你们的政府参加，并且我很高兴我们的总干事将在此事中发挥关键作用。

我国在国家医疗服务方面的投资正在加强普及初级保健的基础设施。我们工作的重点是发展预防性的服务、早期干预，减少不必要的住院治疗。在国家医疗服务制度改革中，我们授权医院负责人向患者交出结果，给予医疗服务提供者更多的自主权，并使他们对结果负更多的责任。

我们正在改革我们的公共卫生体系，以确保我们有能力处理健康问题的社会决定因素，因为政府的责任是提高人口的健康水平。我们正在针对就业、教育、住房和环境对健康的影响方面采取行动。

我们的做法是在人生的关键时刻最大限度地施展我们的影响力，例如在怀孕期和婴幼儿期给予支持。我们还在肥胖、烟草、毒品、酒精和性健康方面开展工作。

我们将有效控制烟草。我们正与食品、饮料和零售行业组建合作伙伴关系，达成共识：公众健康是每个人的事情，合作将会为消费者创造健康的环境，使他们获得健康的生活方式。

我们今天的日程安排突出了世界卫生组织关于做到最好的号召。我们需要世界卫生组织在成员国之间进行协调，就建立强大的全民医疗体系分享思路和策略。

世界卫生组织的改革将使我们取得更大的进步。世界卫生组织强大起来，随时准备好面对21世纪的挑战，这是至关重要的。

Text 2

加拿大公共卫生署及其使命

加拿大公共卫生署（PHAC）于2006年12月由加拿大公共卫生署法案批准，是一个法律实体，是加拿大的主要政府机构，负责加拿大公共卫生事宜。加拿大公共卫生署的目标是加强加拿大改善人民健康状况的能力，协助减轻保健系统的压力，建立一个有效的公共健康体系，以使加拿大人更加健康、更加幸福。所使用的方式是促进身体健康，协助预防和控制各种慢性疾病和损伤，保护加拿大人免受传染病和其他对健康产生威胁的疾病之苦。该卫生署也致力于减小加拿大最优势和最弱势群体之间的健康差距。

为了应对人类对病原体和毒素的担忧，议会于2009年通过了人类病原体和毒素法案（HPTA）。加拿大公共卫生署负责执行法案，发展计划和监管框架。公众健康是我们共同的责任，卫生署与各级政府密切合作，发挥各自的技能和长处。卫生署也与非政府组织，包括民间社会和企业、其他国家和国际组织密切合作，分享知识、专业技能和经验。

加拿大公共卫生署是构成联邦政府健康联合机构的六个部门之一，通过卫生部长向议会报告。卫生署目前由加拿大首席公共卫生官大卫·巴特勒-琼斯博士负责，他起着双重作用：一方面，他是联邦公共服务的副部长，领导该机构，在公众健康和机构功能方面给卫生部长提供建议；另一方面，领导联邦公共健康专业人士，这些专业人士的任务，是就重要公共健康问题直接与加拿大人和加拿大政府沟通。

加拿大公共卫生署有三个主要分支，各分支都由一名助理副部长负责。这三个分支是：传染病预防和控制部（IDPC）、健康促进和慢性病预防部（HPCDP）、应急管理及部门事务部（EMCA）。

重要顾问和机构办公室与这些助理副部长一起直接向加拿大卫生部部长和副部长汇报。为了保持与研发和交付公共卫生建议、提供加拿大人所要求的手段相关的知识和技能，卫生署依靠其工作人员的敬业和努力。卫生署有约2 700名员工，在加拿大各地工作，专业面很宽，职位包括运营、科学、技术和行政。

加拿大公共卫生署的使命是通过领导、合作、促进、创新和公共卫生行动保护加拿大人的健康。它的愿景是“健康的加拿大人和社区在更健康的世界中生活”。

我们的价值观如下：

领导能力：我们在机构层面上珍视领导的作用。这样的领导人能够做长期规划，能进行战略性思维，能够进行开放式的沟通，能够营造热情的气氛和团队协作的氛围。在个人层面上，我们在日常的工作责任之中采取主人公的态度，对工作负责。

健康的工作环境：我们珍视的机构能够公开承认和认可员工的贡献，支持公平公正、多样性和包容性，鼓励个人工作生活和家庭生活之间的平衡。

伦理道德行为：我们珍视的工作场所能够培养相互尊重，人们以公平和平等相待；各级员工在扮演自己的角色、完成自己的责任以及处理内部与外部的关系之时，展现正直诚信、真诚诚实、值得信赖的品质。

追求卓越：在完成加拿大公共卫生交给我们的任务之时，我们珍视追求卓越，途径是专业的行为、不断学习、职业发展活动、创造和创新、持续承诺遵守公共卫生的原则和科学性。

竭诚服务：对我们日常接触的所有人，我们珍视尊重他人的服务和高质量的服务；我们机构在减少加拿大和世界范围的健康差距方面努力工作并做出了贡献，我们关注自己的工作并为此感到骄傲，也为我们机构对社会的贡献感到骄傲。我们珍视追求卓越的承诺与竭诚服务的行为。

加拿大公共卫生署的作用是：

促进健康；预防和控制慢性疾病和损伤；预防和控制传染病；准备和应对突发公共卫生事件；作为服务中心，与世界分享加拿大的专业知识；将国际上的研究和发展运用到加拿大的公共卫生项目之中；加强政府间在公共健康问题上的合作，协助国家策略在公共卫生政策和规划方面的运用。

公共卫生的重点是全体国民，覆盖个人和社区。公共卫生包括由三级政府（联邦政府、省/地区、市）执行的一系列活动，参与活动的三级政府机构同时与国内各类利益相关者和社区合作。

通过我们的研究、项目和服务，我们的目标是使加拿大人更加健康，减少健康差距，获得提供公共卫生活动、支持公共卫生活动的更强能力。

加拿大公共卫生署使用国家经费和捐赠基金资助社区、志愿者以及非营利机构，以支持政府的政策和优先事项。卫生署目前利用国家经费和社会捐赠资助了全国范围内约1 200个项目，相当于卫生署每年预算的33%。

五、英译汉练习

Text 3

健康、尊严与人权

世界卫生组织总干事在第7次欧盟卫生部长会议上的主旨性发言

挪威奥斯陆

2003年6月12日

秘书长，尊敬的部长们，朋友们和同事们：

你们为今天的会议选择了非常重要的主题，即“健康、尊严和人权”。这三个概念之间有着千丝万缕的联系，对欧洲乃至整个世界卫生系统与卫生服务的发展至关重要。

55年以前，世界卫生组织章程的创立者陈述道，享受可达到的最高健康标准是每个人的基本权利。在我们的日常工作中，包括你们卫生部部长的工作中，我们都在努力使这一权利变成现实，将我们的强烈愿望和政策付诸实践。

这从来都不是一件简单的事，我们大家都面临很大的压力。人口老龄化，技术的迅速发展，持续上升的公众期望值，所有这些因素都给我们带来压力，要我们增加医疗开支。

然而，要说服国库和财政部的同事们很艰难，因为他们首要关注的是宏观经济稳定。

我们必须有能力来信守承诺。归根到底，更健康的结果是最重要的。但是，如何获得健康与谁将是受益人的问题也同样重要。人权、健康权恰好有助于解答这个问题。我们都在讨论医疗融资的未来。我们如何能在资源配置中提高成本效益和提高有效率的支出，并同时维护我们资助服务机构方式上的团结？

这里的关键点是，确保充足的资金固然是关键，然而确保共同负担费用也同样重要。

同样，我们不仅仅关注获得医疗保健的权利，我们也关注人们需要服务时所能得到的对待方式。

我们认为卫生系统对此的回应包括确保自身的可靠性、减少等候时间、参与决定，并且，我们认为这些是卫生系统本身应有的合理目标。

上述目标与人权有直接的联系，因为在对人权的思考和实践中，平等和无歧视的概念包括人的尊严这一概念，人的尊严是每一个人与生俱来的价值。

近年来，我们已经更加清楚地认识到健康权应有的含义。首先，它是一个有广泛内涵的权利：它不只包括医疗保健服务，还包括造成健康欠佳的根本性原因。

这些原因的来源范围很宽，包括能否获得安全的饮用水、足够的卫生设施、食品安全、营养食品、健康的职业环境条件、包括有关性与生殖健康信息在内的知情权。

主席先生，

初级卫生保健和全民健康运动已经在塑造欧洲的健康政策，其核心是对公平的关注。

但是，我们都知道，在与会代表所代表的每一个国家里，还有人群未能得到我们卫生系统所应提供给他们的服务。人权框架可以帮助我们满足这些群体的需求。

社会排斥现象的原因是多种多样的。我们处理全国平均值的时候发现，一些少数民族和经济上的弱势群体被忽视。但是，也有显而易见的需求，然而需求的原因是政治上的不受欢迎。例如非法移民。

重视弱势群体是人权方针的基本要素，因为健康权要求优先重视那些最需要的。这本身是很重要的。人权与健康权是国际公认的法律框架的一部分，这赋予了各国政府责任。

健康权是所有政府、富人、穷人应努力的目标。当然，这不能一蹴而就。所有国家都受到各种制约，而且在很多情况下，是有限的资源制约了我们。因此，逐步实现的原则是实现所有人权的核心。

但是，这个原则不是不作为的借口。健康权还包括立即承担责任以及实施具体的、深思熟虑的、有针对性的步骤，以全面实现目标。为此，我们需要准确的标准和指标。

世界卫生组织回顾全球各国的宪法时发现，欧洲理事会一半以上的国家已将健康权奉为人权。

他们的承诺以各种方式表达——一些国家的宪法要求政府提供最好的、民众能得到的、切实可行的医疗保健；大部分国家承认健康权，并认为这个权利可用不同的词汇表达，比如保护健康的权利、获得健康环境的权利、获得社会保障、医疗保险和医疗服务的权利。

在欧洲联盟内，针对有关欧洲未来和出版宪法条约草案的“公约”正在辩论之中，此辩论将针对社区政策和行动范围内的健康优先级别的问题提到了前台。对概述欧盟基本价值观的宪法草案条约明确提及健康为基本人权的进展，我们表示欢迎。最后，我要谈及欧洲以外的情况作为结语。

现实情况是，公众健康正前所未有地成为全球议程上的优先事项。原因很简单：我们面临的诸多挑战都具有全球影响，要求解决方案，要求全球共同应对。我们生活的世界是一个相互联系和相互依存的世界。

SARS已经敲响了警钟。它向我们展示了国际合作的潜在收益，以及合作失败时遇到的意想不到的困难。

但是，还有诸多其他问题要求我们引起注意。发展中国家人们享受更好健康的权利依赖于所有政府的行动，不管是在北方还是在南方。满足提供发展资金的义务、在贸易谈判中建立信任，以及促进人类发展和制度建设等可能意味着努力建立自己招募健康服务人员的政策，资助监控系统之类的公共设施。这些可以使大家都受益，但我们往往无法单独负担。

最后，让我用简单的几句话作为结语。没有健康的人口就没有实质性的增长。不解决疾病和营养不良就没有可持续性的发展。不帮助危机四伏的国家就不会有国际安全。如果我们不把健康作为一项基本人权，就不会有传播自由的希望、民主的希望和人的尊严的希望。

谢谢大家。

Text 4

2011年美国国家预防战略（节选）

美国国家预防、健康促进与公共卫生委员会

2010年通过的具有里程碑意义的卫生法——平价医疗法案建立了国家预防委员会，并呼吁发展国家预防战略，让所有美国人的健康受益于疾病预防。对于平价医疗法案的预防重点而言，国家预防战略非常关键，因它建立于法律之上，依法降低医疗成本，提高医疗质量，并为没有医疗保险的人提供全覆盖性的选择权。

预防疾病和身体损伤是改善美国国民健康的关键。当我们投资于预防，利益将被广泛地分享。社区、家庭和家庭养育的孩子们会健康成长，人们在工作场所内外都富有生产能力并且身体健康。

1. 我们国家紧迫的健康问题大多是可以预防的。保持健康有多种方法，举几个例子：健康饮食并有规律地锻炼身体，避免吸烟，避免过量饮酒，避免滥用药物，开车使用安全带，接受预防性服务与免疫接种，等等。健康不仅仅是不生病，它是生理、心理的健康以及社会的安康。

2. 投资于预防补充与支持治疗护理。预防政策和方案应成本低，效益佳，我们应降低医疗成本，提高生产率。国家预防战略的核心价值是让美国人通过预防变得更健康、更长寿。许多最能预测健康和福利的预测值都未被包括在医疗保健之内。社会、经济和环境因素都会影响健康。

3. 受过高品质教育、有稳定职业、居住在安全的家园和社区、获得高品质预防服务的人群往往生活得更健康、更长久。当各类组织——无论是政府组织、私人组织，还是非营利组织——成功地满足这些基本需求时，人们参加锻炼、吃健康食品，并寻求预防保健服务的可能性更大。满足基本需求并提供有关个人健康和卫生保健的信息，可以使人们做出健康的选择并为终身健康打下基础。疾病的预防工作不只是为人们多多提供做出健康选择的信息。知识是至关重要的，而社区必须加强和支持健康事业，比如设法使健康选择变得容易得到并且不是太贵。当所有的部门（如住房、交通、劳动、教育、国防）一起推动以预防为主的环境和政策时，才会对健康事业有所贡献。

事实上，一个人一辈子的健康始于出生，它延续于人生的各个阶段。国家预防战略以此为理念。预防始于规划并拥有孕期健康，之后在童年发展良好的饮食习惯和健身的习惯，在生活的各个阶段得到预防性的服务，在年老的过程中保持积极性、独立性以及参与社区事务。身心健全、健康的学生在学校学习会具有求知欲；精神和身体无疾病的员工请病假次数很少，更有工作效率，因此能够巩固经济发展；身体与精神上都积极向上的老年人更有可能独立生活。

4. 确保所有美国人都能分享到预防的好处。国家预防战略的另一个重要工作重心是帮助那些不同程度的因病致贫的人。在美国，健康差距显著，并且这些差距与社会、经济和环境的弱势状况紧密相连。例如，缺乏获得优质实惠的医疗保健、健康食品、进行安全体育锻炼的机会，以及教育和就业的机会。

国家预防战略的目标是用可实现的最有效手段来指导国家改善国民健康福利。该战略通过整合来自于跨行业多个背景的建议和行动来达到预防优先，以改善健康和挽救生命。这一战略的愿景是形成一个以预防为主的社会，社会各界人士都认识到健康对个人、家庭和社会的价值，并为所有美国人变得更加健康而共同努力。该战略侧重于延长人们的寿命，并确保人们身体健康并富有生产力。目前，美国人均寿命为78岁，但其中只有69年身体是健康的。

5. 实施国家预防战略，可以增加生命的长度和质量。为了监测这一目标的进展情况，委员会将跟踪并报告人生关键阶段的生命进程和生活质量。为了实现这一愿景和目标，国家预防战略确定了四个战略方向、七个有针对性的优先重点。四个战略方向为我们国家的预防工作提供了坚实的基础，并且就建立以预防为主的社会提供了必要的核心建议。

这四个战略方向是：

● 建立健康、安全的社区环境。创造、维持并认可通过预防促进社区人民保持健康。

● 建立临床与社区预防服务。确保以预防为主的卫生保健和社区预防工作的实际可用性、综合性和相互加强性。

●赋能力于民众。支持民众做出健康的选择。

●消除健康差距。为所有美国人消除健康差距，提高生活质量。在此框架内，针对可预防性死亡和重大疾病的主要原因，重点优先提供最有可能减少疾病的询证建议。

七个优先事项是：

●无烟草生活

●防止滥用药物和过量饮酒

●健康饮食

●积极生活

●没有伤害和暴力的生活

●性健康与生殖健康

●精神健康与情感健康

六、汉译英练习

Text 5

Prioritize Focus, Strengthen Responsibility and Promote Deeper Change of Healthcare System

A Speech at the Work Meeting for Deepening Reform of Healthcare System

Minister Chen Zhu

17April 2012

The last three years are three extraordinary years in the history of public health development since the founding of People's Republic of China. In the past three years, the in-depth medicare reform that is critical to the health and wellbeing of the 1.3 billion people has obtained remarkable achievements. Standing now on a new starting point, we in the health system must further unify our thoughts, clarify our tasks, and give full play to our organizational and professional advantages. We must earnestly implement the guidance of Vice Premier Li Keqiang's important speech and of this meeting, fully implement the "12th Five-Year" medicare reform plan and 2012 tasks identified by the annual healthcare reform work arrangements, and unswervingly deepen the medicare reform.

1. Focus on major tasks, solve difficult problems, and accelerate medicare reform during "12th Five-Year" period

1.1 Accelerate improvement of the New Rural Cooperative Medicare System (NCMS) by expanding coverage and improving quality

With the continuous improvement of financing, healthcare departments must take rural health risk protection as a focusing means for reinforcing and consummating the new rural cooperative medicare system. The first of this is to consolidate coverage and improve the level of protection. The proportion of payment for hospitalization within NCMS in 2012 must reach about 75% so as to reduce personal burdens of medical expenses for the rural residents. The second is to promote reform of methods of payment. The new payment methods have a role in standardizing medical services, controlling medical costs, and promoting the comprehensive reform of the medical institutions. The third is to explore ways of establishing insurance mechanism for serious diseases. We need to continuously expand coverage of protection, integrate medicaid with commercial insurance for serious diseases so as to reduce burdens on individual patients. The fourth is to improve the level of management and services. We will rely on information technology in accelerating the off-site real-time settlement, and at the same time promote participation and management of the commercial insurance institutions in NRCMS services.

1.2 Consolidate the new mechanism of essential drug system and grassroots administration so as to realize overall development of community healthcare institutions on the basis of previous improvements

Essential drug system will be consolidated from four aspects. The first is to orderly extend essential drug system to village health clinics and non-government-run community health institutions, and meanwhile encourage other medical institutions to prioritize using essential drugs. The second is to modulate the National List of Essential Drugs and regulate local supplementary drugs that are not listed in the national directory. The third is to continuously regulate procurement of essential drugs and promote for the quality of drugs the establishment of a comprehensive evaluation system in line with the developmental law of the industry. The fourth is to strengthen the government's macro-control and guidance and establish a new mechanism of production and supply of essential drugs.

To reinforce and improve the comprehensive reform of the primary healthcare institutions, we must tackle the following key aspects. The first is to implement government responsibility in running primary healthcare institutions so as to guarantee expenditures in the development and construction of the primary healthcare institutions. The second is to establish a stable, long-term, and multi-channel compensation mechanism that coordinates financial sectors in establishing and bringing into budget subvention channels of essential drug system. The third is to create a competitive employment system by setting quotas for posts instead of personnel, practicing competitive employment to posts, and adopting employment by contract. The fourth is to promote the reform of payment system by establishing a payment system that encourages hard work and excellence. The fifth is to enhance efforts in training primary healthcare personnel by giving general practitioners standardized training and by taking implementation of general practitioner system as a key initiative for strengthening primary medicare system.

1.3 Vigorously promote the reform of the county-level public hospitals and realize overall change of public hospitals on the basis of previous local pilot project

The reform of public hospitals is one of the important and difficult tasks in healthcare reform. This year we will choose about 300 counties (cities) for pilot reform of the county-level hospitals. We will take comprehensive measures to abolish the mechanism of medical cost compensation through drug-selling by modulating medical service charge, changing mode of medicare insurance payment, and implementing government investment. At the same time, we will continue to deepen urban public hospital reform, provide better service for the convenience of patients who will finally have better feelings in their hospital experiences.

We will establish a salary system in accordance with the needs of the healthcare professionals by further implementing the allocation principle of "encouraging hard work and excellent performance", so that the income of medical professionals will have a reasonable increase after the reform. We will accelerate formation of a pattern of diversified hospitals by implementing related policies on encouraging social capitals to run hospitals.

Together with accomplishing key medicare reform tasks, we will coordinate equalization of a better level of essential public healthcare services, accelerate development of health information technology, and speed up cultivation of innovative healthcare talents.

2. Strengthening responsibility and working on implementation to ensure a full accomplishment of all medical reform tasks

The first of these is to strictly pin down responsibility. Healthcare departments at all levels must take healthcare reform as their central task, strengthen implementation of responsibility and accountability, and effectively increase the intensity of medicare reform.

The second is to emphasize innovation. The healthcare departments must practically push forward all work by continuously having bold exploration, active innovation, constant responses to challenges from medicare reform, and realistic work on details.

The third is to strengthen guidance for publicity. Healthcare departments must take initiative to publicize good practices, experiences and outcomes in the medical reform, insist on correct guidance on public opinions and actively guide social expectation so that healthcare reform can make steady progress in a relaxed and favorable environment.

Since public health is the main battlefield of our healthcare reform, medical professionals are the main force in the reform. Therefore, it is our responsibility to do the work well. For the next step, we must further concentrate our thoughts and strength, tackle tough problems, work hard, and complete various tasks of the medical reform, so that our healthcare services will have a sound and rapid development.

Text 6

Deepening Medical and Healthcare System Reform and Accelerating Scientific Development of the Healthcare Service

Zhang Mao, Party Secretary of the Ministry of Health of the People's Republic of China
1st August 2012

Since the 16th CPC National Congress, under the conceptual guidance of scientific development, pharmaceutical and healthcare enterprises in China have made remarkable achievements. By the year 2010, China's average life expectancy reached 73.5 years; in 2011, China's maternal mortality rate and infant mortality rate dropped to 261/100,000 and 12.1‰, both of which were close to the level of moderately developed countries. Since the April of 2009 when the CPC Central Committee and the State Council started implementation of deepening the reform of our medical and healthcare system, China's essential medicare insurance coverage expanded from 87% in 2008 to 95% in 2011. By then the framework of universal healthcare insurance was established, which built for 1.3 billion residents a security barrier against economic risks of diseases. In 2011, medical and healthcare institutions treated 6.271 billion people, admitted 150 million in-patients, both of which have reached the highest level in history. Summarizing the achievements made in healthcare enterprises, we find that the keys lay in thorough implementation of the concept of scientific development, adherence to the developmental ways that suit China's healthcare conditions, correct management of a harmonious development of both the healthcare services and economic social enterprises, proper handling of important relations that have influence on scientific development of the healthcare service, and efforts made to explore a Chinese solution to this worldwide problem of medicare reform.

1. Adherence to the scientific development concept and promotion of a coordinated development of both the health service and economic social enterprises.

Health service is a social commonweal enterprise that embodies the most concerned, the most direct and the most practical benefit demands of the people and bears the glorious mission of safeguarding and promoting the health of the people. The party and the government have always attached great importance to the health services and made great efforts in safeguarding people's physical and mental health. Practice has proved that continuous development of our economic and social undertakings, the transformation and upgrading of our consumption structure, and the growing needs of people for health are all momentum and inexhaustible source for the development of health services. They have also laid a solid material foundation for deepening medicare reform. Although the regional and economic gap in the development between urban and rural areas is difficult to significantly narrow down in a short term, we can quickly narrow the developmental gap in social enterprises between the urban and rural areas through implementation of equal access to public services including healthcare, and effectively safeguard social fairness and justice. Scientific development of the health services and substantial growth of people's health have provided a large number of highly qualified labors for economic and social development, relieved people's worries of diseases and hospital visits, and enhanced consumer confidence, which in turn played a critical supporting role for expanding domestic demands, transforming economic development mode, and achieving sound and rapid economic development.

2. Adherence to maintaining the commonweal nature of public healthcare and bringing government's role of guidance and market mechanism into play.

How to well play the role of government guidance and market mechanism have been the major issues of our exploration over the years. The new healthcare reform has put forward the basic principles of "insuring essentials, strengthening services for the grass-roots, and establishing mechanism", clarified that medical and health enterprises are public services, highlighted the dominant role of government in medical and health enterprises, effectively repaired "market failure" in medicine and healthcare, practically maintained the commonweal nature of the essential medicare service, and promoted social fairness and justice.

Three years since the new medicare reform, public finance has unprecedentedly increased investment in healthcare. The country's cumulative financial expenditure in healthcare has reached 1.5166 trillion Yuan. The government has played a full role of guidance in optimizing resource allocation and utilization, strengthening supports to poverty-stricken areas, and reinforcing support to weak procedures and areas. As a result, responsibility of "insuring essentials" has been strengthened. After years of efforts, the world's largest essential healthcare insurance network has been established and essential drug system has been implemented in the government-run primary healthcare institutions. Now the urban and rural primary healthcare service system is healthier, its service capacity has substantially been increased, and public hospital reform proceeds in an orderly way.

3. Adherence to focusing on the rural areas and coordinating harmonious development of health services in both the urban and rural areas.

In the allocation of health resources, utilization of health services, and upgrading the level of residents' health in the urban and rural areas, there are obvious disparity among the urban and rural areas, as well as between regions and groups. Most of health resources concentrate in large cities, high-tech and excellent health professionals concentrate in large urban hospitals, rural and urban primary health service capacity is weak, and a large gap exists in the service received and health indicators shown by the urban and rural residents. Realization of equalization in public health and medical services are encountered with many challenges.

The new healthcare reform has worked on narrowing the gap between the urban and rural areas and between regions and groups by optimizing allocation structure of health resources, so that a balanced development of the health services can promote balanced economic and social development in both the urban and rural areas. The first is that we have significantly increased financial support to the central, western and less developed regions and gradually consummated policies on adjustment and optimization of health resources among regions and between the urban and rural areas. The second is that we have given more support to the under-developed areas in terms of talents, technology, policy, management, and capital. In the past three years, the central government has invested more than 470 billion Yuan in infrastructure construction of 2,233 county-level hospitals, 6,213 township hospitals and 25,000 village health clinics. The third is that we have enhanced support in using excellent urban resources in rural areas as well as primary level institutions, and promoted establishing a mechanism of working both in division and cooperation between public hospitals and primary healthcare institutions. Through establishment of long-distance consultation among hospitals, medical groups and medical consortia, excellent medical resources have reached down to the primary level institutions, fully played their leading role and had multiplier effects.

4. Adherence to taking advantages of Traditional Chinese Medicine and coordinating development of Chinese Medicine and Western medicine.

Traditional Chinese Medicine (TCM) is a treasure of the Chinese nation. Practices have proved that both Traditional Chinese Medicine and Western Medicine have advantages that are mutually complementary and mutually promoting. They can work together in protecting and promoting people's health. Their combination has become a Chinese characteristic and unique advantage in China's medicare enterprises. However, Traditional Chinese Medicine is also facing difficulties in having inadequate support, shrinkage of service areas, fading of its characteristics and advantages.

In 2009, the State Council issued "Opinions on Supporting and Promoting the Development of Traditional Chinese Medicine and Chinese Pharmaceutical Industry" as its supporting document for deepening the medicare reform. This document has systematically brought forward the guiding thoughts, fundamental principles and major tasks for the development of Traditional Chinese Medicine and Chinese pharmaceutical industry. Party committees and governments at all levels then showed obvious better understanding of their own role in support and promotion of the development, and enhanced their work. As a result, the services by Traditional Chinese Medicine and drugs have been increasingly welcomed and recognized by people. Chinese medicine now plays a more important role in prevention and treatment of diseases as well as in health promotion.

5. Adherence to prevention and coordination of the development of public health and medical service system.

Prevention first is our consistent policy on medicare for it is the most economical and most effective strategy. However, due to influence of a variety of factors, prevention-based health policy has not been well implemented over a long period of time. To a variety of degrees, treatment was over-emphasized than prevention.

At present, China's economic and social development has entered a new phase, people's lifestyle has changed greatly, and health problems become more complicated. Of particular concern are chronic non-communicable diseases. Presently China has over 200 million hypertension patients and over 90 million diabetes patients; each year, 2 million people die of cardiovascular diseases and 1.9 million people die of cancer. Chronic non-communicable diseases have become the main cause of death. In the new healthcare reform, we prioritize construction of the public health service system and implement the principle of prevention first through system construction. In prevention strategies, we give equal attention to prevention of both infectious diseases and chronic non-communicable diseases; for prevention institutions, we rely equally on public healthcare professional institutions, medical service institutions and medical research institutions; In terms of prevention mode, we adhere to social mobilization and social participation; for the focus of prevention, we base our work on primary healthcare institutions, encourage general practitioners to play their role, and realize overall health management for the urban and rural residents. Aiming at tackling new features of people's health conditions in the new period, we have started to implement 41 essential public health service projects of 10 categories, including establishment of health records, hypertension management and diabetes management. We gradually increased essential public health services subsidy to 25 Yuan per capita in 2011. In addition, major public health service projects focusing on critical resident groups and critical areas have been successfully implemented. The accumulative total of Hepatitis B catch-up vaccination has reached 67 million, cervical cancer and breast cancer screening have been given for free to 11.69 million and 1.46 million rural women respectively, and folic acid has been given for free as supplement to 23.56 million women of childbearing age.

Although we have made great achievements in the cause of our health and medicare reform, overall shortage of supply of our healthcare resources still exists, in particular, excellent resources is still inadequate in meeting people's needs; Allocation of healthcare resources is still irrational, and the regional imbalance and imbalance between the urban and rural areas still exist. Therefore, we must continue our implementation of the concept of scientific development, follow the fundamental concepts, principles and path of in-depth reform determined by the CPC central committee, speed up consummating our universal health insurance system, further improve construction of the new mechanism of the essential drug system and primary medicare institutions, actively promote public hospital reform, and coordinate all work of in-depth medicare reform. We will salute the CPC eighteenth congress with our excellent achievements.

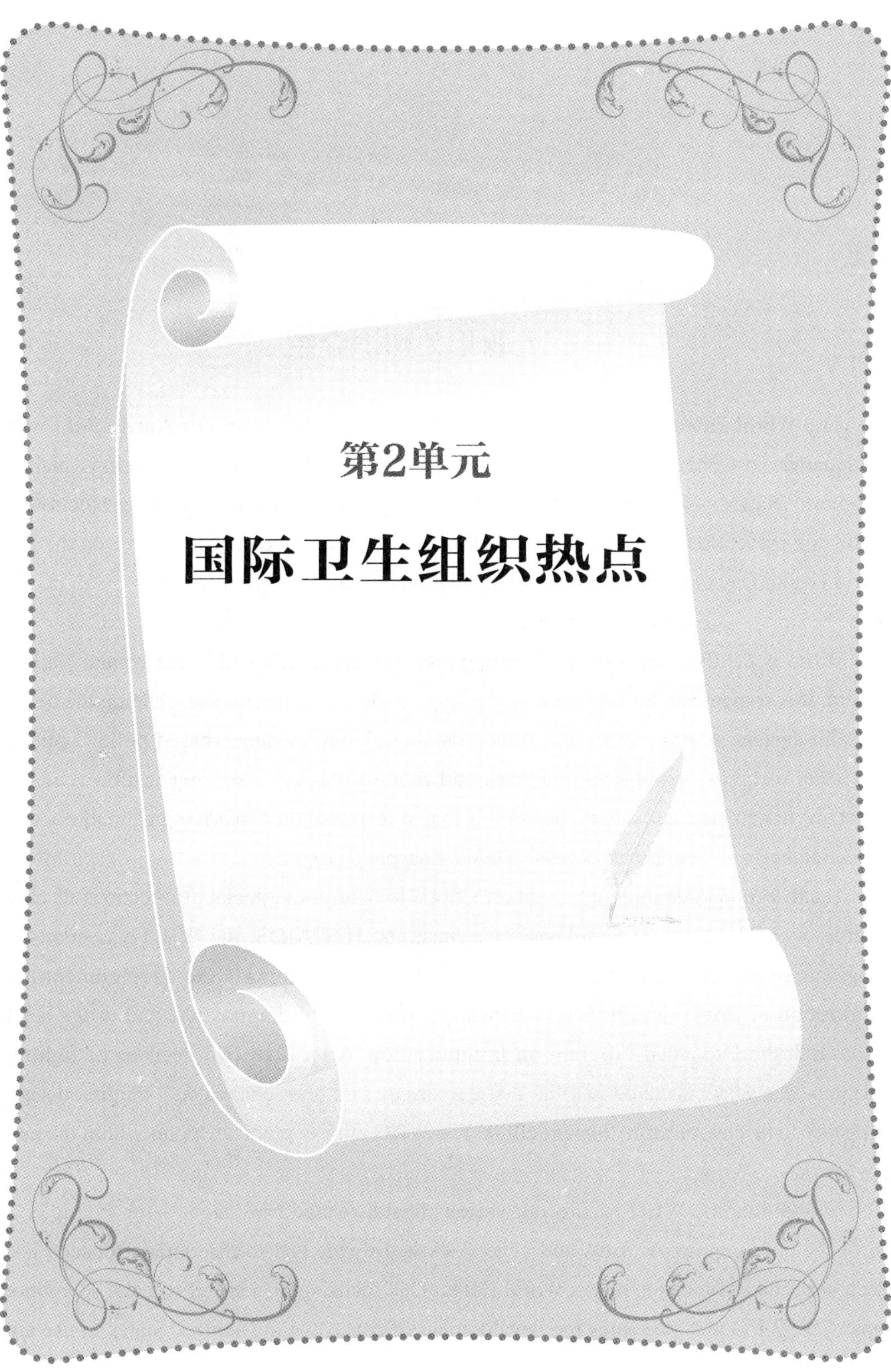

第2单元

国际卫生组织热点

一、主题相关知识介绍

The World Health Organization (WHO) was established on 7th April 1948, with headquarters in Geneva, Switzerland, its origin being traced back to organizations such as League of Nations Health Organization that oversees global efforts for the protection of health and prevention of diseases. WHO's constitution formally comes into force on the first World Health Day (7th April, 1948), stating that its objective "is the attainment by all people of the highest possible level of health".

WHO is the directing and coordinating authority for health within the United Nations system. It is responsible for providing leadership on global health matters, shaping the health research agenda, setting norms and standards, articulating evidence-based policy options, providing technical support to countries and monitoring and assessing health trends. It maintains that in the 21st century, health is a shared responsibility, involving equitable access to essential care and collective defense against transnational threats.

Apart from coordinating international efforts to control outbreaks of infectious disease, such as SARS, malaria, tuberculosis, influenza, and HIV/AIDS, the WHO also sponsors programs to prevent and treat such diseases. The WHO supports the development and distribution of safe and effective vaccines, pharmaceutical diagnostics, and drugs, such as through the Expanded Program on Immunization. After over two decades of fighting smallpox, the WHO declared in 1980 that the disease had been eradicated—the first disease in history to be eliminated by human effort. The WHO aims to eradicate polio within the next few years.

In addition, the WHO carries out various health-related campaigns—for example, to boost the consumption of fruits and vegetables worldwide and to discourage tobacco use. Each year, the organization marks World Health Day focusing on a specific health promotion topic. The WHO also promotes the development of capacities in Member States to use and produce research that addresses national needs.

The WHO has 193 Member states, with six regional offices that enjoy remarkable autonomy. The six regional offices are Regional Office for Africa (AFRO), with headquarters in Brazzaville, Republic of Congo; Regional Office for Europe (EURO), with headquarters in Copenhagen, Denmark; Regional Office for South East Asia (SEARO), with headquarters in New Delhi, India; Regional Office for the Eastern Mediterranean (EMRO), with headquarters in Cairo, Egypt; Regional Office for Western Pacific (WPRO), with headquarters in Manila, Philippines; and Regional Office for the Americas (AMRO), with headquarters in Washington, D. C., USA.

Currently the new WHO agenda has more emphasis on women's health and health in Africa. The agenda includes: 1. Promoting development; 2. Fostering health security; 3. Strengthening health systems; 4. Harnessing research, information and evidence; 5. Enhancing partnerships and; 6. Improving performance.

二、技巧指导：语料类型分析——正式文体之阐释文

语料类型分析这一部分介绍语料特征。了解讲话这种语料类型有助于在翻译中识别主题思想（identification of main ideas），训练如何在理解过程中抓住主题，进而在译入语中根据主题线索重新组织语言内容。鉴于公共卫生口译的特点，本单元着重介绍书面语篇之阐释文。阐释文属于正式文体。公共卫生领域需要口译的场合经常都是正式的讲话，这样的讲话发生在大小型会议室或礼堂。

从译员的角度讲，在充当媒介之时应该做的事是在两种语言对话之间，将一方讲话的意思尽可能完整地传达给另一方。要传达意思首先必须听懂源语言的意思，然后才能用目的语表达源语言的意思。这里不断地重复“意思”一词，就是强调学习者不要孤立地听字、译字。学过一点翻译的读者可能明白，如果只注意词语，只翻译词语，不仅难以传达源语言的意思，译者也会感到非常困难。要进一步学会听懂意思，除了聚精会神地硬听、抓取关键词之外，了解讲稿的构成，了解公共演讲的一些概念，熟悉讲话者的陈述方式，也有助于对讲稿的整体把握，有助于听清发言，抓取关键词，获取中心思想，准确地翻译出源语的意思。

面对公众的讲话可以有不同的形式和场合，但这里只涉及正式场合的讲话，因为需要译者翻译的公共演讲，一般都发生在比较正式的场合。

比较正式的场合通常包括大小会议、讲堂、课堂。政府官员的报告和讲话、各种机构领导的讲话和报告、各级机构上下级或下上级的工作汇报、各种公司对客

户的产品介绍、学校教授的专题演讲等都属于正式场合的演讲。演讲人或代表机构发表讲话，阐明政策、理念，汇报工作方向、工作计划，或工作成果等，或作为学者阐述新知识。这样的演讲多属于鼓动性演讲、传授性演讲（知识讲座、学术报告），以及鼓动加传授性的演讲。

正式的演讲有内容详尽的讲稿，或有幻灯片、影像资料、演示文稿（ppt）等视觉工具辅助。这种讲话的目的是将一个中心点与相关的概念讲清楚，因此内容都经过精心准备，信息丰富、条理清晰、逻辑清楚、语言正式。

从英译汉的角度去理解，需要了解英语写作的方式。在需要翻译的场合，英语正式演讲稿可以按演讲的目的来划分类型。使用频繁的是以告知为目的的发言稿和以说服为目的的发言稿两种。本单元先介绍以告知为目的的发言稿。

斯蒂芬·卢卡斯（Lucas，2001）将告知性的发言分为介绍物品、介绍过程、介绍事件、介绍概念。这种讲稿也被称为阐释文（explanation），其主题一般很明确，讲述方式客观准确，结构步骤清晰，信息全面，阐释详细，逻辑性强。无论是哪一种阐释文，文章的组织方式都可能从时间、空间、分条主题等方面着手。

中文将此类讲稿称为说明文。中文的说明文通常也按照时间顺序、空间顺序、逻辑顺序来陈述，说明方式有连贯式、总分式、并列式、递进式、对照式等；说明方法有举例、比较、定义、诠释、打比方、分类等。这些方法经常会被演讲者综合运用于一篇演讲稿中。

本教材第1单元的主题相关知识介绍是一篇介绍公共卫生概念的阐释文。该文以按条分主题的方式组织，展现了完整的有关公共卫生概念的四点，容易识别。做成口译概括练习时，这四点都应体现出来。概括的结果应该包括相当于该文一半字数的内容：

What Is Public Health?

Public health deals primarily with preventing disease, while medicine is concerned with curing disease in people already ill. Public health deals primarily with the health of populations, while medicine deals with the health of individuals. The difference can be seen in another way. When asked simple question, “What do people die of in the US?” Our medical colleagues will perhaps tell you that 41% die of cardiovascular disease, 24% from cancer, 4% from diabetes and 8% from injuries. We in public health would argue that 19% die of tobacco-related illness, 14% from poor diet and lack of exercise, 5% from alcohol-related disease and 2.5% from gun injuries. For this, people in public health will say that if risk factors for mortality are taken into account, it becomes clear that almost 50% of the 2.3 million deaths in the US each year could be prevented or postponed—that is, 1.1 million lives could be saved each year. Public health is in the business of identifying risks for ill health, and design strategies to enable people to avoid known risks for disease. This role is often described as health promotion, that is, changing our exposure to risks in our environment, or change unhealthy behaviors. Public health, activities, especially schools of public health, have four categories:

1. Research. Research can be defined as the generation of new knowledge, providing scientific evidence for decision-making at the individual or societal level. The discipline of public health embraces a wide variety of approaches to knowledge of the public's health and risk factors for disease. These include epidemiological and statistical sciences to look for disease associations and to design and analyze clinical trials and interventions; laboratory science to elucidate mechanisms of disease and risk; social science to uncover social determinants of illness and behavioral and societal changes that result in better health; and finally policy sciences, particularly to analyze the economic costs of illness, the costs and cost effectiveness of interventions, and the quality of health systems. As Julio Frank says, "A health system is a population's organized social response to its health problems... It represents the common vehicle through which all interventions we talk about are actually delivered to actual populations".

2. Training. Training in public health is a huge mission. Public health training is essential not only for degree students in public health and medicine, but also for police, firefighters, social workers, teachers, national leaders, and most importantly, the public. Decision makers for public health that is less than half of the workforce in the governmental departments have enough formal training. This can be seen in the case of graduates of the Harvard School of Public Health: about one-third serve the public through federal, state, county and municipal health departments; one-third work for the private sector in HMOs, hospitals, consulting companies, and the pharmaceutical industry; and the remaining third become motivated to go into research and academic public health.

3. Communication. Public health is to fulfill its responsibility to prevent death and illness and promote health, so it must have good communication skills in informing risks in a way of informing and motivating, rather than scaring people. The leaders and the public need to have access to accurate information that empowers them but not terrifies them.

4. Practice. All the knowledge from the laboratory needs to be used in practice that improves people's health. Our elected officials and policy makers need to understand and support the work of a large number of people dedicated in public health, because it is currently underappreciated. The achievements of public health in the last century can be seen

in the improved life expectancy that has risen in the US from 47 years in 1900 to 77 in 1999. The Centers for Disease Control and Prevention (CDC) summarized the major achievements of public health in the US during the last century as follows: vaccination and childhood immunization, motor vehicle safety, safer workplaces, control of infectious diseases, decline in deaths from coronary heart disease and stroke, safer and healthier foods, healthier mothers and babies, family planning, fluoridation of drinking water, and recognition of tobacco as a health hazard.

本单元主题的相关知识介绍是一篇大致按照时间、空间顺序排列的说明文。用总分的结构、分类的方式说明世界卫生组织的功能。在这篇英语文章中，每段大致有比较明确的、表明意思层次的主题句或递进关系词。

对本单元主题相关知识所做摘要应包含如下内容：

WHO, established on 7th April 1948, with its headquarter in Geneva. Its objective is “the attainment by all people of the highest possible level of health”. It works under the United Nations system.

WHO provides leadership on global health matters, shapes the health research agenda, sets standards, provides evidence-based policy options, provides technical support, and monitors health trends. It maintains now that health is a shared responsibility which means all people have access to essential care and all countries work together to defend transnational health threats, such as SARS, malaria, tuberculosis, influenza, HIV/AIDS, and others.

WHO also sponsors programs to prevent and treat such diseases by providing safe and effective vaccines, pharmaceutical diagnostics, and drugs through its Expanded Program on Immunization. Through 20 years' efforts, the world has eradicated smallpox in 1980. WHO's next target is to eradicate polio within the next few years.

WHO has other health-related campaigns, such as to boost the consumption of fruits and vegetables worldwide, discourage tobacco use, develop capacities of Member States to research on national needs.

The WHO has 193 Member states that have six autonomous regional offices: AFRO in Brazzaville, EURO in Copenhagen, SEARO in New Delhi, EMRO in Cairo, WPRO in Manila, and AMRO in Washington, D. C.

The current agenda emphasizes on women's health and health in Africa, including promoting development, fostering health security, strengthening health systems, harnessing research, information and evidence, enhancing partnerships, and improving performance.

三、词汇准备

Text 1

interventions 干预
noncommunicable diseases 非传染性疾病
wake-up call 叫醒电话；警钟，警示
wide awake 完全清醒的
epidemiology 流行病学
human and economic wreckage 人性和经济的灾难
chronic diseases 慢性病
cardiovascular disease 心血管疾病
diabetes 糖尿病
jogging lanes 慢跑专用道
fitness centres 健康中心
rudimentary regulatory capacity 基本的监管能力
turn off the tap 关上（水）龙头
resource-constrained settings 自愿受约束的背景
screening and early detection 筛查与早发现
bypass surgery, organ transplantation, chemotherapy, and radiotherapy add to the arsenal
方法中还要加上搭桥术、器官移植、化学疗法、放射性疗法
delivery of chronic care 提供长期护理
the WHO Framework Convention on Tobacco Control《世界卫生组织烟草控制框架公约》
primary health care 初级卫生保健
civil society 公民社会
ciclovias 自行车道

Text 2

financing mechanisms 筹资机制
universal coverage 全民覆盖
financial ruin 倾家荡产
emphasize protection of financial risk 强调经济风险保障

economic downturn 经济低潮
medically induced poverty 因病致贫
coverage of essential health services 基本卫生服务的覆盖面
raising sufficient money for health 筹集足够的卫生资金
generating new funds for health services 开发卫生经费的新来源
tax revenues 征税
universal coverage of insurance 保险全民覆盖
out-of-pocket payments 自付医疗费用
efficiency and equity 效率和公平性
incentive 激励
the New Cooperative Medical Schemes for Rural Populations, and the Urban Residents Basic Medical Insurance Scheme 新型农村合作医疗和城镇居民基本医疗保险
home-grown 由本国产生的
a one-off process 一朝一夕之举

Text 3

antibiotics 抗生素
dramatic advances 巨大的进步
TB (tuberculosis) 结核病
Malaria 疟疾
pneumonia 肺炎
diarrhoea 腹泻
drug-resistant organisms 耐药机制
exacerbate 恶化
resistant infections 抗药感染
impose 强加、强迫
to roll back 使后退、回落
undermine 逐渐削弱
stakeholders 参与方
raise accountability 增加责任心
policy package 一揽子政策
surveillance 监控

Text 4

the WHO Framework Convention on Tobacco Control (WHO FCTC) 《世界卫生组织烟草控制框架公约》

treaty 公约

auspices 支持

Conference of the Parties 缔约方会议

leading preventable cause of death 主要可预防的死因

lung ailment 肺部疾病

confers legal obligations 授予法律义务

vested interests 既得利益

regulate tobacco product disclosures 规范烟草制品宣传的规定

illicit trade 走私

economically viable alternative 经济上可行的选择

the tobacco epidemic 烟草流行病

honour its commitments, obligations and agreements 履行承诺，义务和协定

encompass 包括

sub-national jurisdictions 次国家级管辖区，次国家级行政区

to reach its full potential 充分发挥其潜力

to fully implement its provisions 充分执行其规定

commitment to prioritize the implementation 优先实施的承诺

Text 5

国民保健工程 National Health Project

脑卒中 cerebral apoplexy, stroke

急性脑血管病 acute cerebrovascular disease

致残率 disability rate

死亡率 mortality rate

死因调查 death inquiry

偏瘫、失语等残疾 hemiplegia, aphasia and other disabilities

溶栓治疗 thrombolytic therapy

缺血性卒中 ischemic stroke

颈动脉斑块 carotid artery plaque

常规体检 routine physical examination

颈动脉内膜剥脱手术（CEA） carotid endarterectomy surgery

临床 clinical
复发病例 recurrence case
基础病变 basis of disease
肢体活动障碍 limb movement disorder
视网膜或黄斑病变 retinal or macular degeneration
视力下降 decreased vision
核磁共振影像 magnetic resonance imaging
症状体征 symptoms and signs
脑部低灌注状态 brain hypoperfusion
听诊 auscultation
B超检查 B-ultrasound examination
颈动脉狭窄 carotid narrowness
慢性牙周炎 chronic periodontitis
缺血性眼病 ischemic eye disease

Text 6

海啸 tsunami
飓风 hurricane
同情和慰问 sympathy and condolences
相互联系、相互依存、利益交融 to have mutual communication, interdependence, and converging interests
《共享流感病毒以及获得疫苗和其他利益大流行流感防范框架》 "Pandemic Influenza Preparedness Framework for the Sharing of Influenza Viruses and Access to Vaccines and Other Benefits"
流感病毒 influenza virus
流感疫苗 influenza vaccine
抗病毒药物 antiviral drug
糖尿病 diabetes
患病率 morbidity rate
慢性非传染性疾病 chronic non-communicable disease
疾病防控 disease prevention and control
全球战略行动计划 global strategic action plan
基本医疗卫生服务全民覆盖 universal coverage of basic health services
健康档案 health record

井喷 blowout
核心指标 core indicators
突发公共卫生事件 public health emergencies

四、摘要练习

请听下面英语语篇，第一篇用源语言复述此段主要信息逻辑点及层次，第二篇用译入语复述此段主要信息逻辑点及层次。注意信息点之间的逻辑联系。

Text 1

Chronic Diseases Are No Longer Just a Health Problem

Closing Statement at the Regional High-level Consultation of the Americas on Noncommunicable Diseases and Obesity
Dr. Margaret Chan, Director-General of the World Health Organization
Mexico City, Mexico
25 February 2011

Excellencies, honourable ministers, distinguished delegates, ladies and gentlemen,

I thank the government of Mexico for hosting this event.

Your countries have shown great courage and determination in addressing the lifestyle-related factors that are driving the rise of these diseases.

You have looked at strategies and interventions and reached agreement on some ways forward. The September high-level meeting on noncommunicable diseases is an opportunity that the health sector must seize.

It must be a wake-up call, but not for public health. We are already wide awake.

We know the epidemiology, the global trends, and what the shift from affluent societies to poor and disadvantaged populations means in terms of human and economic wreckage. This is my first point.

My second point is that chronic diseases are no longer just a medical or a public health problem. They are a development problem, and they are a political problem. The pressure not to make the right decisions will be enormous.

Some will question the need for policy change. They will argue that individual choices are responsible for the rise of cardiovascular disease, diabetes, and cancer. People choose to smoke, to consume too much alcohol, to eat junk food, to sit in front of TV sets and computer screens.

In this logic, the responsibility for the world's 43 million pre-school children who are obese or overweight rests with bad parents. No, it is not bad parents. It is bad policies.

More and more people are living in societies that allow the sale of tobacco products and the seductive marketing of foods and beverages that are cheap, convenient, tasty, filling, and very bad for health.

More and more people are living in crowded urban areas with no playgrounds, no bicycle paths, no jogging lanes, and no fitness centres, of course.

Developing countries are soft targets, easy markets. Many lack even the most rudimentary regulatory capacity to address irresponsible marketing and control the products offered to consumers.

The health sector, acting alone, cannot turn off the tap. The measures needed for primary prevention on an adequate population-wide scale lie beyond the direct control of ministries of health. Making a difference will largely depend on action taken by non-health sectors.

My third point is that the challenge of managing these diseases in resource-constrained settings has been almost totally neglected.

In many wealthy nations, deaths from cardiovascular disease and cancer have declined, thanks largely to the success of anti-tobacco campaigns.

Credit must also go to the powerful interventions that are now available, including measures for screening and early detection, and medicines for reducing blood pressure, lowering cholesterol levels, and controlling blood sugar. Bypass surgery, organ transplantation, chemotherapy, and radiotherapy add to the arsenal.

But these interventions are beyond the reach of the poor. Health systems lack the staff, the medicines, the money, the screening and early detection services, and service models for the delivery of chronic care. Thirty developing countries, half of them in Africa, do not have a single radiotherapy machine.

Ladies and gentlemen,

I will close with a few words of advice.

Make primary prevention a top priority. For example, keep pushing for full implementation of the WHO Framework Convention on Tobacco Control.

Use evidence and economic arguments, as you have done, to shape policies at the highest possible level of government and in the international systems.

Continue to make the strengthening of health systems a top priority. Primary health care provides the best model for comprehensive services, from prevention, screening, and early detection, to long-term care that engages communities.

Engage civil society. Civil society can be an especially powerful ally in shaping public views and holding industry accountable for its behaviour.

Engage the private sector. Industry needs to collaborate in making healthy food choices the easy choices and in making medications and other interventions accessible and affordable.

Look at yourselves as leaders. The Latin American "Ciclovias" initiative for promoting physical activity is being copied around the world.

Above all, stand firm, as you have been doing throughout the Americas, and stay loud.

复述要点提示（主要信息逻辑点及层次）

Purpose of the speech:

A wake-up call for governments and people of all sectors around the world to take action, because departments of public heath cannot solve the problem alone.

Three keynotes of the speech:

1. The epidemiology and the global trends alarm us the possible damage chronic diseases are giving to people and society. We must be aware of what it means by shifting from affluent societies to poor and disadvantaged populations.

2. Chronic diseases are no longer just a medical or a public health problem. They are development and political problems.

Supporting ideas: a. Chronic diseases are caused by people's bad habits, such as smoking, alcohol drinking, and junk food. These are easily obtained from uncontrolled market which is a result of wrong policy decision. This situation is especially bad in the developing countries that have no ability to control this market. b. Chronic diseases are also a result of lack of exercises which is partly a result of staying in crowded cities and lack of facilities of fitness building. This also needs to be addressed by public policy.

3. Managing these diseases is difficult in resource-constrained settings and this difficulty is almost totally neglected. In the developed countries, anti-tobacco movement and effective intervention measures have reduced death caused by chronic diseases. The intervention measures include screening, bypass surgery, organ transplantation, chemotherapy, radiotherapy and medicines for reducing blood pressure, lowering cholesterol levels, and controlling blood sugar. However, for many developing countries, these intervention

measures are beyond the reach of the poor. Health systems lack the staff, the medicines, the money, the screening and early detection services, and service models for the delivery of chronic care.

Conclusion:

Call for primary prevention a top priority. Implementing the WHO Framework Convention on Tobacco Control.

Use evidence and economic arguments for policies at the highest possible level of government.

Strengthen health systems.

Engage civil society in shaping public views and holding industry accountable for its behaviour.

Engage the private sector.

Shoulder leader's responsibility. Learn from the Latin American "Ciclovias" initiative.

Text 2

Opening Remarks by Dr. Michael O'Leary, WHO China Representative at the Launch of the *World Health Report 2010*

Beijing, China

29 November 2010

Honorable Vice-Minister Chen,

Professor Ke Yang,

First Secretary Grant Morrison, Australian Embassy,

Colleagues,

Thank you for joining us at this important event. Our purpose today is two-fold. First, we aim to launch the *World Health Report 2010*, which focuses on health financing mechanisms as the path to universal coverage. Second, we aim to provide a forum to think carefully about the messages in this year's report and what they mean for China's national health care reform.

We have all heard about people who fall sick and go into debt to pay their medical bills. Or those too poor to even contemplate seeing a doctor when they need to, or delay treatment until it is too late.

Around the world today, millions of people cannot use needed health services because they are unavailable or are too expensive. Millions more are pushed into poverty each year because they must pay for the health services they use at the time they receive them.

This is unacceptable. No one in need of health care should risk financial ruin as a result.

It may seem impractical to emphasize protection of financial risk in the current economic downturn, at a time when health care costs are rising with ageing populations and there is an increase in chronic diseases. But these challenges only make our task all the more urgent given that protection of financial risks prevents medically induced poverty and promotes security.

This year's *World Health Report* provides countries with some ideas about how to use financing mechanisms to improve coverage of essential health services and provide stronger health security. It emphasizes three main points.

First, the *Report* discusses the importance of raising sufficient money for health. Different countries use different mechanisms to increase health spending. This can include increasing health spending as a share of total government spending—for example, this is being done in China. Other countries are generating new funds for health services. For example, many countries have increased taxes on tobacco, alcohol, and junk food—which have the benefit of reducing consumption of products that are harmful to health while also increasing tax revenues.

Second, the *Report* emphasizes universal coverage of insurance and replacing household out-of-pocket payments with prepayment mechanisms. Even in wealthy countries, such as the United States, people may face financial hardship or go into poverty because they do not have insurance and have to pay directly for health care. In contrast, other countries have made progress in setting up systems to gradually expand universal coverage and reduce the reliance on out-of-pocket payments for health care.

The third point of the *Report* is about efficiency and equity. In these difficult times, it is important to look for opportunities to improve efficiency in the health sector.

While increasing funding to health is crucial, we must also ensure that the funds are well spent and create a healthier population. The *Report* documents many areas in which efficiency can be improved, such as improving rational use of medicines, increasing hospital efficiency, using public funds to pay for the most cost-effective interventions, and making sure that health providers are paid in a way that gives them incentives for high quality care and better health.

This is an interesting time for health finance. Many countries are reforming the way they move towards universal coverage, including two of the most important global economies,

China and the United States.

China has made important progress in health care reform since spring last year, when the government announced plans to provide safe, effective, convenient and affordable health services to all urban and rural residents by 2020. WHO congratulates China on its strong commitment to these reforms. The country is now mid-way through the three-year phase, and is already seeing encouraging results.

At the heart of these reforms are the New Cooperative Medical Schemes for rural populations, and the Urban Residents Basic Medical Insurance scheme. Hard targets have been set. The government aims to reduce dependence on direct payments, and has already increased the proportion of the population covered by rural health insurance system to over 90%. Increased financial risk protection will be done over time.

The reforms in China stand out, partly because of the size of the system involved. But it is not alone in its approach to funding healthcare. Many countries are taking active steps to move towards universal coverage, or to sustain it once achieved.

This global *Report* covers not just successes, but also failures and setbacks, so that other countries can anticipate barriers and challenges and avoid them. No single mix of policy options will work well in every setting. Effective strategies must be home-grown.

Many of these experiences could be useful for China, in making adjustments in the social security system to ensure that everyone in China has access to affordable health services.

We also know from many countries that health care reform is not a one-off process. It requires adjustments along the way. We are pleased to be part of efforts to monitor and evaluate the process of reform in China.

In conclusion, I would like to thank the Ministry of Health for co-hosting this launch, and the China Center for Health Development Studies of Peking University for organizing it. Our appreciation also goes to AusAID, whose support for health systems strengthening in the region has made today's event possible.

I wish you many fruitful discussions ahead.

复述要点提示（主要信息逻辑点及层次）

两个目的：

1. 发布《2010年世界卫生报告》，其核心内容是如何利用筹资机制实现基本医疗全民覆盖。

2. 希望提供一个平台，以便认真思考今年报告中的信息及其对中国医改的

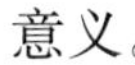

意义。

背景：

1. 数百万人因疾病和医疗费用而负债累累、陷入贫困，数百万人因贫生病无法治疗，或久拖不医酿成大病。但任何人都不应因病而倾家荡产。

2. 由于强调经济风险保障可防止因病致贫和促进安全感，因此在经济处于低潮、人口老龄化、慢性病增多、卫生服务成本不断增加的背景下，我们反而更要尽快完成经济风险保障工作。

围绕第一目的的中心议题：

《世界卫生报告》利用筹资机制来扩大基本卫生服务的全民覆盖面。强调三个要点：

1. 讨论筹够卫生资金的重要性。不同国家采用不同机制来增加卫生支出。例如中国增加政府总支出中卫生支出的比例，其他国家则开发卫生经费的新来源，如提高对烟草、酒和垃圾食品的征税。这样既减少了危害健康产品的消费，又增加了税收。

2. 强调保险全民覆盖和以预付制取代家庭自付支出。即使在美国等富裕国家，也会有人因无保险覆盖，必须直接支付医疗费用而面临经济困难或陷入贫困。同时，其他国家则在建立相应体制、逐渐实现全民覆盖、减少自付医疗费用方面取得进展。

3. 强调效率和公平性。同时要确保资金得到有效使用。《报告》认为多个领域可能提高效率，如合理用药、提高医院效率、用公共资金支付最具成本效益的干预措施等，同时确保薪酬机制能激励医务人员提供高质量的医疗服务。

围绕第二目的的中心议题：

中国医改方面，政府有力承诺2020年向全国城乡居民提供安全、有效、方便和负担得起的卫生服务的计划。三年的时间过了一半，中国已经取得了令人鼓舞的成果。

改革的核心内容为新型农村合作医疗和城镇居民基本医疗保险。政府已经树立了明确的目标，旨在降低对直接付费的依赖程度，并已将新农合的覆盖率扩大到90%以上。强化经济风险保障的目标将逐步得以实现。

中国改革引人注目，部分原因是所涉及体系规模巨大，但中国并非是改革卫生筹资的唯一国家。许多国家都在积极行动，逐步实现全民覆盖，或在实现后保持下去。

全球《报告》并非仅仅记录成功之处，还记录了失败与挫折，以便其他国家参考。没有政策能够通用于各种情况，有效策略一定是由本国制订的。在改革社会保障系统、确保每个中国人都能获得可负担的卫生服务过程中，许多经验都可供中国借鉴。他国的经验表明，医改并非一朝一夕之举，需要不断进行调整。

五、英译汉练习

Text 3

Combat USA Antimicrobial Resistance: No Action Today, No Cure Tomorrow

UN Secretary-General's Message for World Health Day

Ban Ki-moon, New York

7 April 2011

The discovery of antibiotics and other antimicrobial medicines has been responsible for some of the most dramatic advances in human health. Before these drugs were introduced in the 1940s, infectious diseases took the lives of tens of millions of people each year. These medicines helped drive down the infectious disease burden.

Initial gains were primarily in higher-income countries and among wealthier populations in poor countries. But over the past two decades, new public health strategies and financing mechanisms have enabled poorer communities to access medicines that combat major killers, including TB, HIV, malaria, pneumonia and diarrheal diseases. Private sales of medicines for human and animal use have also dramatically expanded.

The gains have been profound, yet we now risk losing many of these precious medicines as drug-resistant organisms emerge. Antimicrobial resistance is a natural phenomenon, but it is exacerbated by the widespread use, overuse and misuse of medicines, and the spread of resistant infections in health-care and agriculture. Trade, travel and migration are increasing the spread of these organisms across communities and borders.

Some of the medicines that saved our parents and grandparents are already unusable today. Drug resistance imposes huge costs on health systems and is taking a growing—and unnecessary—toll in lives, threatening to roll back much of the progress we have made towards the health-related Millennium Development Goals. It could also undermine the gains of other modern medicines and technologies used to fight non-communicable diseases. Perhaps most disturbing is that the pipeline for new antimicrobial medicines to replace those that have been lost has nearly dried up.

The World Health Organization has selected "Combat Antimicrobial Resistance: No Action Today, No Cure Tomorrow" as the theme for this year's World Health Day. The emergence of antimicrobial resistance is a complex problem that involves a range of stakeholders. It needs to be urgently and aggressively addressed through a comprehensive response across sectors, within and across nations.

Today, WHO is calling for action to raise accountability and halt the spread of drug resistance through a six-point policy package: joint planning; surveillance; drug regulation; rational use of medicines; infection prevention and control; innovation and research. Governments, industry and all stakeholders must answer the call. Global health and untold millions of lives are at risk.

Text 4

Remarks by Dr. Mukundan Pillay, Senior Program Management Officer, WHO China, at the Ceremony of the 24th World No Tobacco Day in China

Beijing, China
26 May 2011

Distinguished guests, Ladies and gentlemen,

Good Morning!

The theme of this year's World No Tobacco Day is "The WHO Framework Convention on Tobacco Control".

The WHO Framework Convention on Tobacco Control (WHO FCTC) is the world's foremost tobacco control instrument. The first treaty ever negotiated under the auspices of WHO, it represents a signal achievement in the advancement of public health.

In force only since 2005, it is already one of the most rapidly and widely embraced treaties in the history of the United Nations, with more than 170 Parties.

Today we wish to highlight the treaty's overall importance, to stress China's obligations as a Party to the treaty and to promote the essential role of the Conference of the Parties and WHO in supporting China's efforts to meet those obligations.

Tobacco use is the leading preventable cause of death, in the world and in China. Every year in China, about 1 million people die from tobacco-related heart attack, stroke, cancer, lung ailment or other disease. That does not include the people—more than a quarter of them children—who die from exposure to second-hand smoke.

The annual death toll from the global epidemic of tobacco use could rise to 8 million by 2030. Having killed 100 million people during the 20th century, tobacco use could kill 1 billion during the 21st century.

As with any other treaty, the WHO FCTC confers legal obligations on its Parties including China. Among these obligations are those to:

● Protect public health policies from commercial and other vested interests of the tobacco industry

● Adopt price and tax measures to reduce the demand for tobacco

● Protect people from exposure to tobacco smoke

● Regulate the contents of tobacco products

● Regulate tobacco product disclosures

● Regulate the packaging and labeling of tobacco products

● Warn people about the dangers of tobacco

● Ban tobacco advertising, promotion and sponsorship

● Offer people help to end their addiction to tobacco

● Control the illicit trade in tobacco products. Ban sales to and by minors

● Support economically viable alternative to tobacco growing

WHO would like to congratulate China on the inclusion of tobacco control in the 12th five-year plan. China's leadership recognizes the importance of stopping the tobacco epidemic in this country and that the Government intends to honour its commitments, obligations and agreements under the WHO Framework Convention on Tobacco Control.

By implementing the WHO Framework Convention on Tobacco Control, in line with the 5 years plan, China can save millions of lives, and avert massive costs both economic and humanitarian. In this way, China is part of a global movement to end the burden of death and disease caused by tobacco.

WHO would also like to congratulate the Ministry of Health on their issuance of the revised implementation guidelines for the regulation on public places health management.

WHO encourages implementation of this Rule to encompass all indoor public places, workplaces including offices, and public transport. Indoor smoke should fade into history—as it has done in more than 17 countries and countless sub-national jurisdictions around the world.

More must be done—in China and among all the Parties—for the treaty to reach its full potential, as the Parties themselves recognize. At the Parties recent meeting in Punta del Este,

Uruguay, the Parties urged all countries to ratify the treaty, to fully implement its provisions and to adopt its guidelines.

Furthermore, the Parties reaffirmed their commitment to prioritize the implementation of health measures designed to control tobacco consumption.

On World No Tobacco Day 2011, and throughout this year, WHO will continue to support China to control the epidemic of tobacco use and reduce the toll of tobacco-related diseases and deaths in line with treaty obligations.

Thank you.

六、汉译英练习

Text 5

脑中风筛查及防控——一项被忽略的国民保健工程（节选）

全国人大常委会委员、原卫生部副部长　王陇德

脑卒中是一种急性脑血管病，具有发病率高、致残率高和死亡率高的特点。目前，我国每年用于治疗脑血管病的费用估计约120多亿元，再加上各种间接经济损失，每年用于本病的总支出近200亿元。

我国居民第三次死因调查结果显示，脑血管病已成为国民第一位的死因，死亡率高于欧美国家4至5倍，是日本的3.5倍，甚至高于泰国、印度等发展中国家。根据北京安贞医院20年脑卒中病例资料分析，致死性中风仅占27%，大部分卒中病人存活且遗留偏瘫、失语等严重影响生活质量的残疾。脑卒中已对国民的生命健康造成严重威胁，并将大幅度增加疾病负担。

对血管已有基础性病变的人群来讲，及早筛查出病因及病变程度，并给予适当的干预，即脑卒中的二、三级预防，仍应是一项重要的防控措施。

对缺血性卒中的治疗，虽然超早期溶栓治疗（中风后3小时之内实施）能够显著降低患者的病死率和残疾率，但由于诸多原因，即使是在欧美等发达国家，及时溶栓率仍然相当低。近年来，我国缺血性卒中的比例快速上升。在以往的心脑血管病防控工作中，我国对高血压的筛查和控制比较重视，但对引致缺血性脑卒中重要原因之一的颈动脉斑块造成的狭窄注意不够，甚至在常规的干部体检中也没有颈动脉筛查项目。因此，大量卒中前期的患者没有被及时发现并给予有效的干预。目前，

美国已建成了脑卒中移动筛查网络，每年开展颈动脉内膜剥脱手术（CEA）约20万例，中风的死亡率大幅度下降，而我国目前仅有极少数医院能开展此类手术，年手术仅百余例。我国学者对临床资料的分析表明，门诊的脑卒中患者中约40%为复发病例，说明如造成中风的基础病变不被去除或予以控制的话，会再次或多次反复出现中风。

近几年，我国专家在脑中风筛查及干预试点中发现，许多病人由于颈动脉狭窄引致的中风体征，如肢体活动障碍、失语、听力减退甚至丧失、视网膜或黄斑病变以及视力明显下降等，在颈动脉狭窄解除后，均得到了明显改善或恢复。甚至在核磁共振影像上已显示脑功能区部分坏死的病人，在解除颈动脉狭窄后，其已丧失的功能又出现恢复的奇迹。这些案例说明，我们以往对脑中风的形成机理认识得还不甚清楚，部分中风病人的症状体征，包括视觉、听觉的部分问题，可能是由于颈部大动脉的狭窄而造成的脑部低灌注状态所引起的。

通过对颈动脉状况的筛查，既可对狭窄不甚严重的患者及早给予行为指导或药物干预，延缓其狭窄进展，又可对狭窄严重的患者采取介入或手术治疗，去除其发生中风的病源，减少中风的发生及伤残。

颈动脉筛查的方法比较简便，是一种非创伤性且费用不高的检查。狭窄严重的患者通过颈部听诊就可发现；使用颈部B超检查，可发现绝大部分狭窄患者并判定其狭窄程度，但筛查技术需要经过专门培训。

颈动脉狭窄的主要危险因素有高血压、高血脂、高血糖、长期吸烟史、长期大量饮酒、慢性牙周炎病史、缺血性眼病史、45岁以上男性、55岁以上女性。具有以上两项危险因素者应接受颈动脉筛查。

为尽快改变脑卒中严重威胁国民健康的状况，我国应尽快拟定出筛查规范、干预原则以及颈动脉内膜剥脱手术标准与相关要求，并争取三年内能在全国各省、区、市至少建立起一所脑卒中筛查及干预中心或基地，对高危人群进行普遍筛查，以降低我国脑血管病的发病与死亡率。

Text 6

慢性非传染性疾病防控刻不容缓
陈竺部长出席第64届世界卫生大会所作一般性辩论发言

瑞士日内瓦

2011年5月16日

尊敬的主席先生、尊敬的总干事女士，各位部长、各位同事：

首先请允许我对主席先生的当选表示祝贺。我相信在您的领导下，本届大会一定能够取得圆满成功。

我愿借此机会对在日本地震和海啸、美国飓风灾害中失去亲人，遭受不幸的家庭表示同情和慰问。这些事件说明在遭遇自然灾害时，人类是如此脆弱，因此，我们需要在人与自然、发展与环境间实现和谐。当前，全球化使各国相互联系、相互依存、利益交融达到前所未有的程度，携手合作、同舟共济符合各国共同利益。在此，我祝贺成员国政府间工作组历时四年就《共享流感病毒以及获得疫苗和其他利益大流行流感防范框架》达成共识。对广大发展中国家将不仅只提供流感病毒，并且在《框架》的安排下，将合理、合法、公平地分享流感疫苗和抗病毒药物的利益。这充分体现了各国的团结与合作，必将为今后国际社会共同应对威胁人类自身安全的公共卫生挑战树立一个典范。

女士们、先生们，

根据中国最新的人口普查数据，中国60岁及以上人口占13.26%，人口老龄化进程加快。中国已成为世界上首个“未富先老”的发展中大国。中国有2亿高血压患者，每年新发280万癌症患者，糖尿病患病率已达到9%。慢性非传染性疾病占中国人群死因构成升至85%，每年约370万人因慢性非传染性疾病过早死亡。慢性非传染性疾病已经给社会经济发展造成了巨大的威胁。防控慢性非传染性疾病，任重道远。

中国政府高度重视慢性非传染性疾病防控工作，参照世界卫生组织的“全球战略行动计划”，坚持预防为主，降低发病率；坚持早发现，减少经济负担；坚持以人为本，提高生活质量；坚持政府主导，全社会共同参与。中国当前进行的医药卫生体制改革正在实现基本医疗卫生服务全民覆盖，包括为全民建立健康档案，为35岁以上人群提供高血压、糖尿病健康管理服务，为65岁以上老年人提供健康检查服务等。中国政府已在“十二五”经济社会发展规划中将人均期望寿命提高1岁列为核心指标。我们深知，要实现这一目标，实现慢性非传染性疾病的有效防控是关键，为此，我们还将以创建健康城市为抓手，积极开展健康促进、控烟、提高社会服务综合管理能力，并进一步加强以全科医师为重点的基层医疗卫生队伍建设，提高综合服务能力。卫生改革正在为人们带来看得见、摸得着的实惠。

主席先生、各位同事，

慢性非传染性疾病防控是一项刻不容缓的工作。如果控制不好，未来20至30年，全球将会出现慢性非传染性疾病的“井喷”。必须重视导致慢性非传染性疾病的健康社会决定因素。国际社会必须增强使命感和紧迫感，必须坚定地实施慢性非传染性疾病全球战略行动计划。我在此提出如下建议：

第一，各国将慢性非传染性疾病防控纳入衡量本国社会经济发展状况的核心指标，国际社会进一步推动将慢性非传染性疾病防控指标纳入千年发展目标。慢性非传染性疾病是“社会传染病”，各国政府要像重视GDP一样重视慢性非传染性疾病预防控制工作，将其纳入当地经济社会发展总体规划，建立部门间协调机制，加强社会动员，共同参与。国际社会要积极筹措资金，保障经费投入。

第二，进一步加强卫生体系建设。强有力的卫生体系不仅是应对传染病以及突发公共卫生事件的基础，更是防控慢性非传染性疾病的关键。各国政府应将卫生体系建设作为重点工作内容。发达国家和国际组织应将加强卫生体系建设作为对外援助的一个重要领域，增加援助力度，帮助发展中国家建设卫生体系。

第三，充分发挥世界卫生组织在全球卫生发展日程中的领导作用，支持陈冯富珍总干事领导秘书处的改革进程。希望世界卫生组织在今年9月联合国关于慢性非传染性疾病峰会的筹备中发挥领导作用，在全球建立统一明确的慢性非传染性疾病防控目标与评价指标，制订清晰的行动路线，协调整合国际资源，建立广泛的国际合作和伙伴关系。

主席先生、各位同事，

在此，我也要对总干事陈冯富珍女士表示祝贺，感谢您带领世界卫生组织秘书处，为全球卫生改革和发展发挥的卓越领导和协调作用。

谢谢大家。

资料来源：

Text 1 http://www.who.int/dg/speeches/2011/NCDs_20110225/en/

Text 2 http://www.wpro.who.int/china/mediacentre/speeches/2013/20130407/en/

Text 3 http://www.who.int/dg/speeches/2011/WHD_20110407/en/

Text 4 http://www.wpro who. inr/china/mediacentre/speeches/2011/WRSP_20110425/en/

Text 5 http://zl.39.net/bj/2009620/906091.html

Text 6 http://www.wfas.org.cn/news/ournews/201105/2661.html

参考答案

四、摘要练习

Text 1

慢性病不再仅仅是卫生问题

在美洲区域非传染性疾病和肥胖症高级别磋商会上的闭幕词

世界卫生组织总干事　陈冯富珍博士

墨西哥墨西城

2011年2月25日

各位阁下、尊敬的各位部长、各位代表、女士们、先生们：

我对墨西哥政府主办这次会议表示感谢。

在处理增加这些疾病的生活方式相关因素方面，你们国家显示出了极大的勇气和决心。

你们已经研究过战略和干预措施，并在某些方面达成了一致。9月份召开的非传染性疾病高级别会议是卫生部门必须抓住的一次机会。

这次高级别会议必须成为一次“叫醒服务”，不是针对公共卫生部门，因为我们已经非常清醒。

我们知道流行病学和全球趋势，知道对人类和经济造成的破坏方面，从富裕社会向贫穷和弱势群体的这种转变意味着什么。这是我要讲的第一点。

我要讲的第二点是，慢性病不再仅仅是医学或公共卫生问题，还是一个发展问题和一个政治问题。而做出不正确决定的压力会是巨大的。

有人质疑改变政策的需要。他们可能会争辩，个人的选择决定了心血管疾病、糖尿病和癌症的上升趋势。人们选择吸烟、喝酒、吃垃圾食品、坐在电视和电脑显示器前边。

以这种逻辑看来，不负责任的家长们应该对全世界4 300万患有肥胖症或超重的学龄前儿童负责。不，不是家长不好，而是政策不对头。

越来越多的人居住在允许烟草产品销售和允许食品和饮料诱导性营销的社区，这些东西廉价、便利、美味，唇齿留芳，却极大地损害身体健康。

越来越多的人生活在拥挤的城市，没有活动场地，没有自行车道，没有慢跑的道路，没有健身中心。

发展中国家是他们的软目标和容易占领的市场。这些国家中的大部分甚至没有对其国内市场的这些产品的最基本监管能力。

卫生部门的独自行动无法切断源头。所需的充足的全人群初级预防措施，则远远超出卫生部门直接控制的范围。而差异在很大程度上取决于非卫生部门的行动。

我的第三个观点是，在资源紧缺环境下疾病管理的挑战几乎被完全忽略。

在许多富裕国家，心血管疾病和癌症引起的死亡正在减少，当然，这在很大程度上要归功于反烟运动的成功。

包括筛查和早期发现以及降低血压、胆固醇水平和控制血糖药物在内的各项有效干预措施均能够得到利用。搭桥手术、器官移植、化疗以及放射治疗均被加入了我们的手段储备。

然而，干预措施目前大大超出发展中国家的能力范围。卫生系统无法应对，工作人员、药物、资金、筛查及早期发现服务以及慢性病保健的服务模式匮乏。30个发展中国家，其中半数位于非洲，连一台放射治疗机都没有。

女士们、先生们，

我希望以几句建议结束今天的讲话。

将一级预防作为重中之重。例如，继续推进《世界卫生组织烟草控制框架公约》的全面实施。

利用你已经掌握的证据和经济论点在可能的政府最高级别及国际系统中影响政策。

将继续加强卫生系统作为重中之重。基础医疗保健为从预防、筛选和早期发现到涉及社区的长期保健在内的综合服务提供了最佳模型。

使民间社会参与其中。在影响舆论和确保行业自负其责方面，民间社会可能成为非常强大的盟友。

使私立机构参与其中。行业需要共同努力，使健康的食物易于选择，使生产的药物和其他干预措施能够获得，且人们负担得起。

把你们自己视为带头人。拉丁美洲旨在促进人们锻炼身体的健身自行车道倡议正在被世界各地复制。

总而言之，脚踏实地，正如我们已经在拉丁美洲所做的那样大声疾呼。

谢谢大家！

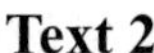

Text 2

世界卫生组织驻华代表蓝睿明博士
在《2010年世界卫生报告》发布式上的致辞

中国北京

2010年11月29日

尊敬的陈副部长、柯杨教授、澳大利亚使馆一秘格兰特·莫里森先生、各位同事：

感谢大家出席今天的重要活动。我们今天有两个目的：首先是发布《2010年世界卫生报告》，其核心内容是如何利用卫生筹资机制实现基本医疗全民覆盖。其次，我们希望提供一个平台，以便认真思考今年报告中的信息及其对中国医改的意义。

我们都听说过有人因疾病和医疗费用而负债累累，还有人因为太贫困生了病想都不敢想去看医生，或久拖不医直至酿成大病。

当今的世界上，有数百万人因缺医少药或无力付费而无法获得所需的医疗服务，还有数百万人每年因在就医时必须支付费用而陷于贫困。

这种情况令人难以接受。任何人都不应因为需要医疗服务而最后变得倾家荡产。

在目前经济处于低潮、卫生服务成本随着人口老龄化及慢性病增多而不断增加的背景下，强调经济风险保障似乎有些不切实际，但由于经济风险保障可防止因病致贫和增加安全感，上述困难只会让我们的任务变得更加紧迫。

今年的《世界卫生报告》就如何利用筹资机制来扩大基本卫生服务的覆盖面、提供更有效的医疗保险，为各国提出了一些想法。报告强调了三个要点：

首先，《报告》讨论了筹集足够的卫生资金的重要性。不同的国家采用不同的机制来增加卫生支出。有些国家增加政府总支出中卫生支出的比例，中国就是一例。其他国家则开掘卫生经费的新来源。例如，许多国家提高了对烟草、酒精和垃圾食品的征税，这既减少了此类危害健康产品的消费，又增加了税收，可谓一举两得。

其次，《报告》强调了保险全民覆盖和以预付制取代家庭自付支出。即使在美国等富裕国家，也会有人因无保险覆盖必须直接支付医疗费用而面临经济困难或陷入贫困。与之相比，其他国家则已在建立相应体制、逐渐实现全民覆盖、减少对自付医疗费用的依赖方面取得了进展。

《报告》的第三点是关于效率和公平性。在困难时期，利用一切机会来提高卫生系统的效率显得十分重要。

增加卫生投资十分重要，同时，还要确保资金得到有效使用，让人民更健康。《报告》阐述了许多可进一步提高效率的领域，如合理用药、提高医院效率、用公共资金支付最具成本效益性的干预措施等，同时还应确保医务人员的薪酬机制能够激励他们提供高质量的医疗服务和更好地促进健康。

我们正逢卫生筹资改革的大好时机。包括全球两个最重要的经济体——中国和美国在内的许多国家，正着手改革其逐步实现全民覆盖的思路。

自去年春季以来，中国已在医改方面取得了重要进展，政府宣布了到2020年向全国城乡居民提供安全、有效、方便和负担得起的卫生服务的计划。世卫组织向中国对上述改革做出如此有力的承诺表示祝贺。三年的时间过了一半，中国已经取得了令人鼓舞的成果。

改革的核心内容为新型农村合作医疗和城镇居民基本医疗保险。政府树立了明确的目标，旨在降低对直接付费的依赖程度，并已将新农合的覆盖率扩大到90%以上。强化经济风险保障的目标将逐步得以实现。

中国的改革引人注目，部分原因是涉及的体系规模巨大，但中国并非改革卫生筹资的唯一国家。许多国家都在积极行动，逐步实现全民覆盖，或在实现后保持下去。

全球《报告》并非仅仅记录了成功之处，还记录了失败与挫折，以便其他国家可以预见到困难及挑战并加以避免。没有哪套政策是能够通用于各种情况的，有效的策略一定是由本国制订的。

在改革社会保障系统、确保每个中国人都能获得可负担的卫生服务过程中，许多经验都可供中国借鉴。

我们还从许多国家的经验中了解到，医改并非一朝一夕之举，需要不断进行调整。在对中国改革过程的监测与评价中，我们很高兴能置身其中。

最后，我要感谢卫生部共同举办和北京大学中国卫生发展研究中心承办了此次发布会。还要感谢澳大利亚国际开发署：正是有了他们对本区域加强卫生系统工作的支持，才有了今天的会议。

预祝会议讨论富有成效。

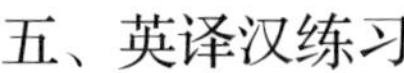

五、英译汉练习

Text 3

战胜抗菌药抗药性：今天不行动，明天无救药

联合国秘书长世界健康日致辞

潘基文
美国纽约
2011年4月7日

抗生素和其他抗菌药物的发现促成了人类健康的一些令人瞩目的进展。在20世纪40年代这些药物问世之前，各种传染病每年都夺去数千万人的生命。这些药物帮助减轻了传染病的负担。

初期成果主要出现在收入较高的国家，也出现在贫穷国家境内比较富裕的人群之中。但过去20年来，新的公共卫生战略和筹资机制使较贫穷地区也能获得防治主要致命疾病的药物，这些疾病包括结核病、艾滋病毒、疟疾、肺炎和腹泻病。人类和动物用药的私营销售量也已显著增长。

这些成果影响深远，但随着抗药性微生物的出现，我们现在面临失去许多这些珍贵药物的危险。抗菌药抗药性是一种自然现象，但药物的广泛使用、过度使用和滥用以及在保健和农业方面各种抗药性传染病的蔓延加剧了这种现象。贸易、旅行和迁徙正增加这些微生物跨越地区和国界的传播。

有些曾挽救过我们父母和祖父母生命的药物今天已无法使用。抗药性给卫生系统带来巨大成本负担，正在造成越来越多的、不必要的生命损失，可能抵消我们在有关卫生千年发展目标方面所取得的许多进展。这种情况还可能破坏用于防治非传染性疾病的其他现代药物和技术所取得的成果。最令人担心的情况也许是：研制新型抗菌药以取代已失去的药物的渠道几乎已经枯竭。

世界卫生组织选择了“战胜抗菌药抗药性：今天不行动，明天无救药”作为今年世界卫生日的主题。抗菌药抗药性的出现是一个复杂的问题，涉及方方面面的利益相关者，迫切需要在各国国内和各国之间通过跨部门的综合应对措施积极予以解决。

今天，世卫组织呼吁大家采取行动，通过以下六点政策加强问责制并遏止抗药性的蔓延：共同规划、监测、药物监管、合理用药、预防和控制传染、创新和研究。各国政府、企业界和所有利益相关者都必须响应这个号召。全球的健康和无数的生命正面临威胁。

Text 4

世界卫生组织驻华代表处高级项目管理官员裴雷博士
在第24个世界无烟日主题活动上的讲话

中国北京

2011年5月26日

尊敬的各位来宾，女士们、先生们：

早上好！

今年世界无烟日的主题是《世界卫生组织烟草控制框架公约》。

《世界卫生组织烟草控制框架公约》（WHO FCTC）是世界上最重要的烟草控制手段，是在世卫组织主持下完成的第一个全球性的公约，也是公共卫生发展的标志性成就。

《世界卫生组织烟草控制框架公约》自2005年生效至今，已有170个缔约方，是联合国历史上在最短时间内获得最广泛认同的协议之一。

今天，我们想从整体上强调该公约的重要性，重申中国作为缔约方应履行的公约义务，以及在中国努力履行这些义务时，缔约方会议和世卫组织如何进一步发挥支持作用。

不论在世界范围还是对中国而言，烟草使用都是首位可预防的死因。每年，中国有大约100万人死于烟草相关的心脏病发作、中风、癌症、肺部疾病或其他疾病。另外还有很多人（其中四分之一以上为儿童）死于接触二手烟。

到2030年，预计全球每年因烟草使用而死亡的人数将上升至800万。20世纪，烟草使用已导致1亿人死亡，21世纪将导致10亿人死亡。

如同其他协定一样，《世界卫生组织烟草控制框架公约》要求其缔约方，包括中国，承担相应的法律义务，包括：

- 保护公共卫生政策免受烟草业及其他既得利益方的影响
- 采取价格和税收措施以降低烟草需求
- 保护人们远离二手烟
- 烟草制品成分管制
- 烟草制品披露的规定
- 烟草制品包装和标签的规定
- 警示人们烟草的危害
- 禁止烟草广告、促销和赞助
- 帮助人们戒除烟瘾

●控制烟草制品的非法贸易

●禁止向未成年人或由未成年人销售烟草

●支持经济上可行的活动，替代烟草种植

世卫组织祝贺中国将控烟工作纳入“十二五”规划。中国政府的领导认识到了遏制烟草流行对于国家的重要性；同时，政府将兑现自己的承诺，履行对《世界卫生组织烟草控制框架公约》的义务和约定。

中国履行《世界卫生组织烟草控制框架公约》不仅与五年计划保持了一致，同时还可挽救百万生命，并免于付出经济和人道主义的双重代价。这样一来，在终止烟草引发的死亡和疾病负担的全球运动中，中国做出了自己的贡献。

世卫组织还祝贺卫生部修改并颁布了新的《公共场所卫生管理条例实施细则》。

世卫组织鼓励执行这一规定，将所有室内公共场所、办公场所和公共交通工具都纳入管理范围。如同全世界17个国家和无数次国家级行政区域已经做到的，室内烟草烟雾在中国也将逐渐成为历史。

缔约方有一个共识：要充分发挥该协议的作用，中国和其他缔约方还需要做更多工作。最近缔约方在乌拉圭埃斯特角城召开会议，敦促所有国家批准该公约，完全履行公约规定，并应用其实施准则。

此外，缔约方还重申了各自的承诺，明确会优先执行用来控制烟草的健康措施。

在2011年世界无烟日以及随后的日子里，世卫组织都将继续支持中国履行公约责任，控制烟草使用流行，并减少烟草相关的疾病和死亡。

谢谢！

六、汉译英练习

Text 5

Stroke Screening, Prevention and Control: A Neglected National Health Service Project

Wang Longde, Member of the NDC Standing Committee, Former Vice Minister of Health

Stroke is an acute cerebrovascular disease with high incidence, high morbidity and high mortality. At present, China’s annual costs for the treatment of cerebrovascular disease are estimated to be around more than 12 billion Yuan. With an additional variety of indirect economic losses, the total expenditure of the disease reaches nearly 20 billion Yuan each year.

China's third survey of causes of death of residents shows that cerebrovascular disease has become the first cause of death. Its mortality rate is 4 to 5 times higher than that of Europe and the United States, and is 3.5 times higher than that of Thailand, India and other developing countries. An analysis of cases of stroke documented by Beijing Anzhen Hospital during the past 20 years shows that fatal stroke takes up only 27% of the total cases, while the majority of stroke patients survive but are left with disabilities such as hemiplegia and aphasia that seriously affect the quality of life. Stroke seriously threatens people's life and health, and substantially increases the burden of disease.

To population whose blood vessels already have basic lesions, both early screening of causes and severity of disease and early delivery of appropriate intervention, namely secondary and tertiary prevention, remains an important measure of stroke prevention and control.

In treatment of ischemic stroke, although the ultra-early thrombolytic therapy that is used within three hours after stroke can significantly reduce the mortality and disability rate, due to many reasons, timely thrombolysis rate is still quite low even in Europe, the United States and other developed countries. In recent years, the proportion of ischemic stroke in China increases rapidly. In our previous cardiovascular and cerebrovascular disease prevention and control, we had more emphasis on screening and control of hypertension than attention to the narrowness caused by carotid artery plaque which is the main reason of ischemic stroke. We don't even have carotid artery screening program in our conventional government employee health examination. Therefore, a large number of pre-stroke patients have not been timely found and treated with effective intervention. Currently, the United States has built a mobile screening network for stroke, and conducted about 200,000 carotid endarterectomy surgeries (CEA) every year, having significantly reduced stroke mortality rates. In China, only a very small number of hospitals can carry out such surgery. We have just 100 cases of such surgery each year. An analysis of clinical data done by Chinese scholars shows that approximately 40% of stroke outpatients are recurrence cases. This indicates that if basis of lesion for stroke is not removed and controlled, the patients will have repeated strokes.

In recent years' stroke screening and intervention pilot project, our experts find that many patients with carotid artery stenosis have developed stroke signs, such as limb movement disorder, aphasia, hearing loss, retina macular degeneration, and decreased vision.

These symptoms have obviously mitigated or disappeared after carotid artery stenosis was treated. Patients with partial necrosis in functional areas of brain reflected in magnetic resonance imaging have miraculous recovery of their lost function after carotid stenosis is treated. These cases show that our past understanding of the formation mechanism of stroke is insufficient. The symptoms and signs of some stroke patients, including visual and auditory problems, are probably the result of brain hypoperfusion caused by narrowness of neck artery.

Screening the carotid artery can give early behavioral guidance or drug intervention to patients whose cases are less severe and delay their narrowing process. It can also give interventional or surgical treatment to patients with severe stenosis, remove sources of stroke, and reduce occurrence of stroke and disability.

Carotid screening method is relatively simple. It is a non-invasive and inexpensive examination. Severe stenosis can be detected through neck auscultation; neck B-ultrasound can find most of the stenosis and determine the degree of their narrowness. Screening technique is a specially trained technique.

The major threatening risk of carotid artery stenosis includes the following factors: hypertension, high blood cholesterol, high blood sugar, long time heavy smoking, long term heavy drinking, history of chronic periodontitis, history of ischemic eye disease, men over the age of 45, and women over the age of 55. People who have more than two risk factors must receive carotid screening.

To change as soon as possible the situation that stroke seriously threatens health of people in this country, we must quickly work out criterion for screening, principles of intervention, as well as standards and requirements for carotid endarterectomy surgery. At the same time, we must try to establish at least 1 stroke screening and intervention center or base at the provincial level, autonomous region, and municipality within 3 years. That will enable us to conduct screening to the high-risk groups, so as to reduce the morbidity and mortality of cerebrovascular disease in our country.

Text 6

Chronic Non-communicable Diseases Prevention and Control Are Urgent

Minister Chen Zhu Speaks for General Debate at the 64th World Health Assembly

Geneva, Switzerland
16 May 2011

Dear President, Ms. Director-General, Ministers and Colleagues,

Allow me first of all congratulate the election of Mr. President. I believe that under your leadership, this session will be a complete success.

I would like to take this opportunity to express my sympathy and condolence to those families who have lost their loved ones and suffered misfortune in the earthquake and tsunami in Japan and hurricane in the United States. These incidents tell us that in natural disasters, human beings are so fragile. Therefore, we need harmony between man and nature, and between development and environment. At present, globalization has resulted in an unprecedented degree of interrelation, interdependence, and mutual benefit among countries. To work together with an idea of "being in the same boat" is beneficial for the common interests of all countries. At this point, I congratulate the Intergovernmental Working Group of the member states for their four years' work in reaching a consensus on "Preventive Framework of Sharing Influenza Viruses, Access to Vaccines and Other Benefits in a Pandemic Influenza". The vast number of developing countries will not only provide influenza viruses, but also reasonably, legally, impartially share the benefit of influenza vaccine and antiviral drugs. This fully demonstrates solidarity and cooperation of all countries, and will set an example for the international community to jointly cope with challenges to public health that threatens the security of human beings.

Ladies and gentlemen,

According to the latest census data, the Chinese population aged 60 and over accounts for 13.26% of the total population. In an accelerated population aging process, China has become the world's first big developing country that is "aging before getting rich". China has 200 million hypertension patients, 2.8 million new cancer patients each year, and 9% diabetes prevalence rate. Chronic non-communicable diseases rise to 85% of the cause of death of the Chinese population, and about 3.7 million premature deaths happen each year due to chronic non-communicable diseases. Chronic non-communicable diseases have been a huge threat to China's socio-economic development. Prevention and control of chronic non-communicable diseases will have a long way to go.

The Chinese government attaches great importance to the prevention and control of chronic non-communicable diseases. With reference to the World Health Organization's global strategic plan of action, the government adheres to giving priority to prevention and reducing morbidity. It adheres to early detection, reduction of economic burdens, humanistic treatment and improvement of quality of life. It also adheres to government leadership and full community participation. China's current health care system reform is trying to achieve universal coverage of basic health services, including establishing health records for all people, providing health management services to hypertension and diabetes patients at or over the age of 35, and providing health examinations to people at or over the age of 65. The Chinese government has set increasing 1 year for average life expectancy as its core target in its "12th Five-Year Economic and Social Development Plan". We deeply know that to achieve this goal, effective prevention and control of chronic non-communicable diseases is the key. To this end, we will focus on creating healthy cities by actively carrying out health promotion, tobacco control, and improvement of our capability of integrated management of social services. We will further strengthen our efforts in building primary health care team with general practitioners as its main part, and improve our comprehensive service capabilities. Our healthcare reform is bringing visible and tangible benefits to people.

Prevention and control of chronic non-communicable diseases are an urgent task. If it is not properly managed, the world will have chronic non-communicable disease "blowout" in the next 20 to 30 years. Therefore, we must attach great importance to the societal determinants that lead to chronic non-communicable diseases. The international community must enhance their sense of mission and urgency, and firmly implement the global strategic plan of action for chronic non-communicable diseases. For this I would like to propose the following:

First, countries include prevention and control of chronic non-communicable diseases into their core indicators that measure their own social and economic development, while the international community further promotes to include indicators of prevention and control of chronic non-communicable diseases into the Millennium Development Goals. Since chronic non-communicable diseases are "societal infectious diseases", governments must attach equal importance to prevention and control of chronic non-communicable diseases as they do to GDP. They must include control and prevention into their overall plan of local economic and social development, establish an intersectoral coordination mechanism, and strengthen social mobilization and common participation. The international community need actively raise funds and guarantee investment.

Second, we must further strengthen improvement of our health system. A strong health system is not only the basis of response to infectious diseases and public health emergencies, but also linchpin to prevention and control of chronic non-communicable diseases. Governments must treat health system construction as the focus of their work. Developed countries and international organizations must regard health system construction as an important area of foreign aid, increase efforts of aid, and help developing countries build their health system.

Third, we expect a full play of the leadership role of World Health Organization in global health development agenda by supporting Director-General Margaret Chan and her Secretariat in their reform process. We hope that World Health Organization will play a leading role in the preparations for the United Nations summit of chronic non-communicable diseases in September this year, establish worldwide, unified and explicit objectives and evaluation norms on prevention and control of chronic non-communicable diseases, formulate a clear course of action, coordinate and integrate international resources, and finally establish extensive international cooperation and partnership.

Mr. President, dear colleagues,

Finally I would like to congratulate Director-General Margaret Chan. Thank you for leading the World Health Organization Secretariat that plays an outstanding role of leadership and coordination in global health reform and development.

Thank you.

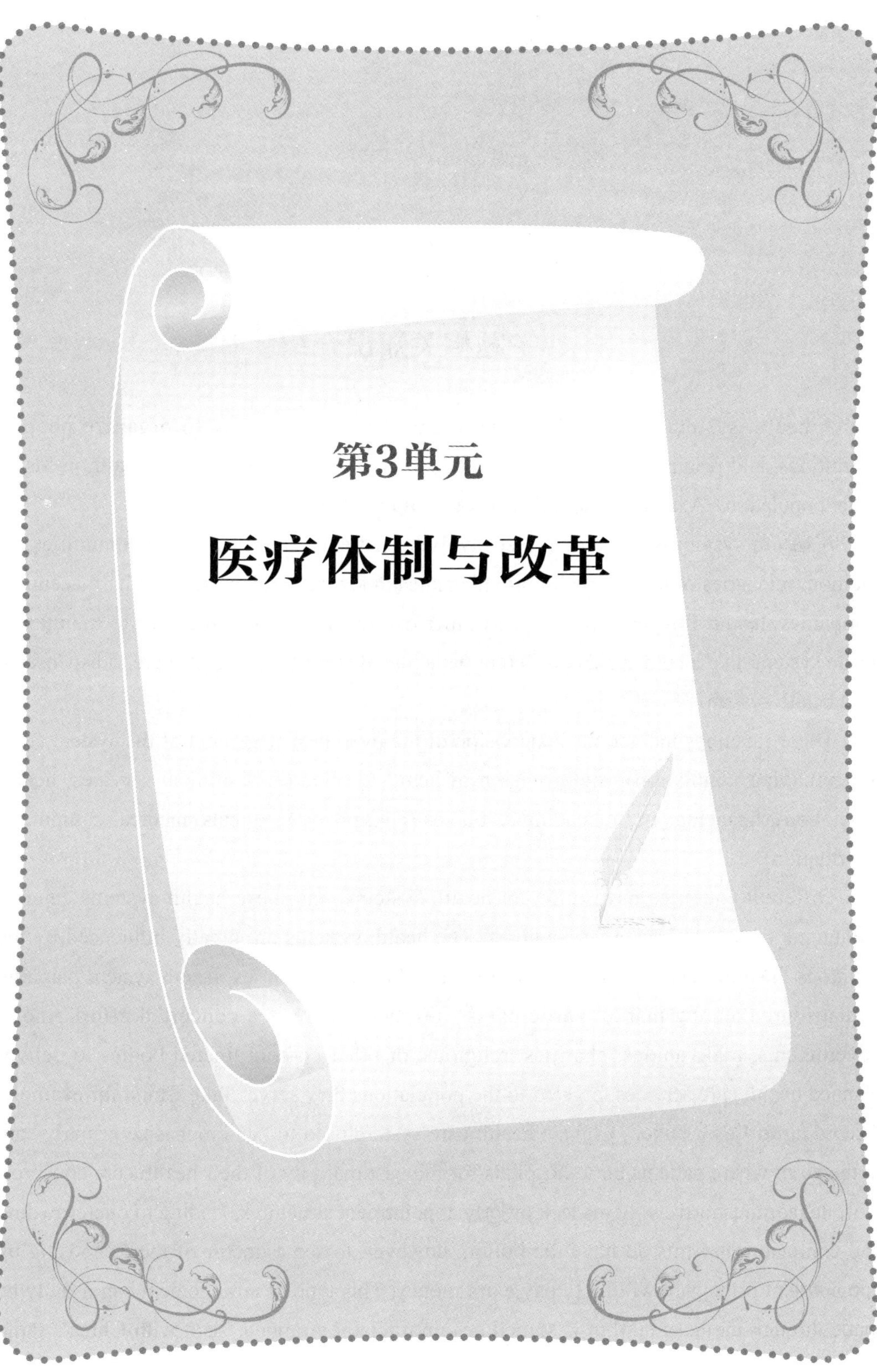

第3单元

医疗体制与改革

一、主题相关知识介绍

A health system, often called health care system, is a way to organize people, institutions, and resources so as to deliver health care services to meet the health needs of target populations. A health system is composed of many different parts.

A health system is more than just involving patients, families, and communities. In addition, ministries of health, health providers, health services organizations, pharmaceutical companies, health financing bodies, and other organizations work together to maintain a health system. In a health system, different parts play different roles, which are indispensable for a health system.

These functions include the supervision of the overall management of the system (e.g., policymaking, regulation), the provision of health service (e.g., clinical services, health promotion), financing, and managing resources (e.g., pharmaceuticals, medical equipment, information).

Different countries have different health systems, and these health systems cater to the unique features of different countries. The health systems are greatly influenced by the countries' histories and organizational structures. In some countries, health system planning is distributed among market participants. In others, there is a concerted effort among governments, trade unions, charities, religious, or other co-coordinated bodies to deliver planned health care services targeted to the populations they serve. Take China for example. According to Laura Dixon, China's health care system used to "de-emphasize primary care to the point where patients go to hospitals for the vast majority of their health care concerns. Hospital administrative systems lack orderly appointment structures, leading to overcrowding and confusion. Patients do have the option, however, to see a doctor of their choosing by appointment if they are willing to pay extra money. This type of arrangement can usually be made through the hospital, but is sometimes unofficially arranged." But with China's rapid development, patients expect "a higher level of care and service and hospitals are adding comfortable, private rooms and more individualized care in order to keep up."

However, health care planning has been described as often evolutionary rather than revolutionary. The goals for health systems, according to the World Health Organization, are good health, responsiveness to the expectations of the population, and fair financial contribution. Progress towards them depends on how systems carry out four vital functions: provision of health care services, resource generation, financing, and stewardship. Other dimensions for the evaluation of health systems include quality, efficiency, acceptability, and equity. They have also been described in the United States as "the five C's": Cost, Coverage, Consistency, Complexity, and Chronic Illness. Also, continuity of health care is a major goal.

二、技巧指导：语料类型分析——正式文体之辩论文

以说服为目的的发言稿，通常用于讲清事实问题、价值观问题、政策问题。以上述目的写出的发言稿或文章，通常称为辩论文（argumentation）。

辩论文的特点是通过诉诸逻辑、情感或伦理，通过正论和反驳，通过翔实的事实证据，对论题进行深入的分析，以理服人，以便听众达成共识，或获得听众内心的支持以参与行动。因此，辩论式的演讲稿通常有明确的题目、鲜明的观点、合情合理的阐述和论证、引起共鸣的角度，以及积极正面的思想，演讲的时候有经验的讲话人语气变化细微。

辩论文的结构顺序也有一些特点。在需要口译的场合，很多讲话都是条分式的，从问题入手。顺序或包括的内容大致有：事情的原委和现状、需要及理由、解决问题的计划与思路、计划与思路的益处、计划与思路的可行性与预期结果。

在论述上，辩论文的主要论点一般会有三到五个。斯蒂芬·卢卡斯（Lucas，2001）认为，论点顺序的组织有几种方式：时间顺序方式、空间顺序方式、因果顺序方式、问题与解决问题方案方式，以及分论题顺序方式。

本书第2单元的摘要练习"Chronic Disease Are No Longer Just a Health Problem"（《慢性病不再仅仅是卫生问题》）一文，是以提出问题与解决问题方案的方法撰写的辩论文，结构是条分式。文章思路清晰，前面部分提出问题及其严重性，中间有分析，最后提出解决方法。

需要注意的是，辩论文的主题与结论应该是一致的，不会得出与主题观点相反的结论。仍以上一单元的摘要练习"Chronic Disease Are No Longer Just a Health Problem"为例。题目本身即为主题。第一个论点是"流行病学与全球趋势对人类

和经济造成破坏，从富裕社会向贫穷和弱势群体的这种转变何等严峻”。接下来是例子。第二点是“慢性病不再仅仅是医学或公共卫生问题，还是发展问题和政治问题。而做出不正确决定的压力会是巨大的”。接下来也是例子。第三点是“在资源紧缺环境下疾病管理的挑战几乎被完全忽略”。接下来也是例子。结论是公共卫生管理应该由各部门相互配合，并呼吁各部门觉醒并参与其中。

以告知为目的和以说服为目的的英文语篇所遵循的方法，在中文写作之中也有体现。在当代社会，涉及学科领域的中文发言稿在目的、功能和内容方面都与英文演讲稿比较接近。中文将辩论文称为议论文。议论文通常也有一个主题，主题提出之后，后面的段落就是从各个方面提出的各种论据。每一个论据提出后，会有进一步的解释，或示例。本书第4单元的第五篇文章，“On How to Ensure the Position of Health in the Future Global Development Agenda”（《如何在未来全球发展议程中确保卫生的地位》），其写作方式就是主题加条分式。首先是原因导致的主题：“健康是经济社会和谐、可持续发展的目标和必要条件。要实现人类社会协调、均衡、可持续发展，必须将健康放在全球政治和发展议程的核心位置，促使各国调动多种资源，加强卫生体系建设，促进健康公平”。接下来是四点论据，每一条后面都附有解释。最后的倡议强化了主题。

三、词汇准备

Text 1

clinical commissioning 临床试用
funding gap 资金缺口
GP (general practitioner) 普通开业医生
NHS (National Health Service) 英国国家医疗服务体系
obesity 肥胖
pensioner 领养老金者
respiratory 呼吸的
the status quo 现状
upfront costs 预付费用

Text 2

Affordable Care Act 平价医疗法案

check-up 体检
constitutionality 合宪性
jacking up rates 上涨保费
mammograms 乳房X光造影检查
premiums 保费

Text 3

deficit 赤字
dissent 异议
Obamacare 奥巴马医疗法案（全称为Patient Protection and Affordable Care Act, PPACA，患者保护与平价医疗法案）
repeal 废除法案
trillion 万亿
the Chamber of Commerce 美国商务部

Text 4

Center for Health Statistics and Information 卫生部统计信息中心
China Medical Board 美国中华医学基金会
Department of Policy and Regulation, Ministry of Health 卫生部政策法规司
evidence-based decision-making 询证
pharmaceutical policies 医药政策
technical backup 技术支持
Workshop on Monitoring and Evaluation for Health Reform 医疗卫生体制改革监测与评价研讨会
UNAIDS (United Nations, Acquired Immune Deficiency Syndrome) 联合国艾滋病规划署
UNICEF (United Nations International Children’s Emergency Fund) 联合国儿童基金会
UNFPA (United Nations Fund for Population Activities) 联合国人口基金会

Text 5

按病种收费 DRG-based payment
报销比例 reimbursement rate
定编定岗 staffing

二级甲等 secondary level A
基本医疗保险制度 medical insurance scheme
基本药物制度 essential drug system
几种采购 pooled procurement
阶段性进展 interim progress
绩效工资 performance-based salary
临床路径管理 clinical pathway management
三级医院 tertiary hospital
统一配送 unified distribution
乡镇卫生院 township hospital
重大疾病 catastrophic disease
卫生资源配置 health resources allocation
新型农村合作医疗系统 the New Rural Cooperative Medical System (NRCMS)
预约挂号 pre-registration system
综合改革 synchronized reform
综合量化考核制度 quantitative assessment
重大公共卫生项目 mega public health programs

Text 6

南丁格尔精神 Nightingale Pledge
护士条例 Nurses Regulation
临终关怀 hospice care
康复促进 rehabilitation
救死扶伤 rescue the sick and the dying
国家卫生计生委 National Health and Family Planning Commission

四、摘要练习

请听下面英语语篇，第一篇用源语言复述此段主要信息逻辑点及层次，第二篇用译入语复述此段主要信息逻辑点及层次。注意信息点之间的逻辑联系。

Text 1

British Prime Minister David Cameron's Speech on NHS Reforms

Ealing Hospital, West London

16 May 2011

Ladies and gentlemen,

The NHS is facing enormous financial pressures in the years ahead—driven by rising demand and the cost of new drugs and technologies.

For the first time ever there are more pensioners in this country than children under 16. And the number of people aged over 85 is set to double in the next twenty years. Every hour the NHS deals with more than 25,000 people... think how many of them are elderly, and then consider with our population ageing at the rate it is...

Already three quarters of the health and care budget goes on long term chronic conditions and the pressure is going to get bigger. Indeed, by 2050, the number of over sixty-fives with one or more long-term conditions is expected to rise by 252 percent. Obesity and poor diets. Drug and alcohol abuse. These public health challenges are getting bigger and bigger.

Take obesity for example: it already costs our NHS a staggering £4 billion a year. But within four years, that figure's expected to rise to £6.3 billion.

Timely interventions with effective new drugs and treatments can of course save money. Our NHS and its patients should get them. But that will only happen if we find a sustainable way to deal with the rising costs. Sticking with the status quo and hoping we can get by with a bit more money is simply not an option. If we stay as we are, the NHS will need £130 billion a year by 2015—meaning a potential funding gap of £20 billion.

There's only one option we've got—and that is to change and modernize the NHS... to make it more efficient and more effective—and above all, more focused on prevention, on health, not just sickness.

But the change will be evolutionary, not revolutionary.

Clinical commissioning has existed in one form or another for the past two decades. Working with others from the independent sector too—that's not new either. The NHS has a long history of this—be it with social enterprises, charities or private companies... and the last government in particular understood the importance of introducing an element of choice to drive up standards. The difference is that we plan to make these changes effective across our NHS.

As I said: evolution, not revolution.

Let me make clear: there will be no privatization... there will be no cherry-picking from private providers... there will be no new upfront costs people have to pay to get care.

Instead, our NHS will be much like what we have today. You'll still be able to call your local surgery, and speak to a receptionist you know to book an appointment with a GP you trust. You'll still be able to go through the doors of an A & E in an emergency, and be seen by a nurse or doctor quickly and effectively. Your parents will still get the healthcare they need, from specialists and nurses on wards or in their homes.

It will be the NHS you love and recognize—only better. An NHS with consistent, high quality care for all—instead of just pockets of excellence. An NHS which addresses the full needs of each person—of their physical and mental health... rather than offering a piecemeal or patchwork approach. An NHS free-from-political control, where what matters is the care you receive not the headlines governments get... A genuine National Health Service, rather than a National Sickness Service... with a greater focus on outcomes and on improving public health—so people don't get sick and ill in the first place. An NHS which makes people healthy—and keeps them healthy.

Thank you.

复述要点提示（主要信息逻辑点及层次）

Purpose of the speech:

British NHS system needs urgent reform to deal with the oncoming financial crisis and offer better service to its people so as to keep people healthy rather than treating them only when they are sick. However, the reform is to improve this system, not to revolutionize it.

Keynotes of the speech:

In this speech, Cameron emphasizes that:

National Health System (NHS) is facing great crisis with the increasing financial burden. More and more ageing people with chronic diseases bring much financial burden to the current NHS system. By 2050, the number of people over 65 years old and with chronic diseases will be more than doubled. The country spends much money on treating these diseases. Besides the ageing group, other population groups also have different health problems. The NHS System is faced with great challenge. This is the background for the NHS reform. NHS will be in great trouble if we do nothing about it.

To help NHS out of trouble, we need to modernize it. We will keep the good things of

NHS and reform only the negative sides of it. For example, we should keep the practice of clinical commissioning, introduce more choices into the system so as to drive up the standard of the service. Patients can still enjoy the great convenience of the old NHS system. On the other hand, the reformed NHS system will not allow privatization, and patients will not need to pay any upfront costs.

The ultimate goal of the new NHS system will not only care about patients' physical health but also their mental health. The NHS will strive to improve the overall health situation of the whole country.

Text 2

American President Barack Obama's Speech on Health Care Reform

28 June 2012

Good afternoon.

Earlier today, the Supreme Court upheld the constitutionality of the Affordable Care Act—the name of the health care reform we passed two years ago. In doing so, they've reaffirmed a fundamental principle that here in America—in the wealthiest nation on Earth—no illness or accident should lead to any family's financial ruin.

This law has a direct impact on so many Americans, I want to take this opportunity to talk about exactly what it means for you.

First, if you're one of the more than 250 million Americans who already have health insurance, you will keep your health insurance. This law will only make it more secure and more affordable. Insurance companies can no longer impose lifetime limits on the amount of care you receive. They can no longer discriminate against children with pre-existing conditions. They can no longer drop your coverage if you get sick. They can no longer jack up your premiums without reason. They are required to provide free prevent care, like check-ups and mammograms, a provision that has already helped 54 million Americans with private insurance.

And by this August, nearly 13 million of you will receive a rebate from your insurance company because it spent too much on things like administrative costs and CEO bonuses and not enough on your health care.

There's more. Because of the Affordable Care Act, young adults over the age of 26 are able to stay on their parents' health care plans, a provision that's already helped 6 million young Americans. And because of the Affordable Care Act, seniors receive a discount on their prescription drugs, a discount that's already saved more than 5 million seniors on Medicare about $ 600 each.

All of this is happening because of the Affordable Care Act. These provisions provide common-sense protections for middle-class families, and they enjoy broad popular support. And thanks to today's decision, all of these benefits and protections will continue for Americans who already have health insurance.

Now, if you're one of the 30 million Americans who don't yet have health insurance, starting in 2014 this law will offer you an array of quality, affordable private health insurance plans to choose from. Each state will take the lead in designing their own menu of options. And if states can come up with even better ways of covering more people with the same quality and cost, this law allows them to do that too.

And I've asked Congress to help speed up that process and give states this flexibility in year one. Once states set up these health insurance marketplaces, known as exchanges, insurance companies will no longer be able to discriminate against any American with pre-existing health condition. They won't be able to charge you more just because you're a woman. They won't be able to bill you into bankruptcy. If you're sick, you'll finally have the same chance to get quality, affordable health care as everyone else. And if you can't afford the premiums, you'll receive a credit that helps pay for it.

Today the Supreme Court also upheld the principle that people who can afford health insurance should take the responsibility to buy health insurance.

This is important for two reasons. First, when uninsured people who can afford coverage get sick and show up at the emergency room for care, the rest of us end up paying for their care in the form of higher premiums. And second, if you ask insurance companies to cover people with pre-existing conditions, but don't require people who can afford it to buy their own insurance, some folks might wait until they're sick to buy the care they need, which would also drive up everybody else's premiums.

The highest court in the land has now spoken. We will continue to implement this law. Now's the time to keep our focus on the most urgent challenge of our time—putting people back to work, paying down our debt and building an economy where people can have confidence that if they work hard, they can get ahead.

But today I'm as confident as ever that when we look back five years from now or 10 years from now or 20 years from now, we'll be better off because we had the courage to pass this law and keep moving forward.

Thank you. God bless you. And God bless America.

复述要点提示（主要信息逻辑点及层次）

主要目的：回顾平价医疗法案将为美国民众带来的福祉。奥巴马总统在演讲中表达了对平价医疗费用法案被最高法院通过的喜悦。他回顾了平价医疗费用法案的中心内容，并鼓舞美国人民将合理医疗费用法案继续下去。

平价医疗费用法案的主要内容：

1. 首先，已经拥有健康保险的美国人不但可以保留保险，而且能够拥有更安全、更优惠的保险。保险公司将再也不能对个人的保险设置限制。比如它们不能利用保险条款来歧视儿童，不能通过提高保费来歧视生病的人。保险公司还必须提供免费的预防保健，如体检和乳房X光造影检查。同时保险公司会将部分保费返还给个人，因为过去保险公司花费过多在行政和为执行总裁分红上。其次，父母的医保可以覆盖26岁以下的青年，这一法案已经帮助了600万美国年轻人。老年人在购买处方药的时候可以得到折扣，美国500万老年人已经人均节约600美金。这项法案将有利于美国的中产阶级，同时为已经拥有保险的美国人提供持续的保障。

2. 对于3 000万没有医疗保险的美国人，法案要求从2014年起每个美国人都将有一系列高质量且能够负担的私人健康保险可选择。每个州可以自主设计适合自己的医疗保险计划。如果每个州能够用更好的方式为更多的人提供同样质量和费用的保险，法律也会允许它们这样做。

3. 但是同时强调，那些能够承担医疗保险的人必须购买医疗保险。如果不强迫能够承受保险的人购买保险，那么在这些人生病的时候，全体人民将不得不为他们的医疗费用买单，这样会变相增加其他美国人所缴纳的医疗费用。另外，也会让保险公司的保费增加。

五、英译汉练习

Text 3

Mitt Romney Remarks on High Court Ruling Upholding Obama Health Care Law

28 June 2012

As you might imagine, I disagree with the Supreme Court's decision and I agree with the dissent. What the court did not do on its last day in session, I will do on my first day if elected president of the United States. And that is I will act to repeal Obamacare.

Let's make clear that we understand what the court did and did not do. What the court did today was say that Obamacare does not violate the Constitution. What they did not do was say that Obamacare is good law or that it's good policy. Obamacare was bad policy yesterday. It's bad policy today.

Let me tell you why I say that. Obamacare raises taxes on the American people by approximately $500 billion. Obamacare cuts Medicare by approximately $500 billion. And even with those cuts and tax increases, Obamacare adds trillions to our deficits and to our national debt, and pushes those obligations on to coming generations. Obamacare also means that for up to 20 million Americans, they will lose the insurance they currently have, the insurance that they like and they want to keep.

Obamacare is a job-killer. Businesses across the country have been asked what the impact is of Obamacare. Three-quarters of those surveyed by the Chamber of Commerce said Obamacare makes it less likely for them to hire people. And perhaps most troubling of all, Obamacare puts the federal government between you and your doctor.

For all those reasons, it's important for us to repeal and replace Obamacare.

What are some of the things that we'll keep in place and must be in place in a reform, a real reform of our health care system? One, we have to make sure that people who want to keep their current insurance will be able to do so. Having 20 million people—up to that number of people—lose the insurance they want is simply unacceptable.

No. 2, got to make sure that those people who have preexisting conditions know that they will be able to be insured and they will not lose their insurance.

We also have to assure that we do our very best to help each state in their effort to assure that every American has access to affordable health care.

And so this is now a time for the American people to make a choice. You can choose whether you want to have a larger and larger government, more and more intrusive in your life, separating you and your doctor, whether you're comfortable with more deficits, higher debt that we pass on to the coming generations, whether you're willing to have the government put in place a plan that potentially causes you to lose the insurance that you like, or whether instead you want to return to a time when the American people will have their own choice in health care, where consumers will be able to make their choices as to what kind of health insurance they want.

This is a time of choice for the American people. Our mission is clear: If we want to get rid of Obamacare, we're going to have to replace President Obama. My mission is to make sure we do exactly that: that we return to the American people the privilege they've always had to live their lives in the way they feel most appropriate, where we don't pass on to coming generations massive deficits and debt, where we don't have a setting where jobs are lost.

If we want good jobs and a bright economic future for ourselves and for our kids, we must replace Obamacare. That is my mission, that is our work, and I'm asking the people of America to join me. If you don't want the course that President Obama has put us on, if you want, instead, a course that the founders envisioned, then join me in this effort. Help us. Help us defeat Obamacare. Help us defeat the liberal agenda that makes government too big, too intrusive, and that's killing jobs across this great country.

Text 4

Speech at the Workshop on Monitoring and Evaluation for Health Reform in Promoting Evidence-based Decision-making

Dr. Michael O'Leary, WHO Representative in China

Beijing, China

1 December 2009

Good morning, dear representatives,

I am very pleased to be here today for the Workshop on Monitoring and Evaluation for health reform in promoting evidence-based decision-making.

The Government of China launched earlier this year its health reform plans, with the aim to achieve universal coverage by 2020. The goals are laudable and ambitious, but they are backed by substantial financial resources for a three-year implementation.

The provinces and regions are now developing implementation strategies for health reform, to take into account local needs. Beyond high political commitment and financial resources, reform depends on how successfully the vision is implemented at provincial and municipal levels.

The major challenge over the next 10 years is to translate health resources into better health, higher risk protection, and greater satisfaction for people across all communities in China.

Monitoring and evaluation systems are critical to this effort, to assess progress and to determine whether the efforts are achieving improved results in terms of access, quality, and outcomes.

In addition, we need to closely examine trends in light of the many policy changes underway. For example, there was a recent announcement to raise medical treatment fees for some clinical services to compensate in part for reduced revenues from drugs. The impact on utilization and health should be monitored closely to see how the people respond to such changes.

In August, the Ministry of Health and WHO jointly held a meeting to discuss monitoring and evaluation for health reform. Impressive progress has since been made. The government has developed a national framework/plan for monitoring and evaluation of health reform. The framework is being used as the basis for identifying a core set of indicators. This builds on international experience, adapted to the unique Chinese context.

During your discussions, it is important to remember the vast differences in economic and human resources across regions in China. Therefore we need to identify not only how the country is doing as a whole but also the differences between provinces, and urban and rural areas. Explaining these variations and trends requires more detailed research. We encourage you to use the government's monitoring and evaluation framework discussed today as the basis for your operational research agenda and to support greater understanding of trends. This will provide information for the government to make better policy choices.

Distinguished colleagues,

WHO maintains a long-standing collaboration with the government on health care reform. We are committed to support national health reform, and specifically to provide technical backup, as requested, in strengthening the systems for public health, pharmaceutical policies, service delivery, and financing and medical security.

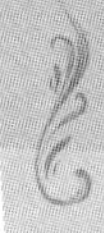

Over the next few years, WHO will actively support systems for monitoring and evaluation of the reform. This commitment includes the establishment of WHO Collaborating Centers to strengthen long-term cooperation in technical areas related to health reform, and to increase capacity in informatics and health information systems.

In conclusion, we thank the Ministry of Health for providing leadership in monitoring and evaluation of health reform, and for organizing this seminar. Dr. Liu Xinming and Dr. Rao Keqin have worked closely together to make this effort successful. We also thank China Medical Board for their support to this workshop. Lastly, we recognize the active participation of many international health partners in Beijing, including UNAIDS, UNICEF, and UNFPA, among others.

I wish you great success in this meeting.

六、汉译英练习

Text 5

中国医药卫生体制改革进展情况介绍

中华人民共和国卫生部部长　陈竺

2012年2月

第11个五年计划期间，中国的医改取得了如下的进展和成效：

首先，基本医疗保障制度基本实现全覆盖。三项基本医疗保险制度覆盖面达95%以上，其中新农合参合率达到97.5%。2011年新农合人均筹资244.6元，其中政府补助207.8元。保障水平不断提高，政策范围内报销比例达到70%以上。提高重大疾病保障水平试点，2011年底已经在93%的统筹地区开展，保障的病种范围不断扩大。

其次，国家基本药物制度取得阶段性进展。在所有政府开办的乡镇卫生院和社区卫生服务机构实施基本药物制度：国家制定307种基本药物目录，30个省份制订了省级增补药品目录，建立了规范的基本药物采购机制，以省级为单位集中采购、统一配送基本药物；不断扩大基本药物制度的实施范围：31个省份在村卫生室启动基本药物制度，10个省份将非政府办基层医疗卫生机构纳入制度实施范围，13个省对二级以上医疗机构配备基本药物的品种数量和使用比例提出要求；同步推动基层医疗卫生机构综合改革：县（市、区）普遍实施了基层综合改革，完成了定编定岗、人员聘用，实行了绩效工资、综合量化考核制度，落实财政专项补助和经常性收支差额补助。

第三，基层医疗卫生服务体系进一步完善。硬件设施条件显著改善：改造2 200多所县级医院和3.3万个基层医疗卫生机构，乡镇卫生院和社区卫生服务中心达到建设标准的比例分别为70%和85%，约70%的县（市）至少有一家县级医院达到二级甲等水平；加强以全科医生为重点的基层医疗卫生队伍建设：累计为中西部地区乡镇卫生院招聘1万名免费定向培养医学生，安排3万名基层在岗人员进行全科医生转岗培训，落实对口支援、卫生支农、招聘执业医师等措施，基层卫生服务利用明显提高，2011年，乡镇卫生院和社区卫生机构门诊量占医疗卫生机构门诊总量的比例达到23.2%。

第四，基本公共卫生服务均等化在加快推进。基本公共卫生服务经费从年人均15元增加到25元，10类基本公共卫生服务项目面向城乡居民免费提供，重大公共卫生项目全面实施。

第五，公立医院改革试点积极推进。确定17个国家重点联系的公立医院改革试点城市和37个省级试点城市，开展重大体制机制改革探索，29个省份部署了推进县级医院综合改革试点，深化公立医院与基层医疗机构分工协作机制，有1 100个三级医院与2 832个县级医院建立了长期对口协作关系；推广惠民便民措施：94%的三级医院开展预约挂号、双休日和节假日门诊，所有三级医院和80%的二级医院开展优质护理服务，78%的二级以上公立医院实施同级机构检验结果互认，34%的三级医院开展按病种收费试点，全国3 467家医疗机构共计2.55万个科室开展了临床路径管理。

总体说来，中国医改使人民群众得到更多实惠，看病难、看病贵问题得到一定程度缓解；国民健康指标继续改善；卫生资源配置、卫生服务利用和卫生总费用均发生重大结构性变化，城乡和地区间卫生发展差距逐步缩小。

Text 6

国家卫生计生委李斌主任在2013年国际护士节护理大会上的讲话

2013年5月14日

女士们、先生们：

在“5·12”国际护士节前夕，我代表国家卫生计生委向全国的广大护理工作者致以节日的问候和崇高的敬意！向长期关心、重视和支持我国护理事业发展的各位领导、各界朋友表示诚挚的谢意！

医疗卫生工作关系到人民群众的健康和福祉，关系到经济社会的全面协调可持续发展，护理工作是医疗卫生事业的重要组成部分，为维护和促进人民群众的健康发挥了重要作用。多年来，我国广大护理工作者秉承南丁格尔精神，始终坚持全心全意为人民服务的宗旨，无论是在日常的医疗护理工作中，还是在重大自然灾害和人民群众健康受到威胁的关键时刻，为保障人民群众生命安全、提高人民群众健康水平做出了重要贡献。

今年3月以来，国家卫生计生委成立之初，就面临着防控人感染H7N9禽流感疫情和四川芦山“4·20”地震卫生紧急救援两大考验，各级卫生计生部门反应迅速有效，广大医务人员奋战在抗击禽流感和抗震救灾的第一线。在救治地震伤员工作中，护理工作者第一时间赶赴灾区，争分夺秒地完成了一项又一项抢救生命、重症救治、医疗康复、心理支持、卫生防疫等任务；在抗击禽流感工作中，护理工作者发扬无私奉献和连续作战的精神，夜以继日，竭尽全力做好患者救治工作。他们以实际行动彰显了白衣天使的本色，诠释了关爱生命、救死扶伤、人道奉献的职业精神，展现出精湛的专业技术和严谨的工作作风，受到了人民群众的高度称赞，也得到了党和政府的充分肯定。我代表国家卫生计生委向所有工作在医疗救治第一线的广大护理工作者和医务人员表示由衷的敬意和衷心的感谢!

党和政府高度重视护理事业发展。近年来，国务院颁布实施了《护士条例》，从法规层面维护护士合法权益；实施了“十一五”时期和“十二五”时期护理事业发展规划纲要，加大了护士队伍建设力度，推动了护理事业健康发展，取得了显著成效：一是护士队伍建设取得了积极成果。全国护士队伍数量快速增长，2012年已达到近250万人，比2005年增长了115万。护士队伍中具有大专以上学历的占56%，比2005年提高了24.4个百分点。二是护理工作者在公立医院改革中发挥了重要作用。广大护理工作者积极推进优质护理，为保障医疗安全、提升服务质量、和谐医患关系做出了重要贡献。三是护理服务领域得到广泛拓展。广大护理工作者以满足人民群众的健康需求为目标，在做好医院患者护理工作的基础上，逐步拓展护理服务领域，走进社区和家庭，为患者提供慢病管理、长期护理、康复促进、临终关怀等服务，满足人民群众多样化、多层次的健康服务需求。

女士们、先生们，“十二五”时期是深化医药卫生体制改革的攻坚阶段，也是贯彻落实党的十八大精神、全面建成小康社会的关键时期。我国的医疗卫生事业已经迈入一个新阶段，我们要从全局角度，顺应时代要求，遵循内在规律，找准发展方向，为促进护理事业又好又快发展，服务于人民群众健康做出新的卓越贡献。

资料来源：

Text 1 http://www.newstatesman.com/uk-politics/2011/05/nhs-health-change-care

Text 2 http://www.shallownation.com/2012/06/28/president-obama-speech-supreme-court-health-care-reform-ruling-video-june-28-2012/

Text 3 http://www.foxnews.com/politics/2012/06/28/transcript-romney-remarks-on-high-court-ruling-upholding-obama-health-care-law/

Text 4 http://www.wpro.who.int/china/mediacentre/speeches/2009/WR20091202/en/index.html

Text 5 http://wenku.baidu.com/view/c479653367ec102de2bd892e.html

Text 6: http://www.moh.gov.cn/lbwz/plxfs/201306/624f1fe898b74b1786e37e05d6ce570f.shtml

参考答案

四、摘要练习

Text 1

英国首相戴维·卡梅伦关于英国国家医疗服务系统的讲话

西伦敦　伊令医院

2011年5月16日

女士们、先生们：

因为人们不断增加的对新药和新科技的需求及其花费，国家医疗服务系统在未来将面临巨大的财政压力。

有史以来英国领取养老金的人数第一次超过了16岁以下未成年人的数量；85岁以上的老年人数量在未来20年内将会翻番；每小时国家医疗服务系统要处理超过25 000人的需求。考虑一下其中有多少老年人，并请再考虑一下如果我们的人口以此种速度老龄化的结果……

我们四分之三的健康预算已经花在慢性疾病上，而且健康压力正在越变越大。到了2050年，年满65岁且患有一种或者多种慢性疾病的老年人将会增加252%。肥胖、营养不良、吸毒和酗酒，这些健康问题越来越挑战人们的生活。

以肥胖为例：每年它耗费医疗服务费用达到难以置信的40亿英镑之巨。但是四年里，这个数字将会上升到63亿。

通过及时有效的药物和治疗进行干预当然能够节省开支。国家医疗服务系统和病人们也应该获得这些帮助。但是这些都只有在我们找到一条可以持续应对不断上涨费用的方法后才有可能。维持现状，希望增加投入就可以渡过难关的想法是不可行的。如果我们维持现状，到2015年国家医疗服务系统每年将需要1 300亿英镑以维持运转，意味着每年的资金缺口将达到200亿英镑。

我们面前只有一个选择——改变和革新国家医疗服务系统，使其更加高效和有效。更重要的是，把更多的重点放在预防上，放在健康保健上，而非治疗疾病上。

但是改革应该是循序渐进，而非一蹴而就的。

临床医生处方权以不同形式存在二十多年了。临床医生和其他独立部门人士合作也不是新鲜事了。国家医疗服务系统和社会企业、慈善机构或者私人公司合作也有很长的历史了。上一届政府尤其了解引入新元素以提高医疗服务标准的重要性。和以前不同，我们现在要使这些改变在整个国家医疗服务系统发生作用。

就像我已经说过的：改革应该是循序渐进，而非一蹴而就的。

让我再陈述清楚一些：我们的医疗服务系统不应该私人化。私人医疗服务提供商不应该挑肥拣瘦。需要接受医疗服务的人们不应该支付新的预付费用。

相反，改革后的国家医疗服务系统和我们现在所拥有的非常相似。你仍然可以给当地的医生打电话，你可以打电话预约你信任的全科医生。紧急情况下你可以在急诊室得到医生或护士迅速有效的服务。你的父母仍然能够得到他们所需要的专业医疗服务，无论是在病房还是在自己家中。

这将是你热爱而且认可的国家医疗系统，而且只会更好。我们的医疗系统将会更强大，更能够发挥作用。这个医疗系统会为所有的人提供持续的高质量的服务。这个医疗系统会考虑每个人全面的需求，无论是身体上的还是精神上的，而非采取一种局部片面或者修修补补的方式。这个医疗系统会不受政治因素的控制，它关心的只是你所受到的照顾而不是报纸头条会如何报道。这将是一个真正的国家医疗系统，而不是一个国家疾病服务系统。它将更多的重点放在改善公共卫生健康上，这样我们首先关心的不是如何治疗疾病，而是如何让人们保持健康。

谢谢!

Text 2

奥巴马总统在最高法院通过医改法案后的讲话

2012年6月28日

各位下午好。

今天早些时候，最高法院维持了平价医疗费用法案——一项我们两年前就已通过的医疗改革法案的合宪性。这样做是最高法院对美国一项基本原则的再次确认——在美国这个世界上最富有的国家，任何疾病或事故都不应该导致家庭的经济毁灭。

正是因为这项法律对众多美国人有直接的影响，我希望借此机会谈谈这项法律对美国人到底意味着什么。

首先，如果你属于超过2.5亿已经拥有健康保险的美国人，你将仍然保留自己的保险。这项法令只会让你拥有更安全和可负担的保险。保险公司将再不能够对个人的保险设置终身限制。他们不能用先提条件来歧视儿童。他们不能在保险人生病的时候终止保险。他们不能无故提高保费。法律要求他们提供免费的预防保健，如体检和乳房X光造影检查，而这项法案已经通过私人保险救助了5 400万美国人。

到今年8月，你们当中将有近1300万人收到保险公司的退费，因为保险公司在行政费用和CEO分红上花费了太多的钱，而在投保人的医疗保健上却缺乏足够的投入。

其次，合理医疗费用法案的好处还不止于此。因为有了合理医疗费用法案，26岁以上的青年人能够继续享用父母的医保计划提供的医疗保障，这一法案已经帮助了600万美国年轻人。也正是因为有了合理医疗费用法案，老年人在购买处方药的时候可以得到折扣，这已经帮助美国500万老年人人均节约了600美金。

所有这些好处都是因为有了合理医疗费用法案。这些条例为美国中产阶级提供了必要的保护，也因此获得了广泛的支持。也正是因为有了今天的决定，这些已经拥有医疗保险的美国人可以继续享受这些福利和保障。

现在如果你是3 000万没有医疗保险的美国人之一，从2014年开始这项法案会为你提供一系列可供选择的高质量且可负担的私人健康保险。每个州可以自主设计适合自己的医疗保险计划。如果每个州能够提出更好的方式为更多人提供同样质量和费用的保险，法律也允许这样做。

我已经要求国会加快审理的过程，在第一年给每个州灵活决定的权力。各州一旦建立了健康保险的交换市场，保险公司就不能对任何人制订先决的健康条件。他们不能因为投保人是女性而提高保额。如果你生病了，你最终会获得和其他人一样的机会得到高质量而且能够支付的健康保险。如果你不能承受保费，你会获得一个信用等级以帮助你支付保险费用。

今天最高法院也坚持了一个原则，就是凡是能够负担健康保险的人都有责任购买健康保险。

这样做之所以重要有以下两个原因。首先，当那些能够负担保险但是却未购买保险的人生病就诊时，其余人就得因这个人的医疗费用而承担更高的保费。其二，如果我们只要求保险公司不设置先提条件却不要求那些能够承受保险的人购买保险，那么一些人可能会一直等到生病了才去买需要的保险，这样也会让每个人的保费增加。

美国最高法院现在发话了，我们将继续实施这项法案。现在是我们集中精力应对最棘手挑战的时候了——让人们重新拥有工作，减少债款，重建经济，让人们相信只要他们努力工作，他们就拥有希望。

但是今天我一如既往地相信，五年、十年或者二十年后，美国一定会因为通过合理医疗费用法案并将此进行下去而变得更加富有!

谢谢你们！上帝保佑你们！上帝保佑美国!

五、英译汉练习

Text 3

美国最高法院通过奥巴马合法医疗法案后
共和党候选人威拉德·米特·罗姆尼的讲话

2012年6月28日

你们也许可以想象，我不赞同最高法院的决定。如果我能够成功当选美国总统，那么我就任第一天要做的事情就是完成法院庭审最后一天没能做的事情。这就是：我将废除奥巴马医疗法案。

让我们明确我们理解法院做了什么、没做什么。今天法院只是说奥巴马法案没有违宪，但并没有说奥巴马法案是一项好法律或好政策。事实上，奥巴马法案昨天是一项糟糕的政策，今天它仍然是一项糟糕的政策。

让我告诉你们我为什么这么说。奥巴马法案让美国人要多交近5 000亿美元的税，而减少近5 000亿美元的医疗保险拨款。但是即使有了这些削减和增税，奥巴马法案仍然让美国增加了上万亿的国家债务，并且把这些负担强加在我们的子孙后代身上。奥巴马法案还意味着近2 000万美国人会失去他们现有的医疗保险，而这份保险正是他们喜欢并想要保留的。

奥巴马法案还让许多美国人失去工作。美国商务部对全国的商业行业进行了一项调查以了解奥巴马法案对他们的影响。四分之三接受调查的商人说奥巴马法案使他们更难雇到合适的员工。更麻烦的是，奥巴马法案让联邦政府成为横亘在美国公民和他们医生之间的障碍。

正是因为所有这些原因，我们才必须废除奥巴马法案，取代以新的法案。

要实现真正的医疗制度改革，我们该做些什么？首先，我们要确保那些希望保留自己医疗保险的人能够真正保住保险。2 000万人失去保险，这一点是完全不能接受的。

其次，必须确保那些患有疾病的人能够得到保险，确保他们不会失去自己的保险。

我们还必须确保我们尽力帮助每个州让每一位美国人能够获得可负担的医疗保险。

所以现在美国人民要做出选择。你可以选择一个更大、影响无所不在的政府，这个政府会把你和你的医生分隔开来，不管你是否满意背上更多的负债、子孙后代负上更沉重的负担，不管你是否愿意这个政府可能会导致你失去喜欢的保险。你也可以选择回到那个美国人民可以自由选择医疗保健方式、消费者可以自由选择医疗保险的时代。

这是美国人民进行选择的时候了。我们的使命很明确：如果我们想取消奥巴马法案，我们必须要取代奥巴马总统。我的使命就是确保我们这样做：把人民一直享有的权利还给他们，确保美国人民能够继续保持他们理想的生活方式，确保我们的子孙后代不会背上沉重的负债，确保我们不会丢失工作。

如果我们希望给自己和孩子一份好的工作和足够的钱财，我们就必须更换奥巴马医疗法案。这是我的使命，也是我们的工作，我在这里呼吁美国人民参加到我们的行列中来。如果你不喜欢奥巴马总统加在我们身上的东西，如果你希望实现国父们的理想，那么和我们一起努力吧。帮助我们！帮助我们击败奥巴马法案！帮助我们击败这项会使政府变得过于庞大、让这个伟大的国家失去更多的工作的自由法案！

Text 4

世界卫生组织驻华代表蓝睿明博士
在推动询证医疗卫生体制改革监测与评价研讨会上的讲话

中国北京

2009年12月1日

各位代表上午好：

我非常高兴今天能来到这里，参加推动询证医疗卫生体制改革监测与评价研讨会。

中国政府今年启动了卫生医疗体制改革计划，目标是在2020年实现人人享有基本医疗卫生覆盖。医改目标雄心勃勃，值得赞赏；实施三年计划所需的资金已经到位。

目前各省各地区正在结合当地需求，开发各自的医改实施战略。医改的成效不仅依赖政治承诺和资金支持，还有赖于医改计划在省市一级的实施效果。

今后十年内，我们面临的主要挑战是：如何利用好各种卫生资源，使人们获得更佳的健康状态、更全面的抗风险保护，以及让全中国民众对卫生服务更加满意。

监测与评价系统对于我们的这项努力至关重要。监测与评价系统可以核定医改的进度，并可以测定我们在医疗服务的可及性、质量和结果方面的努力是否取得了成效。

此外，我们要根据当前的各种政策变化来密切监控医改动向。比如说，最近有一个通知说要提高一些临床服务的诊疗费用来部分补贴药品利润上的损失。我们要仔细监测这个通知对服务使用率及健康的影响，了解人们对这些变化的反应。

卫生部和世卫组织于8月份联合召开了一个会议，讨论医改的监测与评价工作。在那之后我们取得了令人瞩目的进展。中国政府制订出了一个国家级的医改监测与评价框架，在这个框架的基础上确定了一系列核心指标。这个框架以国际经验为基础，结合了中国的特点。

在讨论中，大家应该记住中国各地区之间在经济实力和人力资源方面的巨大差异。因此我们不仅需要了解整个国家的医改状况，还要发现省与省以及城乡之间的差别。要解析这些变化和走向，需要做更细致的研究。我们鼓励大家以今天讨论的政府监测与评价框架为基础，确定运筹研究的日程安排，并支持更深入地理解医改走向。这么做将为政府更好地决策提供信息。

各位同仁，

世卫组织与中国政府在医疗卫生改革上保持长期合作。我们致力于支持国家医疗卫生改革，具体地说，应政府要求提供技术支持来巩固包括公共卫生、药品政策、服务提供，以及资金保证和医疗安全在内的各种系统。

接下来的几年中，世卫组织将积极支持医改监测与评价体系。这个承诺包括建立世卫组织合作中心，推动在医改相关技术领域内的长期合作，并强化信息学和卫生信息系统的能力。

最后，我们感谢卫生部在医改监测与评价工作中起到带头作用，并感谢卫生部组织本次研讨会。正是刘新明司长和饶克勤主任的共同努力，才让这项工作如此成功。我们还要感谢美国中华医学基金会对本次会议的支持。最后，我们非常赞赏很多驻华国际卫生伙伴的积极参与，包括联合国艾滋病规划署、联合国儿童基金会、联合国人口基金会等。

祝本次大会圆满成功！

六、汉译英练习

Text 5

Minister of Health Chen Zhu Introduces the Progress of China's Health Care Reform

February 2012

China's healthcare reform has made the following progress and effects during the 11th Five-Year Plan:

Firstly, China has realized nearly the full coverage of basic health insurance. Three medical insurance schemes covered 95% population, and participating rate of NRCMS reached 97.5%. In 2011, per capita fund pooled for NRCMS reached 244.6 Yuan, of which all levels of governments subsidized 207.8 Yuan. The medical insurance standard is continuously improving. Reimbursement rate for hospitalization increased to over 70%. Pilot projects of medical insurance for catastrophic diseases have been implemented in 93% NRCMS regions by the end of 2011, and have extended to more diseases.

Secondly, essential drug system has made interim progress. Essential drug system has been implemented in all government-run township hospitals and community health institutions, with 307 medicines in national essential drug list. 30 provinces developed provincial-level modified list, standardized essential drug procurement system, and set up pooled procurement and unified distribution of essential drugs at provincial level. Meanwhile, coverage of essential drug system has been expanded. The system has been implemented at village clinics in 31 provinces; 10 provinces brought non government-run grassroots medical institutions into the system; 13 provinces requested certain proportion and variety of essential drugs used in medical institutions at secondary level or above; synchronized reform of grassroots medical institutions has been promoted; counties (cities or districts) have conducted comprehensive reforms, including staffing and recruiting, performance-based salary, quantitative assessment, special financial subsidy, and current account balance subsidy.

Thirdly, grassroots medical service delivery system has been further improved. Grassroots health care facilities have been remarkably improved, 2,200 county hospitals and 33,000 primary health care institutions were renovated, 70% township hospitals and 85% community health centers reached standards, about 70% counties (cities) had at least one county hospital at secondary level A. Grassroots health workforce has been strengthened,

10,000 medical students were recruited accumulatively by township hospitals in central and western regions of China. 30,000 grassroots health workers received training as GPs, cooperative assistance. Urban big hospitals offered cooperative assistance to community and rural hospitals. In 2011, outpatient visits to township hospitals and community health institutions accounted for 23.2% of total hospital outpatient visits.

Fourthly, equal access to basic public health services has been expanded. The per capita budget for basic health services increased from 15 Yuan to 25 Yuan; 10 categories of basic public health service programs have been provided free of charge to rural and urban residents; the Mega public health programs have been implemented.

Fifthly, public hospital reform has made active progress. 17 national pilot cities and 37 provincial pilot cities have been selected to explore institutional reform measures. Pilot reform of county-level hospitals has been promoted in 29 provinces. Collaboration and coordination between public hospitals and primary health institutions has been deepened. Long-term cooperative relations have been established between 1,100 tertiary hospitals and 2,832 county-level hospitals; Convenient medical services have been promoted; 94% tertiary hospitals developed pre-registration system for hospital visits, and outpatient sections are open on both weekends and holidays; Quality care services have been provided in all tertiary hospitals and 80% secondary hospitals; 78% hospitals above secondary level have recognized medical examination results of medical institutions at the same level; 34% tertiary hospitals have implemented pilot of DRG-based payment. 3,467 medical institutions have adopted clinical pathway management in 25,500 departments.

All in all, Health Care Reform has benefited Chinese people in many aspects, and people have more convenient and affordable access to medical services. Health indicators of Chinese people have been improved. Health resources allocation, health service utilization and total health expenditure have undergone significant structural changes and the gap between urban and rural areas has been narrowed.

Text 6

Li Bin, Director of National Health and Family Planning Commission of the PRC, Remarks on the International Nurse Day

14 May 2013

Ladies and gentlemen,

Before the coming of the May 12th International Nurse Day, on behalf of the National Health and Family Planning Commission of the People's Republic of China, I would like to give my sincere respect and greetings to all the nursing workers in China, and give my sincere thanks to every leader and friend who cares about, values, and supports Chinese nursing service.

Medical service is closely related to people's health and benefits as well as the sustainable development of our economic society. And nursing service is an important part of medical service and plays an important role in maintaining and promoting people's health. For many years, Chinese nursing workers have been consistently holding the Nightingale Pledge and serving people whole-heartedly. They've made great contributions in safeguarding people's safety and enhancing their overall health condition no matter in the daily medical service or at the danger of great natural disasters.

Since March this year, at the beginning of its foundation, the National Health and Family Planning Commission has been facing two critical situations: the H7N9 Avian-Flu and the rescue work of April 20th Lushan Earthquake in Sichuan. Health and family planning departments at all levels reacted rapidly to emergency, and nursing workers went to the earthquake-stricken area at the earliest time and seized every minute saving lives, treating patients, offering medical recovery and psychological support, and preventing possible health epidemic. In fighting against H7N9 Avian Flu, nursing workers worked day and night to save every patient. They embodied the professional morality of nursing service, which is the love of life, the rescue of the sick and dying people, and great humanitarianism. Their high skill and rigorous working style have won the high praise of the public as well as the acknowledgement from the Party and the government. On behalf of the National Health and Family Planning Commission, I'd like to offer my sincere thanks and respect to all the medical workers working at the frontier of medical treatment.

The Party and the Chinese government have attached great importance to the development of nursing service. In recent years, the State Council has promulgated the Nurses Regulation, which protects the lawful rights of nurses from the legal aspect. Also, the State Council has implemented the development plans of the 11th and 12th Five Year Periods. All these have contributed greatly to the healthy development of nursing service. Firstly, the nursing team construction has made great progress. In 2012, there are 2.5 million nursing workers in China, which is 1.15 million more compared with that in 2005. Nursing workers with college degree or higher are about 56% of the total team, which is 24.4% higher than 2005.

Secondly, nursing workers have been playing an important role in public hospital reform. Nursing workers use their excellent service to guarantee the medical safety, enhance the service quality, and facilitate the doctor-patient relationship. Nursing workers regard satisfying people's health needs as their goal and gradually expand their service areas based on the quality work at hospitals. They go into communities and families to offer services like chronic disease management, long-term care, rehabilitation, and hospice care to meet the diversified and multi-level needs of people.

Ladies and gentlemen, the 12th Five-Year Period is a crucial state in deepening medical reform as well as implementing the guiding principles of the Eighteenth Party Congress and building a well-off society. The medical service work in China has entered a new stage. We should bear in mind a global view, follow the intrinsic rules, and find the right direction to make new contributions to the public health!

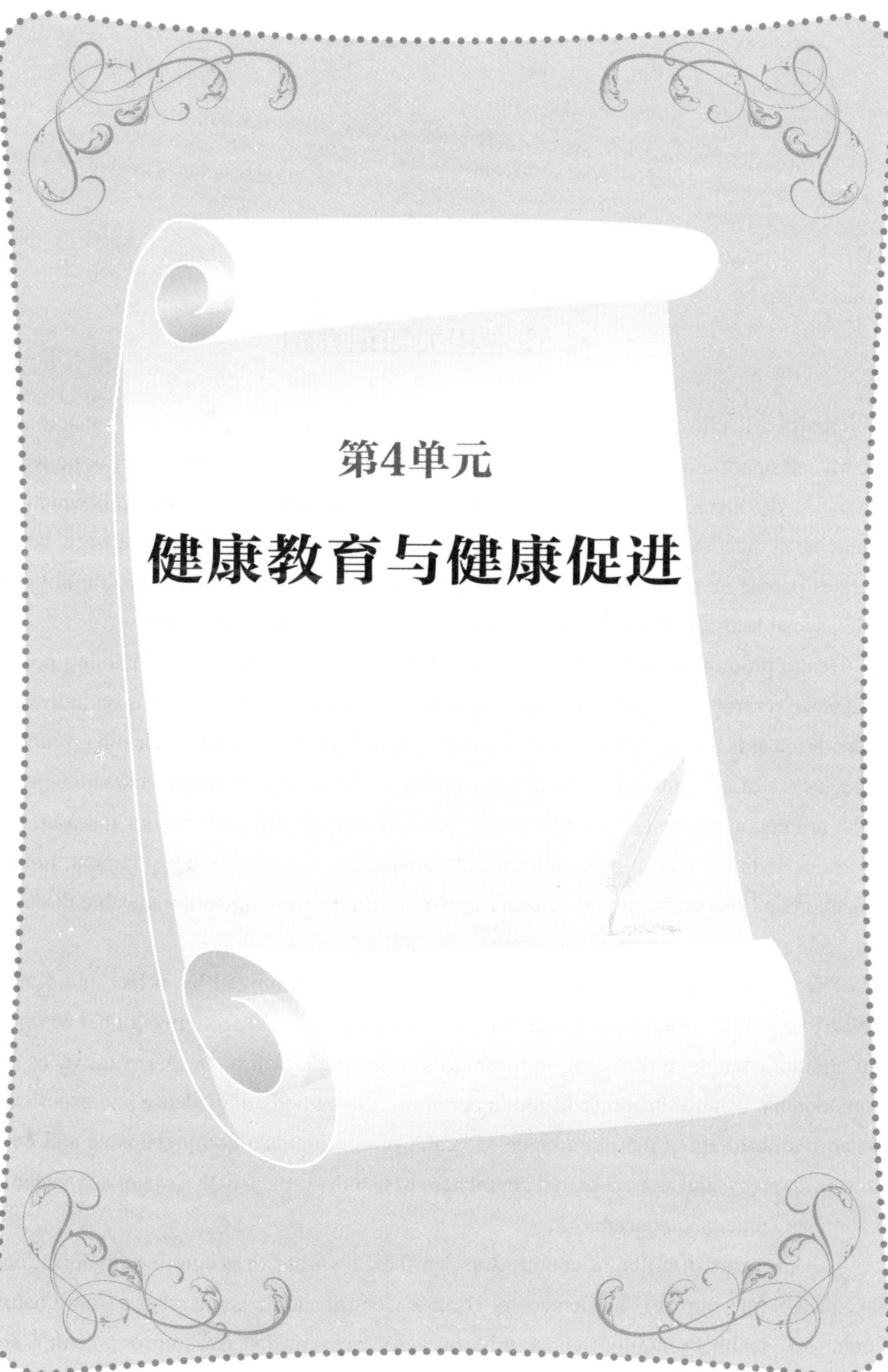

第4单元

健康教育与健康促进

一、主题相关知识介绍

Health education, according to WHO, is defined as "comprising of consciously constructed opportunities for learning involving some form of communication designed to improve health literacy, including improving knowledge, and developing life skills which are conducive to individual and community health." Health education can be a profession, which educates people about how to live a healthy life, including environmental health, physical health, social health, emotional health, intellectual health, and spiritual health.

Health promotion, according to WHO's definition, is "the process of enabling people to increase control over, and to improve, their health. It moves beyond a focus on individual behavior towards a wide range of social and environmental interventions." Health promotion strategies are of complex compositions. According to WHO, the principles and strategies of health promotion can be applied to a variety of population groups, risk factors, diseases, and in various settings. Health promotion, health education, community development, policy, legislation and regulation are all of equal importance in preventing communicable diseases, injury and violence, and mental problems.

The 7th Global Conference on Health Promotion organized by WHO and Kenya Ministry of Public Health pointed out that the worsening of world economy, global warming and climate change are bringing more threats to people's health. In this context, health promotion has achieved unprecedented importance. A large body of evidence and experience has accumulated about the importance of health promotion as a comprehensive and cost-effective strategy, and as an essential component of health systems with a major advantage in dealing with emerging concerns.

Governments in different countries set up their own health promotion organizations. Take the US for example. The Centers for Disease Control and Prevention has a Coordinating Center for Health Promotion whose mission is to "prevent disease, improve health, and

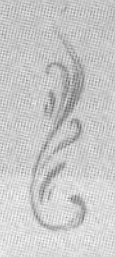

enhance human potential through evidence-based interventions and research in maternal and child health, chronic disease, disabilities, genomics, and hereditary disorders." There are also many non-governmental organizations about health promotion, such as the Public Health Education and Health Promotion Section, the Wellness Council of America, etc., which work together to make people worldwide more healthy.

二、技巧指导：语料类型分析——正式文体的语言特征

理解文体的特征，有助于平时积累词汇与口译时的用词选择。

既然在英语写作方式上有正式文体与非正式文体之分，那么两者的特点必然会在语言上表现出来。英文非正式文体的特点在于其口语性，也就是类似于谈话。非正式文体叙述方式比较个性化，扣题可以不那么紧密；词汇上面允许使用俚语、略缩语和缩写词；句法上以简单句为主，句子短，使用主动句和祈使句，允许省略句和不完整的句法；允许情感的流露，比如对所讲内容的复杂性表示理解。在使用代词上，第一、第二、第三人称都可以用。例如：

I think for an Oral English class you can pick up pretty much any textbook to give you pointers, conversation starters, topics, and perhaps different strategies. However, a halfway decent teacher should be able to use that book as a reference point and then come up with games, skits, and all sorts of activities for the students in order for them to practice their spoken English.

英文正式文体比较职业化，讲究表达策略，适用于官方文章、文件、学术研究、技术报告。特点是：表述方式客观，礼貌，倾向于技术性，具有较明显的书面语特征；在叙述方式上扣题紧密，阐述主要论点时使用明确无误的口吻，每一个论点都会得到介绍，解释并给出结论；客观，主要论点清楚，论据充分。在展示情感方面谨慎，不用表达情感的标点符号；在词汇上不允许使用俚语、缩略语和缩写词（约定俗成的缩略语除外，如WHO，UNESCO）；句法上以用复句与复合句为主，因而句子经常较长，且因为每一点都需要详尽阐述，经常使用被动态句式，少用祈使句，一般不用省略句和不完整的句型；在使用代词方面，为了展示客观性而多使用第三人称，少用第一人称“我”“我们”和第二人称“你”“你们”。因此，上一段口语写成书面语，可能变成下面的样子：

For an Oral English class, a teacher uses various textbooks and selects from them suggestions, conversation starters, topics, and different strategies. An experienced teacher should be able to use those books as reference while preparing games, short drama, and various activities for students to practice their spoken English.

再举一例：

A health system is more than just involving patients, families, and communities. In addition, ministries of health, health providers, health services organizations, pharmaceutical companies, health financing bodies, and other organizations work together to maintain a healthy system. In a health system, different parts play different roles, which are indispensable for a health system.

词汇举例：

口语性表达	非口语性表达
kids	children
guy	man
awesome	wonderful
a lot, loads of	many
I’m, It’s	I am, It is
doesn’t, can’t	does not, cannot
won’t, they’ll	will not, they will
shouldn’t, couldn’t	should not, could not
PHP	Pacific Historic Parks
TV	television
I find	It has been discovered
in recent years	recently
no longer under control	got out of hand

三、词汇准备

Text 1

bilateral investment agreements 双边贸易协定
curb the tobacco epidemic 控烟
graphic health warnings 卫生警示图片
leading preventable cause 主要的可预防死因
lung ailment 肺病
non-compliance 相违背
propagate the sale and distribution 扩大产品的销售和流通
second-hand smoke exposure 二手烟危害
smoke-free public places 无烟公共场所
tobacco related non-communicable diseases 与烟草有关的非传染病
WHO Framework Convention on Tobacco Control 世卫组织《烟草控制框架公约》

Text 2

essential medicines 基本药物
Harmonization for Health in Africa 非洲卫生协调
Health Assembly 卫生大会
improving regulatory control 改进管理控制
International Health Partnership Plus 国际卫生伙伴关系后续程序
malaria 疟疾
mother-to-child transmission 母婴传染
polio eradication 消灭脊灰病
pre-qualified 资格预审
streamlining and integrating health programs 梳理和整合卫生规划

Text 3

addictive 成瘾的
arsenal 武器，工具
comprehensive defense 全面防御
economically viable alternative crops 经济上可行的替代作物
halt the tobacco epidemic 制止烟草流行

illicit trade 违法交易
liability 赔偿责任
minors 未成年人
open for signature 开放以供签署
World No Tobacco Day 世界无烟日

Text 4

chronic nutritional deficiency 慢性营养缺乏
Copenhagen Consensus 哥本哈根协议
ready-to-use therapeutic foods 即食性治疗食物
stunting 发育迟缓
scaling-up nutrition (SUN) movement 扩张营养运动

Text 5

联合国千年发展目标 The United Nations Millennium Development Goals
基本医疗卫生制度 the basic health care system
老龄化 aging
慢性非传染性疾病 chronic non-infectious disease
最不发达国家 the least developed country

Text 6

规范化 normalization
横向联系 lateral connection
行业协会 association
理事 council member
社会平台 social platform

四、摘要练习

请听下面英语语篇，第一篇用源语言复述此段主要信息逻辑点及层次，第二篇用译入语复述此段主要信息逻辑点及层次。注意信息点之间的逻辑联系。

Text 1

Speech on World No Tobacco Day

Dr. Michael O'Leary, WHO Representative in China
At Ceremony of the 25th World No Tobacco Day

Beijing, China
30 May 2012

Honorable Minister,
Distinguished guests,
Ladies and gentlemen,

Good afternoon!

The theme of this year's World No Tobacco Day is "Stop tobacco industry interference in tobacco control". This campaign focuses on the need to expose and counter the tobacco industry's brazen and increasingly aggressive attempts to undermine global tobacco control.

Worldwide, every year tobacco consumption kills nearly 6 million people, of which about 1 million are in China. If current trends continue, by 2030 tobacco will kill more than 8 million people worldwide every year, with 80% of these premature deaths occurring among people in low- and middle-income countries.

Great efforts have been taken by countries to control tobacco epidemic. However, these tobacco control efforts are systematically opposed by the tobacco industry. Historically, the tobacco industry has used its economic power, lobbying, marketing machinery, and manipulation of the media to discredit scientific research and influence governments in order to propagate the sale and distribution of its deadly product.

Recently, in an attempt to halt the adoption of graphic health warnings on packages of tobacco, the industry used the novel tactic of suing countries under bilateral investment agreements, claiming that the warnings impinge the companies' attempts to use their legally-registered brands.

The industry also seeks to interfere with the policy-making process by subverting attempts to ban smoking in enclosed public places and to ban tobacco advertising, promotion and sponsorship.

Therefore, on World No Tobacco Day 2012, and throughout this year, WHO urges countries all over the world to put the fight against tobacco industry interference at the heart of their efforts to control the global tobacco epidemic.

Ladies and gentlemen,

China has made significant progress in tobacco control. China's 12th Five-Year Plan has called for smoke-free public places to contribute to the target of improved life expectancy. Several cities in China such as Harbin and Tianjin are using this World No Tobacco Day as the occasion to launch their revised tobacco control regulations that will ensure more tobacco-free public places and workplaces.

Today, the WHO congratulates the Ministry of Health for launching China's Report on the Health Hazards of Smoking. This marks an important milestone in the history of public health in China in the context of controlling the tobacco related non-communicable diseases affecting so many families and communities.

Following the release of this report, there will be an educational campaign designed to increase the knowledge level on the harms of tobacco. The secondary products which are released will be aimed at healthcare professionals and the general public.

These are all important and significant achievements. But much more needs to be done. In line with Article 5.3 of the Framework Convention, on this World No Tobacco Day, WHO calls for government to be alert to and resist efforts by the tobacco industry to undermine or disrupt tobacco control initiatives; we call for non-governmental organizations to monitor and raise awareness of non-compliance of the tobacco industry with national law; and we also call for individuals to be aware of the tactics of the tobacco industry in interfering with tobacco control.

By implementing the WHO Framework Convention on Tobacco Control, in line with the 12th Five-Year Plan, China can save millions of lives, and avert massive costs, both economic and humanitarian. In this way, China is part of a global movement to end the burden of death and disease caused by tobacco.

WHO will continue to support China in its adherence to Framework Convention obligations, to control the epidemic of tobacco use and to reduce the toll of tobacco-related diseases and deaths. We will work together to improve the health and life of the people of China.

Thank you.

复述要点提示（主要信息逻辑点及层次）

Purpose of the speech:

A call for governments and people to take action to stop tobacco industry's interference in the control of tobacco use. Countries and citizens should follow the suggestions by the WHO Framework Convention on Tobacco Control so as to win the victory against tobacco industry.

Keynotes of the speech:

The use of tobacco brings great health burden to the nations and people worldwide. It is one of the leading preventable causes of death. Every year, about 6 million people died from either directly smoking or second-hand smoke exposure. If we don't control the use of tobacco, by the year 2030, every year 8 million people will die of smoking, and most of this will happen in the underdeveloped countries. So it is highly important to curb the use of tobacco worldwide.

The action of controlling tobacco use is setback by the tobacco industry. 173 countries participate in the WHO Framework Convention on Tobacco Control, including China. However, since these actions prevent the tobacco industry from making great profit, this industry tries to manipulate the public as well as government to protect its market. The tobacco industry either uses money to influence the government or take advantage of the media to advocate its products. Recently, because the government forbids the tobacco industry to put the advertisement on the package, the industry even resorts to laws to win the battle between tobacco use and tobacco control.

China has made great progress in trying to limit the use of tobacco in the public places. China releases a report on the harms of tobacco. China also plans to start a campaign among all the Chinese citizens to educate the health professionals and common people about the harms of using tobacco. Cities in China, like Harbin and Tianjin, are trying to use the No Tobacco Day as a good chance to stop tobacco smoking in the public areas.

Conclusions:

Government, nongovernmental organizations, academia and individual citizens should all act to put an end to tobacco industry interference. It is an important measure in protecting people against the possible harms related to tobacco consumption.

Text 2

Best Days for Public Health Are Ahead of Us

Dr. Margaret Chan, Director-General of the WHO

Speech at the 65th World Health Assembly

Geneva, Switzerland

21 May 2012

Madam President, Excellencies, Honorable ministers, Distinguished delegates, Ladies and gentlemen,

This is the sixth time I have addressed the Health Assembly in my capacity as Director-General. I still get nervous. But I do have some important messages to convey.

Time and time again, we see the importance of national ownership and leadership. India would never have been able to dramatically change the prospects for polio eradication without full government ownership of the program.

Some of these countries need support in upgrading quality standards and improving regulatory control. WHO is providing this support. Last year, after extensive technical collaboration, WHO prequalified China's State Food and Drug Administration. Once individual vaccines are prequalified by WHO, the country's capacity to produce a large number of vaccines at very low prices will revolutionize vaccine supplies and their prices.

These examples give me, personally, great cause for optimism during what many regard as an especially dismal time. They also provide guidance on strategies and approaches that help maintain the momentum for health in the years ahead.

I can suggest three general lines of advice.

First, get back to the basics, like primary health care, access to essential medicines, and universal coverage. Shift to thrift. Develop a thirst for efficiency and an intolerance of waste. When a government commits itself to universal coverage, it takes a hard look at waste and inefficiency. It shifts to thrift.

At the international level, this means making good use of initiatives like the International Health Partnership Plus and Harmonization for Health in Africa. This means streamlining and integrating health programs, as is being done with plans to ensure that every baby is born HIV-free. This means using WHO country offices as a resource for policy dialogue and coordination, and for ensuring that aid for health development moves the country towards self-reliance. Good aid is channeled in ways that strengthen existing infrastructures and capacities. Good aid aims to eliminate the need for aid.

Second, as public expectations rise, costs soar, and budgets shrink, we must look to innovation as never before. These days the true genius of innovation resides in simplicity. This is not rocket science. This is frugal, strategic innovation that sets out to develop a game-changing intervention, and makes ease of use and affordable price explicit objectives.

We are seeing a new wave of innovation that, I believe, the commissioners on Social Determinants of Health would welcome. It looks not just at the causes of preventable deaths, but at the real reasons behind these causes.

My final advice is brief.

Use research. Use science. Shape the research agenda and seize every opportunity

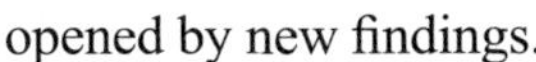

opened by new findings.

WHO does this most conspicuously when it revises policy and technical guidance for HIV/AIDS, tuberculosis, and malaria.

As just one example, evidence indicates that the elimination of mother-to-child transmission of HIV is entirely feasible, and this is now our operational goal.

We must never forget our value system. Never forget the people. Public health is trained in compassion and driven by passion. This will always be our strength, our true comparative advantage.

复述要点提示（主要信息逻辑点及层次）

两个目的：

1. 国家参与和全球疫情警报对全球卫生健康的重要性。

2. 对世卫组织未来工作的三点建议。

围绕第一个目的：

1. 以印度和中国两个发展中国家与世卫组织合作防控疾病的成功案例来证明政府与世卫组织合作对改善全球卫生状况的重要性。

2. 世卫组织分布在全球的疫情警报和反应网络使世卫组织在全球疾控方面的作用不可替代。

围绕第二个目的：

对未来的世卫工作主要有三点建议：

1. 卫生工作最基础的问题就是实现初级卫生保健，获得基本药物以及实现卫生资源的全面覆盖等。要实现这一点，各国政府应该首先落实节约的原则。应该制止对资源的浪费。在国际社会方面，各国需要充分利用“国际卫生伙伴关系后续程序”和“非洲卫生协调”等举措。各国需要梳理和整合自己的卫生资源，进行合理的卫生规划。各国需要在卫生工作中充分发挥主导作用，真正把公民的卫生健康当作工作的重要部分。世卫组织的国家办事处也要充分协调卫生工作和政策资源方面的关系，促进各国更加独立地开展卫生工作。

2. 卫生工作应该注重创新。陈冯富珍博士特别指出，这里的创新重点在于符合实践的需要，是节俭型、战略性创新，是使人们能够享受到更多方便和便宜的卫生产品。

3. 利用研究所取得的成就，制订相关政策，抓住新发现带来的每一次机遇。陈冯富珍博士以世卫组织对有关艾滋病、结核病和疟疾等疾病的技术准则做出及时修订为例，证明明智的政策规定能够有效地实现对疾病的控制，如消除母婴传播艾滋病是完全可行的。

五、英译汉练习

Text 3

UN Secretary-General Ban Ki-moon's Message on World No Tobacco Day

31 May 2011

This year's observance of World No Tobacco Day falls in the midst of preparations for September's United Nations high-level meeting on non-communicable diseases. By controlling tobacco, we can go a long way towards addressing many of these chronic ailments, including cancer and heart disease.

The use of tobacco, which is highly addictive, killed approximately 100 million people in the twentieth century, and unless we act, it could kill up to a billion in this century.

The greatest tool in our arsenal is the World Health Organization's Framework Convention on Tobacco Control. Since it was opened for signature in 2003, more than 170 countries have become parties, making it one of the most rapidly embraced treaties in United Nations history.

From reducing demand through higher prices and taxes to restricting advertising and sponsorship, from warnings on packages to prohibitions against sales to minors, countries are using the Treaty's provisions to protect their citizens. They are sending a clear message that tobacco use makes us poorer—in health and economic terms.

The Treaty's comprehensive defense against industry tactics includes measures to reduce the illicit trade in tobacco products, address issues of liability, support economically viable alternative crops and protect public health policies from undue pressure.

The Framework Convention is clearly working to safeguard health in all countries that have adopted and enforced it. Yet, as the reports from States parties show, we have a long way to go. I urge all parties to fully meet their obligations under the Treaty, and I call on the few countries that have not yet become parties to do so. Together, we can halt the tobacco epidemic and the many problems it brings.

On this World No Tobacco Day, let us push for progress that will cut tobacco-related deaths and enliven the battle against other non-communicable diseases, helping to create a healthier world for all.

Text 4

Speech at the High Level Meeting on Nutrition

Anthony Lake, UNICEF Executive Director

New York, USA

20 September 2011

Ladies and gentlemen,

The emergency in the Horn of Africa has become a catastrophe, where more than 300,000 children are suffering from severe acute malnutrition and are in immediate peril. Their suffering may be receding from our front pages and our television screens... their suffering may be off camera... but each one could soon be dead.

300,000.

And there is another number about global suffering: 20 million.

That is the number of children afflicted with severe acute malnutrition around the world—nearly seventy times the number of severely malnourished children in the Horn of Africa. Imagine if all of those children were in one region. That would be seen as one of the worst child catastrophes ever. And remember, every one of them is a child whose life is in danger and whose parents could, very soon, grieve her or his loss.

They are 20 million reasons why we must lift nutrition higher up our list of global concerns.

20 million.

There is another number... and it represents another silent emergency. Somewhere between 170 million and 180 million children around the world, depending on how you calculate it, are stunted.

180 million.

Stunting is the irreversible outcome of chronic nutritional deficiency during the first thousand days of a child's life. And the damage it causes to a child's development is permanent. That child will never learn, nor earn, as much as he or she could have if properly nourished in early life. What a loss for that child. What a loss for that society.

Just 21 countries account for more than 80 percent of the global stunting burden. In six countries, 50 percent or more of all children under five suffer from this terrible—and preventable—condition. And under-nutrition is not exclusive to the lowest-income countries or the poorest communities. It can occur in children who live in food-secure households and in food-secure countries.

For far too long, this silent emergency has received far too little attention. Even though, in 2008, the Copenhagen Consensus ranked providing young children with micronutrients the most cost-effective way to advance global welfare.

But thanks to the SUN movement and the leadership of many governments represented here today, the global community has begun to recognize that nutrition is—and must be—more than a footnote in the food security debate.

Nutrition security should be an essential element of every national development plan—as critical as clean water, as indispensable as education.

UNICEF is committed to seeing this through. We will continue...

To design programs with governments that improve mother-child nutrition... To provide essential supplies like Vitamin A, zinc and iron supplements, and ready-to-use therapeutic foods... To train more community workers to feed children and keep them healthy... To collaborate with all our partners to monitor these efforts and build on what works... For UNICEF and all those in the SUN movement, this is not only the right thing to do, it is the practical thing to do.

In only one year, the number of countries beginning to implement national strategies to reduce stunting has increased dramatically. Now, we must build on this momentum. We must integrate our efforts and join the forces of the food, health and development communities... for the 300,000 children in the Horn... for the 20 million children, globally, suffering from severe acute malnutrition... and for the nearly 180 million children who are stunted.

Under-nutrition is preventable. And, therefore, inaction is unconscionable.

Thank you very much.

六、汉译英练习

Text 5

如何在未来全球发展议程中确保卫生的地位
国家卫生和计划生育委员会主任李斌在第66届世界卫生大会上的发言

2013年5月20日

尊敬的主席先生，尊敬的总干事女士，各位部长，各位同事：

首先请允许我对主席先生的当选表示祝贺。我相信在您的领导下，本届大会一定能够取得圆满成功。

主席先生，

健康是经济社会和谐、可持续发展的目标和必要条件。要实现人类社会协调、均衡、可持续发展，必须将健康放在全球政治和发展议程的核心位置，促使各国调动多种资源，加强卫生体系建设，促进健康公平。

2000年以来，包括中国在内的各成员国在落实联合国千年发展目标方面取得了巨大进展。随着全球人口快速老龄化，生活方式和疾病模式快速转变，健康和卫生安全问题变得更加复杂，传染病和慢性非传染性疾病的防控形势依然严峻，需要我们共同努力、迎接挑战。为此，我们提出如下倡议：

要确保卫生在全球发展议程中的地位，应强调“在从生至死的生命全程促进健康”的概念。要保留尚未如期实现的千年发展目标，促进孕产妇和儿童的健康；支持纳入糖尿病、心血管疾病、癌症以及精神疾病等慢性非传染性疾病的控制指标。

应将实现全民健康覆盖作为重要实施策略。要突出提高健康公平、缩小人群健康差距、增强卫生服务提供体系等方面的指标。应从健康的社会决定因素角度设定具体目标，动员全社会共同参与、促进健康。应将健康内容融入社会、经济公共政策，完善扶贫和开发政策，加大对卫生和教育领域的投资，促进基本公共服务均等化，以及就业和可持续发展。

应注重加强卫生系统能力建设。今年3月以来，中国部分省份出现人感染H7N9禽流感疫情。4月四川雅安发生强烈地震。中国有效防控人感染禽流感，成功开展地震救援、防疫和灾后恢复建设的实践经验，使我们更加深刻感到“预则立、不预则废”，完备的卫生服务提供，以及卫生应急救援响应机制和保障系统是妥善应对突发公共卫生事件的必要条件。

应加强信息交流和经验分享等国际合作，加强对发展中国家特别是最不发达国家和地区的卫生援助、政策支持和技术支持，制订适合本地的实际、有效、可行的卫生政策，促进卫生体系的公平与效率。

2009年以来，中国政府全面启动深化医药卫生体制改革，逐步建设了覆盖城乡居民的基本医疗卫生制度，有力地促进了千年发展目标的全面、均衡实现。截至目前，基本医疗保险覆盖超过13亿人。2012年5岁以下儿童死亡率下降到13.2‰，已经提前实现了千年发展目标；孕产妇死亡率下降到24.5/10万。

中国愿与各成员国一道，为确保卫生在未来全球发展议程中的地位而努力，促进全球人民的健康和福祉。

谢谢大家！

Text 6

甘肃省副省长咸辉在甘肃省健康促进与教育协会成立大会上的讲话

2010年7月13日

同志们：

今天，我们隆重召开甘肃省健康促进与教育协会成立大会，这是我省健康教育事业发展中的一件大事，必将对我省健康教育事业的发展产生积极的促进作用。发展健康教育事业是政府的职责，也是人民群众的共同愿望。我省因经济欠发达，社会性健康教育工作相对滞后，广大人民群众特别是广大农村群众的自我保健意识和能力还很弱，生活中存在着很多不科学、不卫生的习惯，即使是生活条件较好的城市居民，也存在着不少健康方面的误区和问题。成立健康促进与教育协会，积极开展健康教育，努力满足人民群众日益增长的健康需求，是我省健康教育事业发展的内在要求，对进一步提高我省健康教育工作水平，加快卫生事业发展，保障人民群众身体健康，具有非常重要的意义。

健康教育作为公共卫生的基础性、先导性工作，是一项投入少、产出高、效益大的卫生保健措施，是预防疾病、保护和增进群众健康的治本性措施。多年来，我们的医疗卫生事业已经积累了一条重要的经验，即“健康教育在先，预防为主”，这也是医药卫生体制改革的一个重要理念。

当前，我省医改工作正在深入推进，加强健康促进与教育工作，大力开展健康教育，及时把防病、健身的卫生知识向广大群众普及，帮助他们克服不良的生活习惯，提高健康水平，改善生活质量，已经成为当前推进医改的重要举措。今天，我们成立健康促进与教育协会，就是要依靠行业协会，动员全社会力量广泛开展全民健康教育与健康促进，把健康教育与健康促进延伸到社会各个方面，充分利用协会“横向联系、专家荟萃”的优势，打造健康教育的社会平台，促进健康教育社会化、大众化和规范化，努力引导广大人民群众建立科学、文明、健康的生活方式，不断提高我省人民群众健康的整体水平。

卫生行政部门要在深入开展农村健康教育的基础上，大力组织实施“健康教育进家庭”活动，积极创造条件开设农民健康教育学校，引导农民群众合理健康消费，努力改变不卫生的生活习惯和生活方式。要紧紧抓住城市社区卫生服务体系建设的有利时机，进一步完善社区卫生服务机构功能，着力研究新时期城市社区健康教育工作的方法和途径，逐步建立经济、持续、有效的城市社区健康教育和健康促进工作新机制。各级、各部门要采取多种形式，促进学校、企事业单位和医院健康教育再上新台阶，进一步提高城镇居民文明卫生意识和道德水平。

同志们，我省健康促进与教育协会的成立，标志着我省卫生健康促进和健康教育工作步入了新的发展时期，希望协会的全体理事团结一致，努力工作，把我省健康促进与教育工作提高到一个新的水平，为推动我省医药卫生体制改革深入进行，促进全省经济社会又好又快发展做出新的更大的贡献。

谢谢大家！

资料来源：

Text 1 http://www.wpro.who.int/china/mediacentre/speeches/2012/20120530/en/index.html

Text 2 http://www.docin.com/p-549068126.html

Text 3 http://www.kouyi.org/field/health/1604.html

Text 4 http://www.unicef.org/media/media_59871.html

Text 5 http://www.moh.gov.cn/lbwz/plxfs/201305/589222beca734b4b81c7738fb9cbad6e.shtml

Text 6 http://www.gansu.gov.cn/content/2010-07/2892.html

参考答案

四、摘要练习

Text 1

世卫组织驻华代表蓝睿明博士在第25个世界无烟日仪式上的致辞

中国北京

2012年5月30日

尊敬的部长，
各位来宾，
女士们、先生们：

下午好！

今年“世界无烟日”的主题是“制止烟草业干扰控烟”。

此次活动的重点是揭穿并反击烟草业企图破坏全球控烟活动的肆无忌惮并且日益升级的伎俩。

世界范围内，每年近600万人因吸烟致死，其中中国因吸烟致死的人数约100万。如果这种趋势继续下去，到2030年烟草将会导致全球每年超过800万人死亡。

各国已经采取措施大力控制烟草疫情。然而控烟活动受到烟草业系统性的抵制。长久以来，烟草业一直利用其经济影响力、游说和营销手段，以及对媒体的操纵，诬蔑科研成果，影响政府决策，以便扩大其致死性产品的销售和流通。

为阻止在烟草包装上采用图片健康警语，烟草业最近采取了根据双边贸易协定对国家起诉的新手法，并声称这些图片警语影响了其合法注册商标的使用。

烟草业还通过破坏封闭公共场所内禁烟的努力和禁止烟草广告、促销和赞助活动的努力，试图干涉政策制订的过程。

因此，在2012年“世界无烟日”，以及今年全年，世卫组织敦促全世界将反对烟草业干扰作为全球控烟活动的重点。

女士们，先生们，

中国在控烟上已经取得了显著的成绩。中国的第12个五年计划呼吁实现公共场合无烟化以实现提高人口寿命的目标。包括哈尔滨和天津在内的几个中国城市正在利用“世界无烟日”这个契机施行修订过的控烟条例，以便更多公共场合和工作场合实现无烟化。

今天，卫生部发布了《中国吸烟危害健康报告》，世卫组织对此表示祝贺。在控制危害大量家庭及社区的烟草相关性非传染病方面，它是中国公共卫生史上的重要里程碑之一。

《报告》发布之后，中国将随之开展旨在提高对烟草危害认识的宣传活动。此后的活动重点将针对卫生专业人士和公众。

这些都是重要而富有意义的成就，但控烟工作仍任重道远。值此“世界无烟日”之际，按照《框架公约》第5.3条规定，世卫组织呼吁各国政府警惕并反对烟草业对控烟工作的破坏或干扰。我们呼吁非政府组织对烟草业违反国家法律的活动进行监督并提高认识。我们还呼吁个人了解烟草业干扰控烟工作的各种伎俩。

通过履行世卫组织《烟草控制框架公约》和实施五年规划，中国可以挽救数百万人的生命，并且可以避免吸烟所带来的巨大经济及人道损失。与此同时，中国也成为全球消除烟草相关死亡及疾病负担行动的一部分。

世卫组织将一如既往地支持中国履行《框架公约》的义务，开展控烟活动，从而减少烟草相关疾病及死亡带来的损失。我们将共同努力，提高中国人民的健康和生活水平。

谢谢。

Text 2

卫生工作最光明的日子在我们的前方
世界卫生组织总干事陈冯富珍博士在第65届世界卫生大会上的讲话

瑞士日内瓦

2012年5月21日

主席女士，各位阁下，尊敬的部长们，尊贵的代表们，女士们、先生们：

这是我第六次以总干事的身份在卫生大会上讲话，我还是会紧张。但是，我确实有一些重要的信息要向你们传达。

我们一次又一次地看到国家自主决策和领导作用的重要性。如果政府对规划没有充分的自主决策，印度永远也不会有能力显著改变脊灰消灭工作的前景。印度政府有资格接受我们对这一巨大成就的祝贺。

在这些国家中，有一些需要在提升质量标准和改进管理控制方面获得支持。世卫组织正在提供这种支持。去年，在开展广泛的技术合作之后，世卫组织完成了中国国家食品药物管理局的资格预审。一旦一种疫苗通过世卫组织的资格预审，该国以很低价格生产大量疫苗的能力将使疫苗供应及其价格出现突破性的进展。

在许多人认为情况特别糟糕的时候，这些例子为我个人提供了保持乐观的重要原因。这些例子也对有助于在未来数年中维持卫生工作动力的战略和做法提供了指导。

我可以提出三条总体建议：

首先回到基本问题上来，如初级卫生保健、获得基本药物以及全民覆盖等问题。

需要转向节俭，建立对效率的追求、对浪费的不容忍。政府如果致力于全民覆盖，就会认真考虑浪费和低效问题，就会厉行节俭。

在国际一级，这就意味着需要妥善利用“国际卫生伙伴关系后续程序”和“非洲卫生协调”等举措。

这就意味着梳理和整合卫生规划，一如针对确保婴儿无艾滋病毒计划所做的那样。

这就意味着让各国都坐在主导者的位置上，使它们在为其民众的健康而采取的行动方面拥有充分的自主权。政府正是凭借这些赢得其公民、其选民的信心和信任。

这就意味着利用世卫组织国家办事处这一资源，进行政策对话和协调，确保卫生发展援助有助于推动国家走向自力更生。

有效的援助应以加强现有基础设施和能力的方式来输送。有效的援助旨在消除援助需求。

其次，随着公共期待提高，费用增加，预算削减，我们必须比以往任何时候都更加注重创新，我指的是那类正确的创新。创新如果能够呼应社会关注和需要，而不仅仅是赢取利润的前景，就能带来莫大好处。

当今时代，创新的真谛在于简单。这不是火箭科学，这是节俭型、战略性创新，目的是发展改变游戏规则的创新，将方便使用和价格低廉作为明确的目标。

我们目睹了这一波新的创新，我相信，健康的社会决定因素问题的主管者们将会表示欢迎。它不仅关注可预防死亡的死因，而且关注这些死因背后的真正原因。

我最后的建议很简单。利用研究工作；利用科学；制定研究议程，抓住新发现带来的每一次机遇。

世卫组织在修订其关于艾滋病毒/艾滋病、结核和疟疾的技术准则时，再明显不过地做到了这一点。只需举出一个例子，有证据表明，消除母婴传播艾滋病毒是完全可行的，这是我们现在的工作目标。这是提高效率的一个部分。

科学促成了突破，公共卫生进行了操作，取得了长足进展。

五、英译汉练习

Text 3

联合国秘书长潘基文2011年世界无烟日致辞

2011年5月31日

今年世界无烟日活动适逢为9月联合国非传染性疾病问题高级别会议开展筹备工作期间。通过控制烟草，我们可以在防治许多慢性病方面取得长足的进步，其中包括癌症和心脏病。

烟草很容易使人上瘾，烟草的使用在20世纪导致了约一亿人死亡。如果我们不采取行动，它在本世纪可能造成多达十亿人丧生。

我们现在可以运用的最好的工具是世界卫生组织的《烟草控制框架公约》。自该公约2003年开放供签署以来，已有170多个国家成为缔约国，使之成为联合国历史上获得最迅速接受的条约之一。

各国正在使用该公约的条款保护其公民，包括通过提高价格和税收降低需求，限制广告和赞助，要求在包装上印出警告，禁止向未成年人进行销售，等等。这些国家正在发出一个明确的信息，即烟草的使用会令我们越来越糟糕——在健康和经济方面都是如此。

该条约对烟草行业策略的全面防御，包括规定措施以减少烟草制品的非法贸易、解决赔偿责任问题、支持经济上可行的替代作物和保护公共卫生政策免遭不当压力。

在所有已通过和执行了框架公约的国家中，该公约显然正在发挥保障健康的作用。然而，正如一些缔约国报告所显示的那样，我们还有很长的路要走。我敦促所有缔约方充分履行条约所规定的义务，我也呼吁为数不多的尚未成为缔约方的国家成为缔约方。我们齐心合力，就可以制止烟草的流行及其带来的诸多问题。

值此世界无烟日，让我们推动进步以减少与烟草有关的死亡和加强防治其他非传染性疾病的斗争，帮助创造一个让所有人都更加健康的世界。

Text 4

联合国儿童基金会执行主任安东尼·雷克在营养问题高层会议上的讲话

美国纽约

2011年9月20日

女士们、先生们：

非洲之角的危机已经成为一场灾害，它导致超过30万儿童严重营养不良、生命垂危。也许不久这些处于痛苦中的孩子们就会从我们的报纸、我们的电视报道、我们的视线中淡去，但是我们不要忘了，这些孩子中的任何一个都可能因为灾难而很快死去。

30万儿童!

全球还有另外一个数据：2 000万。

这是全世界遭受严重营养不良的儿童的数量——几乎是非洲之角这些孩子的70倍。设想一下，如果所有的这些孩子都处在一个区域，这将是有史以来最可怕的儿童的灾难。让我们记住，这2 000万儿童中的每一个都面临生命的危险，而他们的父母会为他们的离去而深深痛苦。

我们有2 000万个理由要把营养问题列入全球关注问题的首位。

2 000万!

这里还有一个数字，它代表着另外一种沉默的危机。全世界大约有1.7亿到1.8亿的儿童（根据计算方式的不同）因为营养不良而发育迟缓。

1.8亿!

发育迟缓是儿童出生后的1 000天内因为长期缺乏营养而造成的一种不可逆转的结果。它对儿童的生长发育造成了永久的伤害。发育迟缓的孩子无法在学习和工作上和那些在出生后1 000天内吸收了良好的营养的孩子们相比。这对孩子是怎样的一种伤害！这对社会又造成了怎样的一种损失!

仅仅21个国家的儿童发育迟缓数量就占了全球总量的80%。在六个国家里，有50%（甚至更多）的5岁以下的儿童正在承受这种可怕的但是可预防的疾病。而且营养不良并不只限于低收入国家或者最贫困的社区。发育迟缓也发生在那些食物充足的家庭和国家的孩子身上。

太长的时间里这个沉默的危机没有受到人们的注意，尽管2008年哥本哈根会议曾将为幼儿提供微量营养元素列为推进全球人类健康工作中最有效的方法。

但是因为有了扩张营养运动和出席会议的各国领导层的努力，国际社会开始渐渐认识到，营养必须在食品安全辩论中发挥更重要的作用。

营养安全应该是每个国家发展计划中必不可少的一部分，就像干净的水和教育一样不可或缺。

联合国儿童基金会致力于这一切的实现。我们会一直继续下去……

我们将和各国政府合作制定项目，改善母婴营养……

为孩子们提供必要的维生素A，锌和铁，以及即食性治疗食物……

我们将培训更多的社区工作者，帮助照看孩子们，让他们健康……

我们将继续和我们的合作伙伴一起监督这些努力，使之生效……

对于联合国儿童基金和所有参与扩张营养运动的成员而言，这些不仅是正确的，而且是可行的。

仅仅一年时间里，开始实施全民计划以减少生长发育问题的国家的数量大幅增加。现在我们必须抓住这个机会。我们必须把我们的努力和食品、健康以及发展等领域的力量相结合，为了非洲之角30万挨饿的孩子，为了世界上2 000万遭受严重营养不良的孩子，也为了近1.8亿遭受发育迟缓的孩子。

营养不良是可以预防的，因此，不作为是不明智的。

非常感谢大家！

六、汉译英练习

Text 5

On How to Ensure the Position of Health in the Future Global Development Agenda

Remarks on the 66th World Health Assembly by Li Bin, Director of China National Health and Family Planning Commission

20 May 2013

Respectful Mr. president, respectful Madam director-general, ministers and colleagues,

First, please allow me to give my sincere congratulations to the election of your honorable president. I believe that this assembly will achieve a great success under your leadership.

Mr. President,

Health is the requisite and goal of social economic harmony and sustainable development. To realize the balance and sustainable development of human society, we have to put health at the core position in global political and developmental agenda, promote every country to motivate multi resources and strengthen the construction of health system so as to promote the overall health equity.

Since 2000, every membership country, including China, has made tremendous progress in implementing The United Nations Millennium Development Goals. With the rapid aging of global population and the rapid change of people's living styles and the modes of diseases, health issue has become more complicated, and the control and prevention situation of infectious as well as chronic non-infectious diseases is still grim. It needs us to work together to meet the challenge. Therefore, we'd come up with the following proposals:

To ensure health's core position in the global development agenda, we should emphasize the concept of "promoting health from birth to death", regard the unfinished Millennium Development Goals as our future goals and promote the health of pregnant women and children, and support to include in the control index chronic non-infectious diseases such as diabetes, cardiovascular diseases, cancers, and mental illnesses.

Regard universal health coverage as an important implementing strategy. We should enhance health equality, bridge the population health gap, and strengthen the index of health care service system. We should set a concrete goal from a healthy social determining factor, motivate the whole society to participate in and promote health work. We should include health in social and public economic policies, improve the poverty alleviation and development policy, step up the investment in health and education, and promote the equality of basic public services, employment and sustainable development.

Strengthen the capability construction of health system. Since March this year, H7N9 Avian Flu epidemic occurred in some provinces in China. In April, a strong earthquake hit Ya'an, Sichuan. China's experience in controlling the H7N9 epidemic, earthquake rescue, epidemic prevention and after-earthquake recovery construction makes us keenly aware that "Preparedness ensures success, unpreparedness spells failure". Complete health care supply, health emergency response, and provision mechanism are the prerequisites for the proper treatment of public health emergencies.

Reinforce the international cooperation in the exchange of information and experiences, step up the efforts in health care, political and technical support for developing, especially the least developed, countries, and design practical and efficient health policies that suit local conditions, and promote the equality and efficiency of health care system.

Since 2009, the Chinese government has been deepening medical health reform in an all-round way. We have gradually built up the basic health care system which covers both urban and rural populations, and powerfully promoted the comprehensive and equal realization of the Millennium Development Goals. Till now, the basic medical insurance has covered over 1.3 billion people. In 2012, the mortality rate of children under 5 years old was reduced to 13.2‰, which means that we had realized the Millennium Development Goals before schedule; the mortality rate of pregnant women was reduced to 24.5 in every 1000,000.

China would like to work with every member country to ensure the important position of health in the future global development agenda and promote the health and benefits of people all over the world.

Thank you!

Text 6

Remarks by Xian Hui, Deputy Governor of Gansu Province at the Foundation Ceremony of Gansu Healthcare Promotion and Education Association

13 July 2010

Comrades,

Today we gather here to celebrate the establishment of Gansu Healthcare Promotion and Education Association. This is an important thing in Gansu Healthcare Education development and will actively promote the development of Gansu healthcare education. The development of healthcare education is our government's responsibility and the common wish of the public. Gansu is underdeveloped, and the social healthcare education work is comparatively lagging behind. The public, especially the rural population, lack the self protection consciousness and ability, and many of their habits are not scientific nor healthy. Even the city population that enjoy better living conditions have many misunderstandings about health issue. Therefore, to establish the healthcare promotion and education association, actively conduct health education, and try hard to satisfy the daily increased health needs of the people are the internal needs of Gansu's health education work. It is of great significance to further improve the health education level of our province, speed up the health development, and guarantee the health of the public.

Health education is a basic and pioneering work in public health, and is a health care prevention which means little input, high turn out and great benefits. It is the basic measure in disease prevention and the protection and promotion of public health. For many years, there is an important experience in our health care project, that is "health care first, prevention the focus", and this is an important concept in healthcare reform.

Currently, the healthcare reform of our province is progressing. Strengthening health promotion and education, popularizing the health knowledge of disease prevention and body building, helping people overcome the unhealthy living habits, enhancing healthcare, improving living quality, etc, have become the important measures of current healthcare reform. Today we established the healthcare promotion and education association in the hope to rely on the association to mobilize social efforts in conducting health education and promotion among people. We should extend the health education and promotion to every aspect of society, take full advantage of "lateral connection and the expertise of experts" of the association to build a social platform of health education, promote the socialization and normalization of health education, lead the public into a scientific, civilized and healthy living style, and constantly enhance the overall level of the public health of our province.

The healthcare administration should strongly promote the conduction of "healthcare education going into family" at the basis of deepening health education in the rural areas, actively create conditions to set up health education schools for farmers, guide farmers into healthy consumption, and try to change the unhealthy habits and living style of farmers. We should catch the opportunity of urban community health service construction, further improve the function of community healthcare service, study the methods of current urban community healthcare education, and gradually establish a new working mechanism that is economic, sustainable and effective in health education and promotion. Departments at all levels should take a variety of methods to facilitate the health education in schools, enterprise and public institutions, and hospitals, and enhance citizens' consciousness and morality of health and civilization.

Dear comrades, the foundation of Gansu Health Promotion and Education Association means that the healthcare promotion and education of our province have entered a new period. I hope every council member can work together to elevate the health promotion and education in our province to a new level and make greater contribution to the development of Gansu province!

Thank you all!

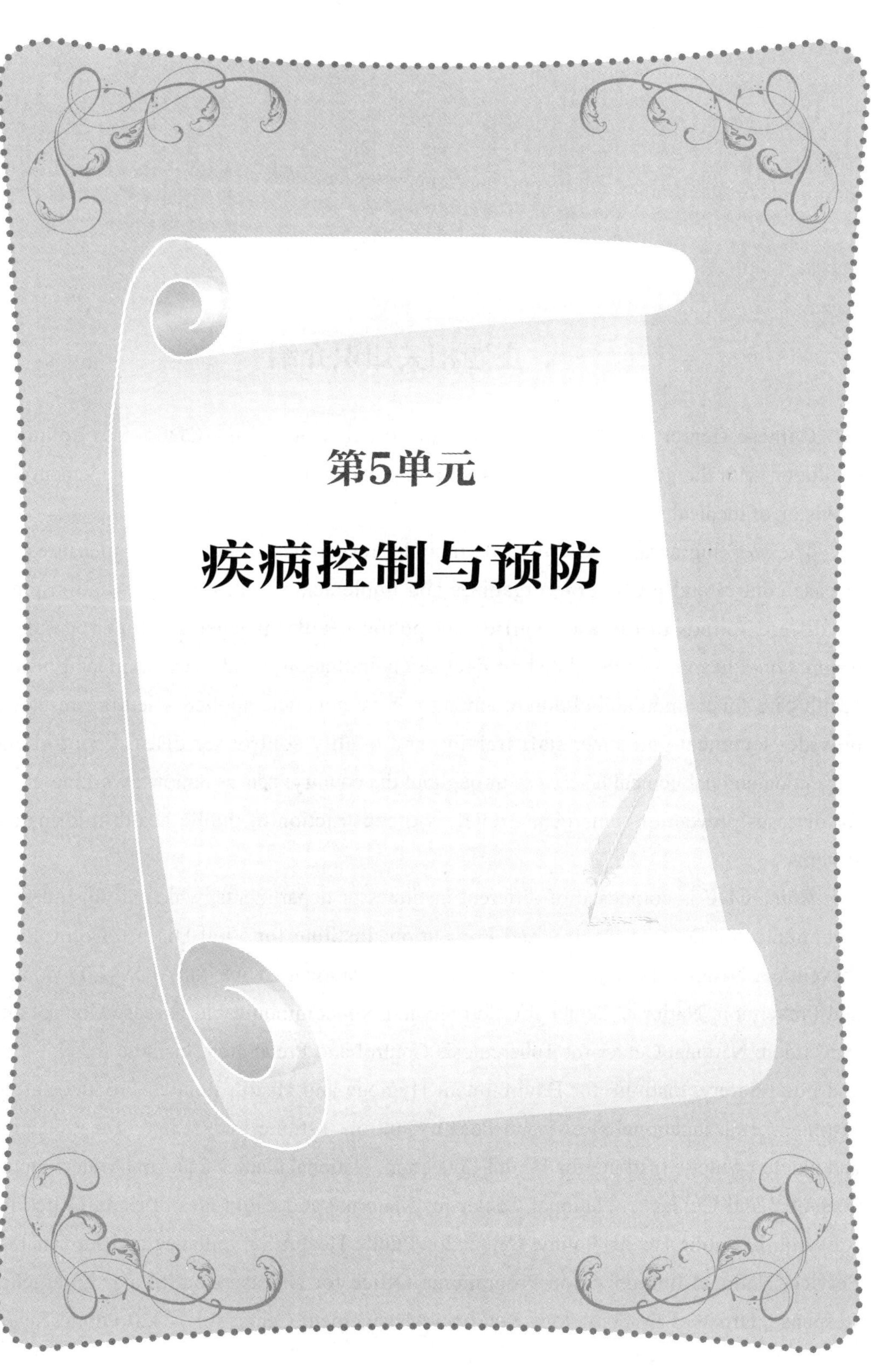

第5单元

疾病控制与预防

一、主题相关知识介绍

Chinese Center for Disease Control and Prevention (China CDC), is a nonprofit institution with the goals of disease control and prevention, public health management and provision of medical service.

The working areas of China CDC include: researches strategies and measures for disease control and prevention; organizes and implements control and prevention plans for different kinds of diseases; carries out public health management for food safety, occupational health, health related product safety, radiation health, environmental health, health care for women and children, among others; conducts applied scientific research; provides technical guidance, staff training and quality control for disease control and prevention and public health services throughout the country; acts as national working group for diseases prevention, emergency relief, and construction of public health information systems.

China CDC is composed of different institutes or departments, which are Institute for Communicable Disease Control and Prevention, Institute for Viral Disease Control and Prevention, National Institute of Parasitic Disease, National Center for AIDS/STD Control and Prevention, National Center for Chronic and Noncommunicable Disease Control and Prevention, National Center for Tuberculosis Control and Prevention, Institute for Nutrition and Food Safety, Institute for Environment Hygiene and Health Related Product Safety, Institute for Occupational Health and Poison Control, Institute for Radiological Protection and Nuclear Safety, Institute for Health Education, National Center for Rural Water Supply Technical and Guidance, National Center for Maternal and Child Health Care, Office for Research in Public Health Policy, Center for Public Health Surveillance and Information Service, National Immunization Programme, Office for Disease Control and Emergence Response, Office of Epidemiology, National Management Center for 12320 Public Health

Hotline.

China CDC is currently carrying out the following projects: Rapid Assessment of Drinking Water Quality, IDD Intervention Programme in Western and Inshore District, MON-WHO-UNICEF Accelerating Meals Control and Strengthening Routine, Immunization Services Project Guizhou Province, Expended Program on Immunization Strengthening Project in China, Surveillance for Creutzfeldt-Jacob Disease in China, Discovery and Identifying Genetic Susceptibility or Resistance Genes Associated with NP, Urban Health and Poverty Project, Accelerated Actions to Increase TB Care Detection in China, Chemical Constituents of Decreasing Lipid in Blood from Chinese Medicine, Prevention and Control of Occupational Diseases in Small and Medium Scale Enterprises in China, etc.

二、技巧指导：解析信息与逻辑整理——语篇的逻辑组织方式

要识别讲话稿的主题思想，先要明白语篇的逻辑组织方式。在所有的语言材料中，信息均按特定的逻辑组织成一个语篇整体。逻辑加表述顺序是语篇结构的基本点，是构成段落的根本原则。在思维结构、逻辑顺序、信息布局方面，英文的中心思想一般都在一开始就提出，这种开门见山的思维习惯有时候甚至体现在诗歌、小说、散文里面。大多数讲稿或演示文稿（PPT）的标题就是主要论点，比如“母乳喂养的益处”“酗酒的害处”“吸烟有害健康”等。这些介绍概念的题目通常会用条分式的方法，将“益处”与“害处”一一解释清楚。接下来的每一个自然段也多遵循这个顺序：先有一个主题句，用以表述主要论点，紧接主题句的后面通常会解释主题句的意思，并提供证据。例如：

One major change that has occurred in the Western family is an increased incidence in divorce. This change is borne out clearly in census figures. For example, thirty years ago in Australia only one marriage in ten ended in divorce; nowadays the figure is more than one in three (Australian Bureau of Statistics, 1996). An interesting issue is why this change has occurred—a question that has been considered by a number of sociologists. In this essay, I will seek to critically examine a number of sociological explanations for the “divorce phenomenon” and also consider the social policy implications that each explanation carries with it. It will be argued that the best explanations are to be found within a broad socio-economic framework.

（Source: http://www.monash.edu.au/lls/llonline/writing/general/essay/drafting-essay/3.xml）

这一段的主题句为：

One major change that has occurred in the Western family is an increased incidence in divorce.

解释句为：

This change is borne out clearly in census figures.

证据句为：

For example, thirty years ago in Australia only one marriage in ten ended in divorce; nowadays the figure is more than one in three (Australian Bureau of Statistics, 1996).

与汉语文章相同，英文文章也讲究前后一致（coherence），因此文章中的每一个论点都与中心论点相关，包括篇末的结论。一个语篇开始立论为正面或肯定的，那么得出的结论也是肯定的；开始立论为否定的，那么结论也是否定的；立论为正反两方各有利弊，那么结论也会支持正反两方各有利弊的观点。如果立论为肯定，结论为否定，则文章无逻辑性，因为写一篇论说文，就是为了证明中心论点。与以阅读为目的的文章不一样，会议讲稿一般都开门见山，很少有到了结尾才点出主题的，因为时间有限。

一般各条信息之间都表现出一定的逻辑关系模式，如分门别类（division/classification），因果（cause-effect），对比对照（compare/contrast），按照时间、空间、步骤、重要性的顺序排列（sequencing）或列举（simple listing），提出问题－解决问题（problem-solution）等。

分门别类（**Division and classification**）

有时，我们将一个概念细分成若干小的构成部分，以表示其区分，例如：一间房有墙、天花板、地面、门、窗户。有时，我们将同样的事情放在同一概念下表达其相同之处，例如大学里有生命科学院、医学院、化学工程学院、环境科学院、水利电力学院、纺织工学院、文学院等各种学院。但是如果说“最近十年我们学校招了很多外国学生，有印度学生、尼泊尔学生、美国学生、非洲学生、韩国学生”，这句话的逻辑就有问题。这里本是以国家来区分学生的，但是非洲的概念比国家的概念大，因此这句话逻辑上有瑕疵。

原因结果（Cause and effect）

原因结果关系在演讲中用得最多，也体现在“提出问题－解决问题”（problem-solution）式的讲稿中。通常这类关系解释事物的原因或事情的结果，表达见解看法。一页半纸以内、十分钟以内的篇幅短的讲话则可能少有同时既讲原因又分析后果的，而长篇的演讲才有可能两者都讲，比如《空气污染的原因与后果》。

这一关系体现在段落与句子中，便是表达因果关系的关联词。这些关联词显性地或隐性地表达因果关系。进一步从因或果的层面上区分，这些关联词可划分为：表原因的关联词，如because, since, on account of, as, for；表结果的关联词，如therefore, so that, hence, thus, thereby, consequently, accordingly, as a result；原因导致结果的关联词，如cause, trigger, make, generate, lead to, spur, contribute, bring about, give rise to, result in, render, stimulate, produce, be responsible for；结果来自某原因的关联词，如result from, derive from, originate from, initiate from, stem from, be attributable to；结果反映某原因的关联词，如show, demonstrate, reflect, present, suggest, imply；条件导致结果的关联词，如when, once, as soon as, given, as long as, rely on, depend on, resort to, considering, in view of, according to, thanks to。

对比对照（Comparison and contrast）

从表意来看，对比对照的目的是将两者进行比较，以找出高低；或区分相同与不同，形成正反关系、差异关系、升降关系、比较关系等；或用熟悉的概念来类比不熟悉的概念以便理解后者。依次例如，《公共服务中的公心与私心》《正史与野史的区别》《也谈旧瓶装新酒》《家庭作业的多与少》《完成工作的两种方式：个人与团体》《机遇像条河》。

在段落与句子的层面上，同样有提示比较关系的词，如like, likewise, in like manner, similarly, similarly + adj., not only... but also..., in the same way, in the same sense, as well as, in comparison with, in common with, when compared with, compared to/with, both... and..., rather than等；提示对照或转折关系的词，如however, but, yet, although, though, rather, whereas, unlike, instead, nevertheless, while, otherwise, conversely, notwithstanding, on the other hand, be the other way around, neither... nor..., in contrast, contrary to, different from, as opposed to等。

顺序排列（Sequencing）

顺序排列即按时间、空间、步骤或者重要性的顺序列举。表示顺序的词汇有

first，second，furthermore，before，preceding，during，when，finally等。顺序排列的方式在当今的各种讲稿中广泛使用。从其语言特征来看，以顺序排列方式组织的讲稿一般结构紧密，传达非常具体的信息，观点明白无误，所有相关信息都陈述清楚。在这点上，中、英文文章类同，尤其是技术层面的中文讲稿与英文讲稿有很大的相似性。很多中文讲稿在一段开场白后，直接进入一、二、三等若干要点。

三、词汇准备

Text 1

aerophobia 怕风
cardio-respiratory arrest 心跳呼吸衰竭
hydrophobia 恐水
hyperactivity 多动
immunoglobulin 免疫球蛋白
incubation period 潜伏期
inflammation 发炎
multi-site intradermal regimen 多点皮内注射法
post-exposure preventive regimen 暴露后预防治疗
rabies 狂犬病
tissue culture 细胞组织培养
spinal cord 脊髓
zoonotic disease 人畜共患疾病

Text 2

aromatase inhibitor 芳香化酶抑制剂
breast cancer 乳腺癌
European Association for Cancer Research (EACR) 欧洲癌症研究协会
follow-up 跟进治疗
inflammatory breast cancer 炎性乳腺癌
leverage 为达目的所运用之力量
paradigm 范例
remission 疾病的缓解期

taxanes 它莫西芬
translational research 转化性研究
triple-negative cancer 三阴性乳腺癌

Text 3

anti-retroviral therapy 抗病毒治疗
bilateral organization 双边组织
multi-drug resistant TB 多发抗药性结核
scourge 导致痛苦的祸端
TB and HIV co-infection 结核病和艾滋病重合感染
tuberculosis 肺结核

Text 4

cardiovascular disease 心血管疾病
cholesterol 胆固醇
cardiac bypass surgery 心脏搭桥手术
dialysis 透析
diabetes 糖尿病
intake 摄入
kidney failure 肾衰
prevalence （疾病）流行
stroke 中风

Text 5

艾滋病感染者和病人 people living with HIV/AIDS (PLHIV)
艾滋病相关死亡 HIV/AIDS related death
艾滋病致孤儿童 children orphaned by AIDS
葛兰素史克公司 GSK
男男性行为者 men who have sex with men
全球艾滋病、结核和疟疾基金 The Global Fund to Fight AIDS, Tuberculosis and Malaria
四免一关怀 Four Exemptions and One Care
血液管理 blood management

Text 6

H7N9禽流感 H7N9 avian flu
病原体 pathogen
毒株 virus strain
疾病变异 variant
（疾病）散发的 sporadic
冠状病毒 corona virus
裂解 split
流行病学调查 epidemiological investigation
密切接触者 close contact
器官衰竭 organ failure
佐剂 adjuvant

四、摘要练习

请听下面英语语篇，第一篇用源语言复述此段主要信息逻辑点及层次，第二篇用译入语复述此段主要信息逻辑点及层次。注意信息点之间的逻辑联系。

Text 1

WHO Expert Talks about Rabies

September 2011

Ladies and gentlemen,

Rabies is a fatal disease, and worldwide, more than 55,000 people die of rabies every year. The incubation period for rabies is typically 1 to 3 months, but may vary from less than 1 week to more than 1 year. The initial symptoms of rabies are fever and often pain or an unusual or unexplained tingling, pricking or burning sensation at the wound site. As the virus spreads through the central nervous system, progressive, fatal inflammation of the brain and spinal cord develops.

Two forms of the disease can follow. People with furious rabies exhibit signs of hyperactivity, excited behavior, hydrophobia and sometimes aerophobia. After a few days, death occurs by cardio-respiratory arrest. Paralytic rabies, which is less dramatic and usually runs a longer course, accounts for about 30% of the total number of human cases. The muscles gradually become paralyzed, starting at the site of the bite or scratch. A coma slowly develops, and eventually death occurs. The paralytic form of rabies is often misdiagnosed, contributing to the underreporting of the disease.

Dogs are the main host and transmitter of rabies. They are the major source of infection in all of the estimated 55,000 human rabies deaths annually in Asia and Africa. Transmission can also occur when infectious material—usually saliva—comes into direct contact with human mucosa or fresh skin wounds. Human-to-human transmission by bite is theoretically possible but has never been confirmed.

Post-exposure prevention can effectively prevent infections and deaths. It consists of local treatment of the wound, administration of rabies immunoglobulin (if indicated), and immediate vaccination. Recommended first-aid procedures include immediate and thorough flushing and washing of the wound for a minimum of 15 minutes with soap and water, detergent, povidone iodine or other substances that kill the rabies virus.

Dog rabies potentially threatens over 3.3 billion people in Asia and Africa. People most at risk live in rural areas where human vaccines and immunoglobulin are not readily available or accessible. And children aged under 15 are the group at particular risk.

Rabies is a vaccine-preventable disease. The most cost-effective strategy for preventing rabies in people is by eliminating rabies in dogs through vaccination. Preventing human rabies through control of domestic dog rabies is a realistic goal for large parts of Africa and Asia, and is justified financially by the future savings of discontinuing post-exposure prophylaxis for people.

Safe, effective vaccines also exist for human use. Pre-exposure immunization in people is recommended for travelers to high-risk areas in rabies-affected countries, and for people in certain high-risk occupations such as laboratory workers dealing with live rabies virus, and veterinarians and animal handlers in rabies-affected areas. As children are at particular risk, their immunization could be considered if living in or visiting high risk areas.

WHO promotes wider access to appropriate post-exposure treatment using modern tissue culture or avian embryo-derived rabies vaccines through: use of the multi-site intradermal regimen to reduce the cost of post-exposure treatments; increased production of safe and efficacious rabies biologicals, which are in critical short supply globally, particularly rabies immunoglobulin; continuing education of health and veterinary professionals in rabies prevention and control; and immunization of 70% of the dog population to stop circulation of the virus at source.

复述要点提示（主要信息逻辑点及层次）

Purpose of the speech:

To draw people's attention to rabies, a fatal disease, and give people a brief introduction of the causes of rabies, its harms, its prevention, and its immediate treatment so that people can know how to prevent and control this lethal disease.

Keynotes of the speech:

1. Simple facts about rabies: Rabies is a common disease which happens in many parts of the world, and every year it kills over 55, 000 people. And dogs are the main source of this disease.

2. Symptoms: People infected with rabies usually have an incubation period ranging from several days to over one year. People with rabies often show some of the following symptoms: fever, tingling, pricking or burning sensation. There are usually two kinds of rabies: the furious rabies and the paralytic rabies. The previous one develops more rapidly than the latter one.

3. Transmission: Dogs are the major source of transmission. There are also other ways of transmission, though much less frequent. For instance, the direct contact between the patient's saliva and other people's wound will possibly cause rabies.

4. Treatment: First-aid treatment of the wounded area is highly recommended. In-time vaccination effectively prevents the disease. So it is vitally important for the person being bitten or scratched to receive timely treatment.

5. People with higher risks: Usually people living in remote areas or poverty tend to have much higher chances of infecting rabies because they lack easy access to in-time vaccination. In addition, for people traveling to rural areas or remote areas, they are also faced with the danger of rabies. But generally speaking, children under 15 years old, especially boys, are the group that is most susceptible to the danger of rabies.

6. Prevention is the best method: The most cost-effective way of preventing rabies is to give dogs vaccination so as to prevent the spreading of rabies. Besides vaccination on dogs, vaccination should be available to people who need it. For travelers to high-risk areas or people living in high-risk areas, they should be given vaccination before hand.

What did WHO do?

WHO supports experiments to reduce the cost of post-exposure treatments; increases production of safe and effective medicines for rabies; continues to educate health professionals to deal with rabies control and prevention; has given immunization to over 70% dog population so as to effectively prevent the spreading of rabies virus.

Text 2

Nancy Brinker's Speech on the 22nd Biennial Congress of the EACR

Nancy Brinker, Founder as well as Ambassador of Susan G. Komen for the Cure Foundation

Barcelona, Spain

July 2012

Thank you, Professor Celis, for that introduction and for inviting me here for this historic Congress.

I'm always excited to be in Spain, though it's also bittersweet. My sister Suzy and I had a wonderful time touring here many years ago, and we agreed at that time that we would come back again. But ten years later, Suzy was diagnosed with breast cancer. And a few years after that, she died. Before her death, Suzy made me promise to do everything in my power to ensure that other women didn't have to suffer and die from this disease. That promise became the foundation of Susan G. Komen for the Cure.

In the thirty years since Suzy died, we have made some remarkable progress.Thanks to groups like EACR and the research that has been done, we have a much better understanding of breast cancer.

For starters, we now know that breast cancer isn't a disease, but rather many diseases. Different groups of women are susceptible to different forms of the disease.

For that reason, Susan G. Komen for the has invested more than $52 million dollars over the past four years into research that could help us predict who will or will not respond to certain therapies. This includes our Promise Grants that go toward research that will hopefully:

- Tell us who will experience the most devastating side effects from taxanes; and
- Who will respond to tamoxifen over aromatase inhibitors (or vise versa); and
- Help us to develop a personalized breast cancer DNA vaccine.

These are exciting developments, but also just one piece of the puzzle. Our increased understanding of breast cancer must go hand in hand with better forms of screening and treatment. Last month, Susan G. Komen for the approved funding for a grant to develop a blood test that, when combined with mammography, could detect aggressive forms of breast cancer very early.

And since 2008, we have supported more than 120 clinical trials to look at the safety and efficacy of new treatments. These trials look to answer some of the most challenging questions in breast cancer, such as treatments for inflammatory breast cancer and triple-negative cancer.

But though we've made remarkable advancements, we must remain mindful that most of our work still lies in front of us. Today, over 60 percent of cancer deaths occur in the developing world, yet only 5 percent of world cancer resources are dedicated there. This lack of resources and lack of attention is going to cost millions of people their lives. It shouldn't be this way.

At Susan G. Komen for the Cure, we believe that focus should be on the continuum of care. The continuum of care is the chain of events that begin with education and screening, and carry a patient through diagnosis, treatment, follow-up and hopefully remission. Today, in too many instances, women are getting lost along this continuum for a variety of reasons—lack of awareness, lack of money, lack of child care/transportation or lack of access to quality care.

We must start by bridging the gap between basic research and clinical application. For researchers, that means thinking about how your work is applied down the continuum, how it can be delivered to patients. That's why Susan G. Komen for the Cure is focused on supporting translational research, bringing the gap from basic research to clinical application. And in the past five years, we have begun to see a true translational component to our work.

Conquering cancer will require more than a cure, it will require new global paradigms that leverage resources, and foster innovation, interactions and consensus. If we can find ways to work together, we will be stronger, better and faster. And we can finally reach our shared vision of a world without breast cancer.

复述要点提示（主要信息逻辑点及层次）

主要目的：警惕乳腺癌对女性的危害，号召全世界的人们团结合作，共同对抗这个顽疾。

演讲的主要内容：

1. 该基金的主要目的：帮助全世界更多女性远离乳腺癌的威胁。

2. 该基金的主要成绩：首先，乳腺癌绝不是一种单一疾病。不同的女性群体容易患上不同类型的乳腺癌。这个发现让我们能够集中资金来研究适于不同人群的抗癌药物，如哪些人群不适合使用紫杉类药物，它莫西芬和芳香化酶抑制剂这两种药物分别对哪类人群效果更好等。我们还着手于开发针对性更强的抗乳腺癌DNA疫苗。近期苏珊·可门基金又批准基金投入开发一项血液检查，希望和乳腺X光造影检查术配合，在早期诊断出侵袭性乳腺癌。

3. 面临的问题：癌症仍然是世界上对人类威胁最大的疾病，而发展中国家或者贫穷地区因为严重缺乏医疗资源，那里的女性面临更大的威胁。苏珊·可门基金相信抗癌的重点应该在于关怀的持续。首先应该是教育、筛查，然后是对病人进行具体诊断、治疗、跟进，直到疾病得到控制。而因为贫穷，许多地方的女性无法得到必要的知识和医疗帮助。

4. 专注支持转化性研究的原因：希望填补基础研究和临床运用方面的空白，使更多的女性能够得到必要的医疗服务。同时，我们呼吁全球共同行动起来，平衡资源，推进创新，进行互动，达成共识。如果我们能够共同协作，就会变得更加强大，获得更快更好的解决方法，最终实现全球消灭乳腺癌的理想。

五、英译汉练习

Text 3

Talk on the World Tuberculosis Day

Dr. Luis Gomes Sambo, WHO Regional Director
24 March 2013

Dear everyone,

Today, 24th of March 2013, is World Tuberculosis Day. It is a day when the whole world is reminded about the suffering that Tuberculosis (TB) continues to exert on people although effective control measures are available. This year's slogan for World TB Day is "Stop TB in my lifetime."

TB remains a major public health problem in the African region, which accounted for over 26% of notified TB cases globally in 2011. It is estimated that TB killed over half a million people in the African Region and only 62% of existing TB cases were detected in that year. The situation is further worsened by the threat of drug-resistant TB and multi-drug resistant TB which continue to be serious problems complicating TB treatment.

It should be noted that the TB epidemic in Africa is largely driven by factors related to poverty and the negative effects of TB and HIV co-infection. People living with HIV are more likely than others to become sick with TB. According to the Global Tuberculosis Report of 2012, 46% of those who had TB in 2011 were HIV positive and sadly, only 46% of them received the WHO recommended anti-retroviral treatment.

On a positive note, over the last five years, African countries have been increasingly using new rapid TB detection methods which significantly reduce diagnostic delays and increase the detection of TB cases. As a result, the rising trend of TB cases has been halted as treatment success rate improves. Equally the death rate as well as the number of people who fail to complete their TB treatment continues to decline.

In spite of these achievements, there is no place for complacency and I would therefore like to stress the importance of early diagnosis as the most effective way of preventing the spread of TB. Anyone with persistent cough for more than two weeks is advised to seek medical attention.

Stopping TB in our lifetime will require governments and development partners to increase and sustain political and financial commitments for TB control. This is vital to ensure that everyone has access to TB prevention and treatment services in all countries of the region. Strong strategic partnerships between governments, communities, bilateral and multilateral organizations, and the private sector are essential to control the scourge of TB.

Together, let us join forces to stop TB in our lifetime.

Thank you!

Text 4

World Health Day Message on Blood Pressure

Dr. Margaret Chan, Director-General of the WHO

Geneva, Switzerland

3 April 2013

Distinguished guests, staff, ladies and gentlemen,

Let me extend a warm welcome to this World Health Day event, where we are drawing attention to the problem of hypertension, or high blood pressure.

The problem is huge. WHO estimates that more than one in three adults worldwide has high blood pressure. In some parts of Africa, nearly half of all adults have high blood pressure.

High blood pressure is one of the most important contributors to premature death from cardiovascular disease worldwide. It contributes to nearly 9.4 million deaths due to heart disease and stroke every year. Together, heart disease and stroke are the number one cause of death worldwide.

High blood pressure also increases the risk of kidney failure, blindness, and several other conditions. It often occurs together with other risk factors, like obesity, diabetes, and high cholesterol, increasing the health risk even further.

For all these reasons, high blood pressure contributes substantially to the escalating costs of health care.

In wealthy countries, strong public health policies, preventive programmes, and widely available diagnosis and treatment have led to a reduction in the prevalence of high blood pressure. Unfortunately, in many developing countries, the disease burden caused by high blood pressure has increased over the past decade.

Our aim today is to make people aware of the need to know their blood pressure, to take high blood pressure seriously, and then to take control. In doing so, they will need support from responsive health services.

High blood pressure must be taken seriously. It is a strong and reliable warning signal that health is at risk and that something needs to be done.

But high blood pressure is also a silent warning signal, usually showing no symptoms for years or even decades, even when values are dangerously high.

That vital early warning signal will go unheard, and unheeded, unless people have a chance to take a simple, inexpensive, and rapid blood pressure test. When symptoms of high blood pressure do appear, cardiovascular disease is usually advanced and the risk of sudden acute events, like a heart attack or a stroke, is greatly increased.

Getting the warning signal early on is by far the better option. The actions that can be taken early on are far less costly, and less risky for patients, than interventions, like cardiac bypass surgery and dialysis, that may be needed when hypertension is missed and goes untreated.

High blood pressure is preventable, and it is treatable. For both, knowing blood pressure levels is the first critical step.

For prevention, reduce salt intake. Keep fit, trim, and active. Know your ideal body weight, and aim for it. Eat more fruits and vegetables and less highly processed foods, especially junk foods.

Go easy on the sugary beverages. Do not use tobacco, and stay away from tobacco smoke. Drink alcohol only in moderation, or not at all.

For many people, these lifestyle changes are sufficient to control blood pressure. For others, medication is required. Hypertension can be treated with safe and inexpensive medicines. Doing so greatly reduces the risk of heart disease, stroke, and kidney failure.

My advice to the public is this: be safe, know your blood pressure, act smart, shape up your lifestyle, follow recommendations for medication and safe-care meticulously.

Your health is in your hands. Don't let an invisible, silent killer steal years of your life away.

Thank you.

六、汉译英练习

Text 5

全面预防、积极治疗、消除歧视
——卫生部部长陈竺谈我国艾滋病防治工作

2011年11月30日

根据卫生部和联合国艾滋病规划署、世界卫生组织联合评估结果，截至2011年底，估计我国现存活艾滋病感染者和病人约78万人，其中病人约15.4万人；2011年新发感染者约4.8万人，因艾滋病相关死亡约2.8万人。

我国艾滋病疫情总体形势向好。从全球来看，我国的感染者和病人数约占全球的2%，仍属于低流行国家。党中央、国务院历来高度重视和关心艾滋病防治工作。近年来，中共中央总书记胡锦涛多次到医院、疾病预防控制中心、社区考察艾滋病防治工作，看望艾滋病患者，慰问医务人员和志愿者。国务院总理温家宝坚持每年深入基层和疫情严重地区考察艾滋病防治工作，与艾滋病患者座谈，同艾滋病致孤儿童和老人共度除夕夜，邀请艾滋病致孤儿童和患儿，以及医生和教师到中南海做客座谈。李克强副总理先后3次召开国务院防治艾滋病工作委员会全体会议，并视察中国疾病预防控制中心性病艾滋病预防控制中心。党和国家领导人的实际行动，充分体现了党中央、国务院对人民健康的关心和坚决遏制艾滋病在我国流行的决心。

中央财政加大了防治经费投入，近年来，中央财政艾滋病防治专项经费投入进一步加大，2007年为9.4亿元，2008年10.7亿元，2009年12.2亿元，2010年增加到20.7亿元，2011年增加到22亿元，地方财政也在逐步增加财政支持力度。

我国艾滋病防控任务艰巨而复杂，面临着一系列新问题和挑战。

一是“四免一关怀”等政策落实不平衡，防治措施覆盖面还需提高；二是艾滋病病毒感染者进入发病和死亡高峰，耐药人群增多；三是抗机会性感染的费用较高，病人因无力负担而不去就诊，影响抗病毒治疗的覆盖面和效果；四是国际合作项目进一步减少，需加大投入，弥补经费缺口；五是社区组织参与不够；六是社会歧视比较严重，消除社会歧视困难较大；七是防治工作风险高、任务重、压力大、待遇低，队伍不稳定。

“十二五”期间，我国艾滋病防治工作目标是减少艾滋病新发感染、降低艾滋病病死率、减少社会歧视、提高感染者和病人生存质量，到2015年将艾滋病感染者和病人数控制在120万人左右。

下一步，我们要在总结和推广防治经验的基础上，从实际出发，继续推进深化医药卫生体制改革，完善防治工作机制，健全防控网络，在深入落实“四免一关怀”政策的基础上，全面落实扩大宣传教育、监测检查、母婴传播阻断、综合干预和抗病毒治疗的覆盖面，加强血液管理、医疗保障、关怀救助、权益保护、组织领导和防治队伍建设的“五扩大、六加强”的防治措施。

疾病无国界，艾滋病防治备受当今世界关注。卫生部与世界卫生组织、联合国艾滋病规划署等国际组织及全球艾滋病、结核和疟疾基金保持密切的合作关系，与英国、美国、澳大利亚等国开展了良好的双边合作，许多国际非政府组织和企业，如克林顿基金会、盖茨基金会、葛兰素史克公司等也参与到我国艾滋病防治工作中来。

我国积极承担国际义务，已向全球艾滋病、结核和疟疾基金捐款2 000万美元；为非洲国家的艾滋病防治人员开展培训，积极与周边国家合作开展区域艾滋病防治项目；出席国际和区域艾滋病会议，与其他国家交流、分享防治经验。

Text 6

梁万年就H7N9禽流感答凤凰卫视记者问

2013年4月8日

凤凰卫视记者：能否给一个H7N9疫苗生产的准确时间？另外，过渡期间我们的解决方案是什么？

梁万年：从病原体到生产出疫苗的时间周期来说最短是6到8个月，现在我们正在启动疫苗的制备工作，它的过程非常复杂，首先要筛选疫苗的毒株，哪一类毒株适合做疫苗，有些毒株可能毒性相当大，要经过处理程序。筛出来以后才能决定这种疫苗的形式，全病毒的好还是裂解好，是不是要添加佐剂，然后决定什么样的工艺和流程，现在我们启动的疫苗研究是基础性的研究。

以后，假如说这个疾病变异，导致人之间的传播，尤其是大人群传播，那疫苗就要生产，现在我们正在做准备。现在还没有明确证据证明有人际传播，如果是一种散发的，主要来源于动物的，那么病人的发生数只是点状的，这时候没有必要注射疫苗，从成本效率、防疫效果来说也不需要对散发的病例都施行注射疫苗来防控。

疫苗当然是有效手段，但不是唯一手段，我们一系列的措施同样可以有效防控。现阶段从联防联控机制到卫生计生委，我们主要采取几方面的工作：一是溯源。也就是大家关心的疫情发生的可能范围有多大，它的根本标志是看动物携带这种病原体的范围有多大，理论上说，只要动物尤其是和人类接触的动物带有这种病原体，就有潜在发生人类疾病的可能。

溯源的第二个方面，就是要尽快判定有没有人传染，如果有的话，人传染的能力有多强。现在我们正在做大量的流行病学调查，包括病例之间的关联、病人的密切接触者是否有相应的感染，到现在为止还没有发现这方面的证据。

二是加强病例救治。目前看，这种疾病主要是呼吸道感染、发热、呼吸道症状、呼吸道肺炎，重症患者会出现多器官功能衰竭，临床上我们是强化密切接触者，对这一部分加强救治。这个疾病防范的最大难点和H5N1相比，H5N1是动物发病，人群就跟上去。而如果动物不发病或者发病状况较轻，我们要有效防范人感染的可能，这个难度就大了。

为了做到这一点，我们特别强化了监测，在全国有500多家医院、400多家实验室都开展了这项工作，同时从2004年开始就要求全国各地医疗机构必须报告不明原因肺炎，一旦发现了肺炎，体温超过38度，现有的已知病原体不能解释这种症状，排除SARS、排除H5N1、排除新型冠状病毒，符合肺炎判断标准，就必须报告。现在每天监测各地的报告数字，一旦发现，当地卫生部门必须进行排查。从2004年以来这个工作一直在做，现在我们在进一步强化这项工作。

另外要关注老百姓的需求，加强健康教育，及时、准确、全面地公布疫情防控的各方面工作。这些方面是当前的重点，我们有信心能够控制疫情。

资料来源：

Text 1 http://www.who.int/mediacentre/factsheets/fs099/en/print.html

Text 2 http://www.aacr.org/home/public-media/multimedia-/supplemental-material-and-photos/ambassador-nancy-brinkers-eacr-biennial-congress-speech.aspx

Text 3 http://www.afro.who.int/en/rdo/speeches/3799-message-of-the-regional-director-on-the-occasion-of-world-tuberculosis-day-2013.html

Text 4 http://www.who.int/dg/speeches/2013/world_health_day_20130403/en/#

Text 5 http://money.163.com/11/1130/20/7K4S715400253B0H.html

Text 6 http://firefox.huanqiu.com/china/politics/2013-04/3806757_2.html

参考答案

四、摘要练习

Text 1

世界卫生组织专家谈狂犬病

2011年9月

女士们、先生们：

狂犬病是一种致命性疾病，全世界每年有超过5.5万人死于狂犬病。狂犬病潜伏期通常为1到3个月，短则不到一周，长则一年以上。狂犬病最初症状是发热，伤口部位常有疼痛，或有异常或原因不明的颤痛、刺痛或灼痛感（感觉异常）。随着病毒在中枢神经系统的扩散，发展为致死的进行性脑脊髓炎。

然后可能出现以下两种情况。狂躁性狂犬病患者的症状是机能亢进、躁动、恐水，有时还怕风。数日后患者因心跳和呼吸衰竭而死亡。早瘫性狂犬病约占人类死亡病例总数的30%。与狂躁性狂犬病相比，其病程不那么剧烈，且通常较长。从咬伤或抓伤部位开始，肌肉逐渐麻痹。然后患者渐渐陷入昏迷，最后死亡。早瘫性狂犬病往往遭误诊，造成狂犬病低报现象。

犬类是狂犬病的主要宿主和传播者，是造成亚洲和非洲每年大约5.5万例人类狂犬病所有死亡病例的感染源。该病也可通过感染性物质（通常为唾液）直接接触人体黏膜或新近皮肤破损处传染。因咬伤而出现人传人的情况虽有理论上的可能性，但从未得到证实。

暴露后预防可以有效地防止出现症状和死亡。暴露后预防措施是，对伤口进行局部处理，按医嘱注射抗狂犬病免疫球蛋白，并立即接种疫苗。建议采用的急救程序包括立即用肥皂和水、洗涤剂、聚维酮碘消毒剂或可杀死狂犬病毒的其他溶液彻底冲洗和清洗伤口15分钟以上。

狂犬病威胁着亚洲和非洲超过33亿人口。那些在可能不太容易立即获得适当医疗服务的农村地区从事密集户外活动的旅行者，不论停留多久，也应被视为高风险者。在狂犬病疫区生活或停留的15岁以下儿童面临的风险尤其高。

可以通过接种疫苗预防狂犬病。为犬类接种疫苗以消除犬类狂犬病是预防人类狂犬病的最具成本效益的战略。在亚洲和非洲大多数地方通过控制人工驯养的犬只预防狂犬病是完全可行的。而且因为能够节省暴露后预防的花费，在经济上也是合理的。

同时已有供人类接种的安全、有效疫苗。建议对在狂犬病发生国高风险地区旅行的人以及从事某些高风险职业者（例如处理狂犬病活病毒以及其他狂犬病毒的实验室工作人员和狂犬病疫区的兽医和处理动物者）进行接触前免疫接种。由于儿童面临特别大的风险，可以考虑为在高风险地区生活或停留的儿童接种疫苗。

世卫组织促进采用先进的组织培养法或源自鸡胚的狂犬病毒，更广泛地提供适当的接触后治疗。世卫组织促进采取以下措施：采用多点皮内注射法，以降低接触后的治疗费用；扩大全球紧缺的安全有效的狂犬病生物制品（尤其是抗狂犬病免疫球蛋白）的生产；继续向卫生专业人员和兽医提供狂犬病预防和控制培训；以及为70%的犬类接种疫苗，从源头堵住狂犬病毒的传播。

Text 2

苏珊·可门基金创始人及大使南茜·布林克尔在欧洲癌症研究协会第22届双年会上的讲演

西班牙巴塞罗那

2012年7月

西里斯教授，谢谢您邀请我参加这次历史性的会议。

我一直期待着来到西班牙，虽然西班牙对我不仅意味着快乐，也意味着痛苦。多年以前，我和姐姐苏西一起在西班牙度过了快乐的假期，我们还约定以后再回来。可10年后，苏西被诊断患上了乳腺癌，几年后就去世了。她去世前要我答应她，尽我所能让其他女性不再遭受这种疾病的侵袭。苏珊·可门基金就是我对她的承诺。

苏西去世后的30年里我们在抗击乳腺癌方面取得了不小的成就。感谢欧洲癌症研究协会这样一些组织的努力以及医学上的研究成果，让我们对乳腺癌有了更深入的了解。

首先，我们现在知道乳腺癌不是一种单一病种，而表现为多样性。我们知道不同的女性群体容易患上不同类型的乳腺癌。

出于上述原因，苏珊·可门基金在过去的四年内投入了超过5 200万美元用于研究相对应的治疗方法。这包括：

- 研究紫杉类药物对哪类人群副作用最大；
- 它莫西芬和芳香化酶抑制剂这两种药物分别适用哪类人群；
- 以及开发更针对个体的抗乳腺癌DNA疫苗。

这些研究成果都让人兴奋，但是它们仅仅是等待我们破解的问题中的一小部分。随着我们对乳腺癌了解的不断增加，我们也必须在检查和治疗方面投入更多。上个月，苏珊·可门基金又批准投入经费研发一项血液检测方法，这种检测和乳腺X光造影检查术结合在一起，可以在早期诊断出侵袭性乳腺癌。

从2008年开始，我们资助了超过120次临床试验，检验新的治疗方式的有效性和安全性。这些试验有望解决乳腺癌研究中最具有挑战性的一些问题，如对炎性乳腺癌和三阴性乳腺癌的治疗。

虽然我们取得了巨大进展，但是我们必须记住，我们面临着更多的问题。当今，超过60%的癌症死亡案例发生在发展中国家，而世界上只有5%的抗癌资源用于这些国家。这种资源和关注的缺乏会剥夺上百万的生命。事情不应该是这个样子。

苏珊·可门基金相信，抗癌的重点应该在于关怀的持续。首先应该进行疾病筛查和健康教育，然后对病人进行具体诊断、治疗、跟进，直到疾病得到控制。当前女性因为不同的原因（意识的缺乏，缺钱，担心无人照顾子女，或者没有合格的医疗条件等）没能获得这种持续关怀。

我们必须着手弥补基础研究和临床实践之间的差距。对于研究者来说，这意味着要考虑如何将自己的研究运用到整个对癌症病人的关爱过程中，怎样直接用到病人身上。这就是苏珊·可门基金专注于支持转化性研究的原因。我们希望填补基础研究和临床运用方面的空白。在过去的五年里，我们开始看到我们的工作取得了一定的成果。

征服癌症需要的不仅是一剂药方。它需要新的全球性的策略，平衡资源，推进创新，进行互动，达成共识。如果我们能够一起协作，我们会变得更加强大，找到更快更好的解决方法，我们才能最终实现全球无乳腺癌的理想。

五、英译汉练习

Text 3

世界卫生组织非洲地区负责人路易斯·戈麦斯·桑博博士在世界肺结核日的讲话

2013年3月24日

大家好!

今天，2013年3月24日，是世界肺结核日。它提醒我们，尽管有了有效的控制手段，但是肺结核仍然在影响着全世界的人们。今年肺结核日的口号是“遏制结核，奋斗终生”。

肺结核病仍然是非洲的主要公共卫生疾病。2011年非洲的肺结核发病率占全世界的26%。据估计，仅2011年，在非洲就有超过50万人死于肺结核，而已经发现的结核病例只占现存病例的62%。此外，抗药性肺结核和多发抗药性结核病的威胁使结核病防治的形势更加复杂。

值得注意的是，非洲普遍的贫困以及结核病和艾滋病重合感染是导致结核病疫情的主要原因。艾滋病感染者比常人更容易感染结核病。据2012年全球肺结核报告，2011年46%的肺结核患者也同时表现为艾滋病阳性。不幸的是，其中只有46%的病人接受了世界卫生组织建议的抗反转录病毒治疗。

好的一方面是，在过去的五年里，非洲国家越来越多地使用新型的快速结核检测方法，极大降低了诊断延迟，提高了结核发现率。随着成功治愈率的增加，结核发病率的上升趋势也得到了遏制。同样的，因为没能完成结核治疗而死亡的人数也持续减少。

然而尽管有这些成就，我们却不能自满。在这里我想强调结核早期诊断在有效防止结核病扩展态势方面的重要作用。凡是持续咳嗽两周以上的人都应该及时就医。

“遏制结核，奋斗终生”需要政府和开发伙伴们对结核控制持续的政治和资金投入。这种投入对于确保该地区所有国家人民获得结核防治是至关重要的。政府、社团、双边和多边组织和私有行业强大的战略合作伙伴关系在控制结核疫情方面缺一不可。

让我们一起“遏制结核，奋斗终生”!

谢谢!

Text 4

世界卫生组织总干事陈冯富珍博士在世界健康日谈高血压防治问题

瑞士日内瓦

2013年4月3日

尊敬的各位来宾，同事们，女士们、先生们：

首先让我对此次世界卫生日的活动致以热烈的欢迎。今天我们关注的是高血压问题。

高血压是个大问题。世界卫生组织预计全世界超过1/3的成年人面临高血压问题。非洲的一些地方，几乎每两人中就有一人患有高血压。

高血压是全球心血管病致死的主要原因。每年近940万人死于因高血压导致的心脏病和中风。心脏病和中风也是全球致死的最主要原因。

高血压也增加了肾衰、失明和其他一些病变的风险。它常常与其他一些危险因素，如肥胖、糖尿病和高胆固醇一起，加大了人们的健康风险。

基于以上这些原因，高血压大大增加了医疗保健的花费。

在富裕国家，其强有力的公共卫生政策、有效的预防措施，以及广泛又方便的诊断和治疗途径在一定程度上遏制了高血压的广泛传播。可是在众多发展中国家，由高血压所导致的负担在过去十年里呈上升趋势。

我们今天的目标是帮助人们意识到血压问题，重视并且控制高血压。而这些都需要反应性卫生系统的支持。

高血压必须要得到重视。高血压是健康处于危险状态的强烈而可信的预警信号。

但是高血压同时也是一个沉默的预警信号。通常几年甚至数十年都没有任何症状，哪怕血压指数已经处于危险状态。

除非人们有机会接受一次简单、低价、快速的血压监测，否则这种早期的重要预警信号就不会为人所知，也不会被人警惕。与后期的治疗（如因为忽视和没有及时治疗导致后期需要接受心脏搭桥手术和透析等）相比，早期的措施其费用和风险都要低得多。

高血压是可预防且可治疗的疾病。其预防和治疗最重要的第一步是要了解自己的血压。

要预防高血压，请减少食盐摄入量。保持健康、苗条和积极的生活状态。了解自己理想的体重并为之努力。多吃水果和蔬菜，少吃深加工食品，特别是垃圾食品。少吃含糖量高的饮料。不要抽烟，避免吸入二手烟。适量或者完全不饮酒。

对于许多人而言，改变生活方式足以控制血压。而对于另外一些人而言，则需要药物治疗。高血压可以通过安全和便宜的药物来治疗。这样可极大地减少心脏病、中风和肾衰的危险。

我对公众的建议就是这些。为了生命安全，了解自己的血压。理智行为，构建良好的生活方式。严格遵守医师的用药建议。

你的健康自己掌握，别让这个无形的沉默的杀手夺去你的岁月。

谢谢。

六、汉译英练习

Text 5

Comprehensive Prevention, Active Treatment and Eradication of Discrimination

Chen Zhu, Minister of Health Talks about China's AIDS Prevention and Treatment

30 November 2011

According to the united survey by China Ministry of Health, UNAIDS, and WHO, by the end of 2011, there are about 780,000 people living with HIV and AIDS (PLHIV) in China, among which the number of AIDS patients is about 154,000. In 2011 alone, there are about 48,000 new infections and about 28,000 HIV/AIDS related deaths.

The HIV/AIDS epidemic situation in China keeps improving. Globally, the number of Chinese PLHIV is about 2% of the total world infection cases, which means that the overall HIV prevalence in China remains low. Chinese government and leaders have always attached great importance to HIV/AIDS prevention and treatment. In recent years, General Secretary of the CPC Central Committee Hu Jingtao inspected many times hospitals, CDCs and communities to investigate HIV/AIDS prevention and treatment. Every year, Premier Wen Jiabao investigated HIV/AIDS prevention and treatment work at the epidemic areas in person, held talks with PLHIV, and spent the Lunar New Year's Eve with HIV/AIDS orphans and elders. He also invited the HIV/AIDS orphans, medical professionals, and teachers to visit Zhong Nanhai. Vice Premier Li Keqiang conducted three State Council AIDS Working Committee meetings and also visited the China CDC AIDS Center. The leaders' actions fully demonstrated Chinese government's determination to control HIV/AIDS prevalence in China.

The central financial input in HIV/AIDS prevention and treatment keeps increasing. It was 0.94 billion in 2007, 1.07 billion in 2008, 1.22 billion in 2009, 2.07 billion in 2010, and 2.2 billion in 2011. Meanwhile, local governments are also gradually increasing the input.

However, the HIV/AIDS prevention and treatment in our country is still an arduous task facing a series of challenges. Firstly, the implementation of "Four Exemptions and One Care" is imbalanced, and prevention and treatment coverage should be extended. Secondly, China arrives at a critical moment when many PLHIV are dying and drug-resistant cases are increasing; thirdly, the high cost of anti-opportunistic infection treatment makes it difficult for patients to receive in-time treatment, which affects the coverage and effect of ARV treatment; fourthly, the number of international projects is further reducing, and the government needs to put in more money to meet the financial needs; fifthly, community participation is far from enough; sixthly, there is serious social discrimination against PLHIV; seventhly, the current HIV/AIDS prevention and treatment faces the problems of high risks, heavy burden, low salary and unstable health professional team.

During the 12th Five-Year period, the goal of China's HIV/AIDS prevention and treatment is to further reduce the new cases of HIV/AIDS infection, lower the casualty rate, reduce social discrimination, and enhance the living quality of PLHIV. By 2015, we will try to limit the number of people with HIV/AIDS to about 1.2 million.

Next, we will learn from our experiences and proceed from reality to promote the medical health reform, improve the system and strengthen the network of prevention and treatment. Based on the implementation of "Four Exemptions and One Care", we should extend our HIV/AIDS education, expand the coverage of HIV/AIDS screening, comprehensive intervention and ARV treatment, prevent mother-to-child transmission, reinforce the blood management, medical care, the protection of the rights of PLHIV as well as reinforce the construction of leadership and health team.

The HIV/AIDS epidemic is not limited to just one country. HIV/AIDS prevention and treatment is drawing the attention of current world. China Ministry of Health keeps close cooperation with WHO, UNAIDS, and the Global Fund to Fight AIDS,Tuberculosis and Malaria. We also have conducted bilateral cooperation with the UK, America, and Australia. Besides, many international NGOs and enterprises, such as Clinton Foundation, Gates Foundation, and GSK, have also been actively participating in China's HIV/AIDS prevention and treatment.

China has always been highly responsible for its international obligations. We donated $ 20 million to The Global Fund to Fight AIDS, Tuberculosis and Malaria, provided training for African HIV/AIDS health professionals, conducted HIV/AIDS prevention and control projects with neighboring countries, and attended international and regional HIV/AIDS meetings to share and exchange experiences in HIV/AIDS prevention and control.

Text 6

Liang Wannian's Response to Reporter from Hong Kong Phoenix TV Station on H7N9 Avian Flu

8 April 2013

Reporter from Hong Kong Phoenix TV Station: My question is: Is there a timetable about when the H7N9 vaccines will be available? Also during this period, what are the main measures for the prevention and control of this epidemic?

Liang Wannian: Usually it takes at least 6-8 months for a vaccine to be developed. Now we have already started the preparation for the vaccine. It is a complicated process. First we need to filter the virus strain and decide which strains can be the vaccine and which strains are more poisonous and need to be processed. Only after filtration can we decide on the form of the vaccine, should it be whole virus vaccine or split vaccine, and whether we need to add adjuvant into the vaccine. Then we will decide on the production process of the vaccine. Now what we have done on vaccine research is still basic.

In the future, if H7N9 flu develops into any variants which lead to human-to-human transmission, especially mass transmission, we will start the mass production of H7N9 vaccine. Now we are still preparing for it. And there is no specific evidence which proves that H7N9 can be transmitted from human to human. If the disease is sporadic and mainly comes from animals, then it is not necessary for people to receive vaccination. Also, considering the factors of cost efficiency and the effect of prevention, it is not necessary to prevent sporadic diseases with vaccines.

Vaccination is an effective method, but not the only method. We have a series of measures to control and prevent diseases effectively. Currently, from the joint prevention and control mechanism to the National Health and Family Planning Commission, there are several major works that we are implementing now. The first is to trace the source of H7N9 Avian Flu. It is to find out the possible scope of this epidemic and to find out the possible transmission scope of this animal-borne virus. Theoretically, as long as animals, especially animals that have direct contact with human beings, carry this virus, then there is potential danger for human beings to catch this disease.

The other reason to trace the source is to find out whether there is human-to-human transmission. If so, to determine how bad this transmission can be. Now we are doing extensive epidemiological investigation, including the connection between cases and the possible infection between patients and the patients' close contacts. But till now we haven't found any proof yet.

On the other hand, we need to strengthen the treatment of patients. Now the symptoms of this disease are mainly the respiratory infection, fever, respiratory symptoms, and respiratory pneumonia. In severe cases patients can develop into multiple organ failure. Clinically we emphasize the patients' close contacts and focus on the treatment of these close contacts. If we compare H7N9 with H5N1, the latter is highly infectious between animals and human beings. But H7N9 is more difficult to prevent and control because animals usually do not show any symptoms, which makes it more difficult to detect among people.

To ensure early detection, we especially emphasize surveillance. Over 500 hospitals and over 400 labs nationwide are doing this surveillance work. Meanwhile, ever since 2004, we have been requiring medical organizations nationwide to report unexplained pneumonia cases. After excluding the possibility of SARS, H5N1,or novel coronavirus infection, medical organizations are required to report any pneumonia case that has the body temperature over 38 degrees and cannot be explained by any known pathogen and fits the criteria of pneumonia. Now we are monitoring the surveillance number daily. Once any suspicious case is detected, local health department has to screen. We have been doing this work since 2004, and now we are further strengthening this work.

In addition, we need to pay close attention to people's need and concerns, to reinforce our work in health education, and guarantee the in-time, accurate and thorough publicity of H7N9 Flu. These are the focus of current work. We are confident that we can control this epidemic.

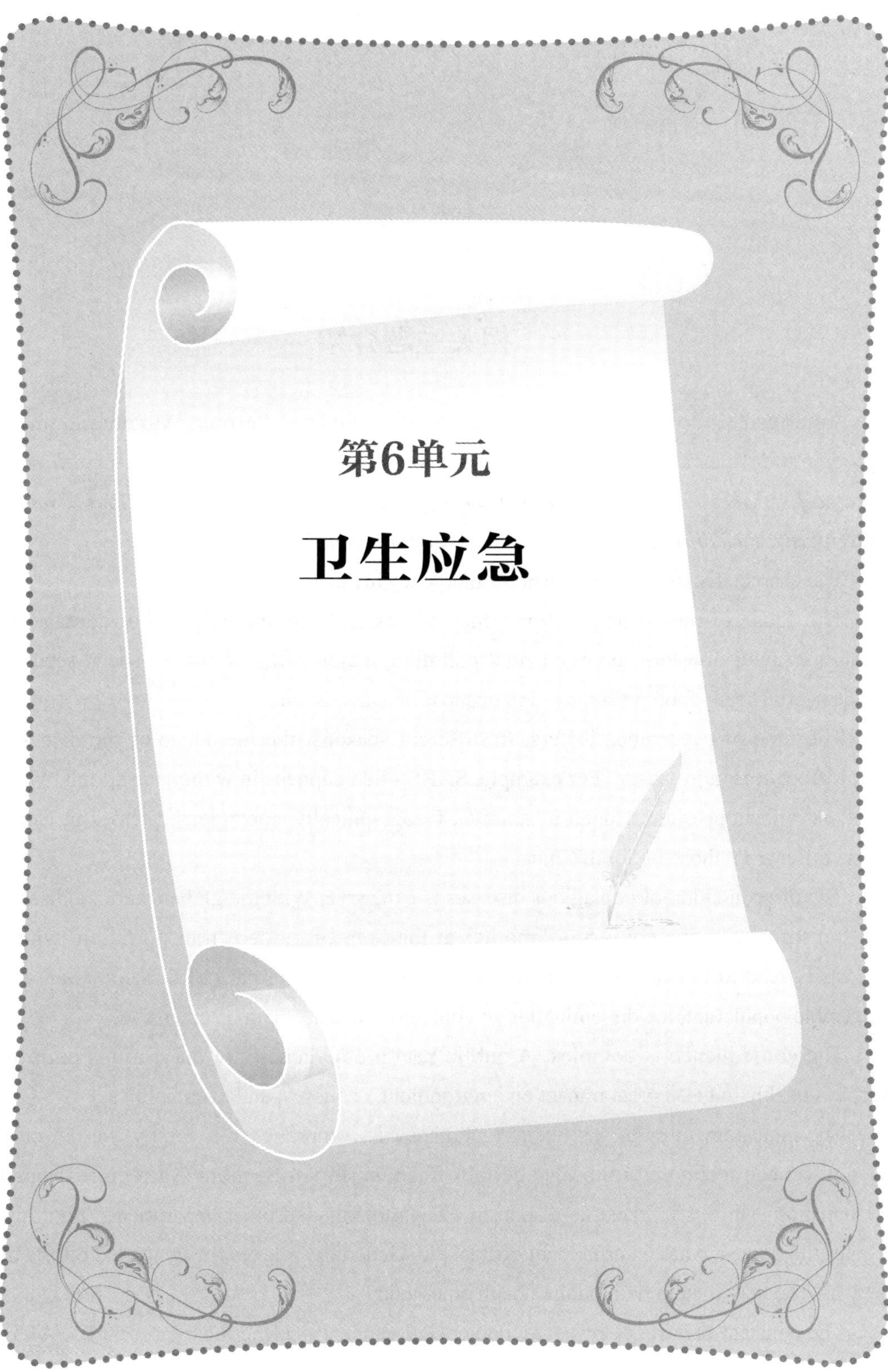

第6单元

卫生应急

一、相关主题介绍

American National Disaster Medical System Federal Partners Memorandum of Agreement defines a public health emergency as "*an emergency need for health care [medical] services to respond to a disaster, significant outbreak of an infectious disease, bioterrorist attack or other significant or catastrophic event*."

The characteristics of Public Health Emergency are as follows:

The cause of public health emergency varies, such as the eruption of contagious diseases, natural disasters, environmental pollution, major traffic accidents, social security accidents, drug risk, food poisoning, and occupation hazards, etc.

The time of occurrence differs. In different seasons, the incidence of the diseases differs from season to season. For example, SARS often happens in winter and spring, while intestinal infections often happen in summer. Geographically, contagious diseases in North China differ from those in South China.

The dissemination of contagious diseases is extensive. With the globalization, a disease can transmit from one country to another at the help of modern transportation, which can easily lead to global transmission. So with the source, the path of dissemination and vulnerable population, the dissemination of contagious diseases can be extensive.

The consequence is complex. A public health emergency not only brings harm to people's health, but also great impact on environment, economy, and even politics.

The management of public health emergency is comprehensive. Firstly, we not only need advanced technology but also certain financial input. Secondly, it requires social participation. Thirdly, it takes the responsible departments and other departments. Fourthly, it takes the domestic and international efforts, etc. Generally, it takes the concerted efforts of the whole society to help with public health emergency.

The constant recurrence of new emergencies. Since 1985, the incidence of HIV/AIDS keeps rising and seriously endangers people's health. In 2003, the SARS caused people's great panic.

Food borne diseases and food poisoning are getting more serious. For example, in China, Hepatitis A eruption happened in 1988 in Shanghai, EHEC-caused food poisoning happened in 2001 in Jiangsu and Anhui Provinces, and Sanlu Milk Power Scandal happened recently. These are all serious health emergencies.

二、技巧指导：综合信息与信息重组——短时记忆与笔记

说笔记之前，需要简单了解记忆的特征。记忆分瞬时记忆、短时记忆、长时记忆。瞬时记忆持续的时间以秒计算，短时记忆最多不超过一分钟，而且这两种记忆的容量有限。长时记忆可以持续几分钟乃至终身，容量大。不管是哪种记忆，记忆方式都是重复。

复述也是一种重复。在交替传译中，演讲人说话的时间如果在30秒到1分钟以内，那么译者可以马上以译语加以复述。但是如果这样的程序持续发生，讲者的内容大量涌入译者的脑海，或者讲话人说话超过1分钟，译者的大脑工作起来便不那么顺畅了。

本科阶段的口译培训经验告诉我们，口译人员单凭瞬时记忆是无法很好地完成口译任务的，口译笔记是不可或缺的一项辅助功能。有效的笔记能够补足瞬时记忆的缺漏，能够帮助口译人员在较长时间里有效地工作。

笔记是脑记的延伸，因此口译笔记的原则是以记忆为主，笔记为辅。口译笔记既不是速记，也不是会议记录。它有时候像课堂笔记，既反映要点也有一些细节，有时又像关键词，能刺激记忆。无论哪种记法，都需要译员自己建立一套可行的方法，以满足速度和精确度，且字迹必须清晰可辨。

口译笔记的能力是系统培训的结果。这种培训或自我培训所需时间因人而异，但有一点是确切无疑的，即口译课的一学期训练时间远远不够。有的学生发现自己笔记上的信息量与翻译好的同学相比差不多，但自己的译语却还有支离破碎感；也有学生只能翻译记下来的东西而丢失了其他信息。这些情况说明，学生在抓取信息、理解主要信息点上有问题。因此这里就涉及笔记应该记什么的问题。

口译笔记具体记录什么？不是记字和句子。虽然具体操作上因人而异，但是大线条的概念应该是记何人、何时、何地、何事、如何。具体内容包括关键词、主题句、逻辑关系。关键词反映了讲话的主题概念和中心内容。关键词可以是名词主语、主句动词、主句宾语等。关键词的特点是易记、易回忆。主题句一般在一段话

或一个意群的开始，反映了对主题概念或中心内容的支持。逻辑关系则如前文所示，包含因果关系、正反关系、升降关系、差异关系、比较关系、前后关系等。再加上英语中的时态、各种名称或专有名词、数字（后两种属于高难度的信息），所有这些因素构成完整的信息概念和逻辑顺序。因此在做笔记或做改写练习的时候，要有意识地捕捉文章的主题，有意识地以意群为单位记录，并用斜线将各个意群分开。

口译笔记使用的语言因人而异。技术好的译员的笔记一般都是源语言、译入语、略缩语、首字或首字母、标准符号、某些速记符号、某种形象简笔画、个人自创符号的混杂体，并且这些符号已在重复使用中逐渐固定下来。例如：

The job of public health preparedness has never been more challenging than it is today. We face a wider range of public health threats than ever before in our history. It could be a dirty bomb set off in a subway car, or a contaminated food outbreak that originates outside our borders. Or we could face a new strain of flu that targets our children, like the novel H1N1 virus. America's families are counting on us to prepare for all of these threats—and to be as prepared as possible even when we face a new threat that we haven't seen before.

这一段话的笔记可以是这样的：

nev challen now
    more thre histr
        eg bom car, fd 污, new flu→chil eg HINI
            Ame rely prep, pre'd at new

也可以是这样的：

备挑
    今多thre 比历
        eg sub bb, fd污，流virus
            民求备，∴ even new，也必

还可以是这样：

php nev !! 今

wider thre cf史
eg sub bm, fd毒，flu virus→儿
Ame依, ∴mst备未见

在如何依循相关原则记录句子、段落的主旨大意上，译员都会有自己方式，因此要逐渐固化自己的记录习惯和符号。其余未记录的信息，译员仍需用瞬时记忆同时心记下来。

三、词汇准备

Text 1

antiviral dose 抗病毒剂
Food and Drug Administration (FDA) 美国食品及药物管理局
National Institutes of Health (NIH) 美国国家卫生研究院
pandemic （全国或全球）流行的疾病，大流行病
Strategic National Stockpile 国家战略储备
the White House Situation Room 白宫情报室

Text 2

concession card 优惠卡
Divisions of General Practice 全科部门
emergency response 危机反应
Medicare 全民医疗保险（澳大利亚）
mind boggling 让人极为震惊的

Text 3

Ambassador Extraordinary and Plenipotentiary of the United States of America 美国特命全权大使
Dengue Outbreak 登革热疫情
law enforcement officer 执法官员
mitigate 减轻
public infrastructure 公共基础设施

Public Health and Hospital Emergency Preparedness Summit 公共卫生和医院应急准备峰会

Text 4

a flash appeal 紧急呼吁
besiege 隔断；阻隔
Central Emergency Response Fund 中央应急基金
civilian staff 文职人员
initial reports 初步报告
United Nations Stabilization Mission in Haiti (MINUSTAH) 联合国海地稳定部队
Office for the Coordination of Humanitarian Affairs (OCHA) 联合国人道协调厅
Special Representative of the Secretary-General (SRSG) 秘书长特别代表
United Nations Population Fund (UNFPA) 联合国人口活动基金会
UN Entity for Gender Equality and the Empowerment of Women (UNIFEM) 联合国妇女发展基金
UN Environment Program (UNEP) 联合国环境规划署
UN World Food Program (WFP) 联合国粮食计划署

Text 5

非择期手术 non-selective operations
国药集团 sinopharm group
个体化治疗 personalized treatment
高原病 high attitude disease
环境消杀 disinfect the surrounding environment
救灾物资 relief materials
批次 batch
食品药品监管局 Food and Drug Administration
收治伤员 hospitalize
药品快速检测车 rapid drug test vehicle
预备队 reserve team
质检总局 General Administration of Quality Supervision
致残率 disability rate

Text 6

病因溯源平台 the etiology tracing platform

放射性物质 radioactive materials
国际食品法典委员会 CAC
禁用农药与兽药 prohibited pesticides and animal remedy
食品安全风险监测与评估 food safety risk assessment and monitoring
食源性疾病 food-born disease
食品安全法 Food Safety Law
食品中非法添加物 illegal food additives
食源性致病微生物 food-borne Pathogenic microorganism

四、摘要练习

请听下面英语语篇，第一篇用源语言复述此段主要信息逻辑点及层次，第二篇用译入语复述此段主要信息逻辑点及层次。注意信息点之间的逻辑联系。

Text 1

Speech of Kathleen Sebelius, the 21st United States Secretary of Health and Human Services, at the Public Health Preparedness Summit

16 February 2010

Ladies and gentlemen,

The job of public health preparedness has never been more challenging than it is today. We face a wider range of public health threats than ever before in our history. It could be a dirty bomb set off in a subway car, or a contaminated food outbreak that originates outside our borders. Or we could face a new strain of flu that targets our children, like the novel H1N1 virus. America's families are counting on us to prepare for all of these threats—and to be as prepared as possible even when we face a new threat that we haven't seen before.

The 2009-2010 H1N1 flu was one of those crises that put every aspect of our public health system to the test. I was sworn in as Secretary just as we were recognizing the first wave of the disease. Less than an hour after I became Secretary, I was taken to the White House Situation Room to get briefed. I've been involved in the H1N1 response from my first day on the job. And what's been striking about this flu is that like so many public health crises, it hasn't evolved the way we planned. We had planned for a pandemic that was more deadly and emerged far away from our shores. The flu that presented was less lethal—thank heavens—and already present in several states. This confirmed the wisdom of our flexible, "all hazards" approach to public health preparation. The most dangerous public health threat is often the one you're least prepared for, so we tried to be prepared for everything.

When the H1N1 flu hit in April, these preparations paid off. One of the first steps we took after identifying the flu was to release 11 million antiviral doses, 13.5 million surgical masks, and more than 25 million respirators from our Strategic National Stockpile. Having these countermeasures on hand allowed us to ensure that commercial shortages didn't slow our response.

Another example of preparation paying off is our Hospital Preparedness Program. Since 2002, we've sent more than $3 billion to state, local, and territorial public health departments, which have been invested in strengthening our medical surge capacity. Because of this investment, many of our hospitals had actually conducted pandemic flu exercises before H1N1 hit, so they knew what to do when their emergency rooms and ICU beds started filling up.

Steps like these allowed our public health response to hit the ground running. Working with partners in government, industry, and around the world, we rapidly characterized the virus, developed a candidate vaccine, made sure it was safe, and began production. By acting quickly, we made the first doses of the vaccine available in October, less than six months after the flu was identified.

At the same time, we launched an unprecedented multimedia communications campaign, first to educate Americans about how to recognize the flu and how to prevent it from spreading and then to encourage them to get vaccinated. We taught an entire generation of kids how to sneeze and built an incredibly powerful one-stop web site called flu.gov that served as a resource for millions of people.

All these successes had one thing in common: they were made possible by our unified public health response. In some cases, that meant partnerships between agencies within our own department, for example when the CDC, NIH, FDA and others worked to develop a safe vaccine. In other cases, it meant partnership with other departments in the federal government, like when we worked with the Education Department to develop a school closing plan that balanced health risks with the value of time in the classroom.

Most often, it meant partnership with state, local, tribal and territorial public health officials like all of you. In any public health emergency, you are both our eyes and ears on the ground and our first line of defense. That was certainly true with the H1N1 flu. And what we also saw with H1N1 was that these partnerships pay off. When we spoke with one voice, our message was clearer. When we responded together, our efforts were more effective. One good example was our vaccine locator tool on *flu.gov*, which used information you collected about clinics in your neighborhoods to make it incredibly easy for any family to find the nearest vaccine site.

We can't predict when or how the next public health emergency will hit. But by building on the success of our H1N1 response and applying the lessons we learned, we can be even more prepared next time. So thank you for inviting me here today. Thank you for your partnership. And I look forward to working with you in the months to come to keep Americans safe and healthy.

复述要点提示（主要信息逻辑点及层次）

Kathleen Sebelius emphasized the importance of a sound public health preparedness system and the important role health professionals play in safeguarding people's health.

1. Remind people of the unprecedented danger American people face so as to draw people's attention to the importance of public health response.

2. 2009 H1N1 flu is a good example, which demonstrates how an effective public health linearedress and public health system can do to save people and benefit society. In this flu, American National public health released 11 million antiviral doses, 13.5 million surgical masks, and more than 25 million respirators from the strategic National Stockpile for any American who needed help.

3. The importance of public health education. Public health system also conducted extensive education among Americans so as to give them knowledge about flu and its prevention. Also, they educated children to live a healthy life. In addition, they created a powerful website *flu.gov* as an easy access for Americans to gain knowledge of H1N1.

The important role public health professionals can play in helping American citizens. When professionals at state, local, tribe levels all work together, they can successfully prevent the spread of diseases. If all health professionals work in concerted efforts, the health message will be more clear and the results will be more effective. The *flu.gov* website is a good example. With the information collected by health professionals at different levels, this website becomes an easy and accessible approach for American citizens to get knowledge of flues and diseases.

Text 2

Hon Mark Butler MP Talks about Federal Government Assistance for Queensland Flood Victims

13 January 2011

Well, the scale of this disaster, as you say, is just mind-boggling, and the health implications that come from a disaster like this equally are very, very significant. Not only, obviously, the tragic loss of life and the serious injury that some have suffered, particularly in the Lockyer Valley, but there is the potential for widespread significant health implications, which we at a Commonwealth level are very conscious of.

So yesterday we activated the National Incident Room, which is, I guess, an emergency response to make sure that we are providing all the support that we can, particularly with the Queensland health authorities, but also to help professionals on the ground—GPs, allied health professionals, pharmacists—to make sure that the health of Queensland, as far as possible, is looked after.

There are some particular areas of responsibility we also have at a Commonwealth level. One of the things is that people who need medicines may well have lost their scripts, their Medicare cards, their concession cards. Their pharmacist that they usually go to might well be flood-affected themselves. So we have put arrangements in place to make sure that people are able to go to any pharmacy—with or without their cards or their scripts—and get the medicines that they need on an emergency basis for the next several days.

We know from previous disasters that there are emergency counseling needs that people have, particularly family members who are suffering grief. But there are quite broad, long-term implications that people have for long-term psychological support, which can go on for weeks and months.

So today I have announced some extra funding arrangements to make sure that when the time comes—which will be fairly soon, we imagine—those people who need ongoing psychological support will be able to access it. And we are already in contact with the coordinators of that support, which are the Divisions of General Practice, to make sure that that will be available.

Hospitals are certainly doing it tough, but they have all got their own independent electricity supplies, obviously, through generation. So those hospitals in areas that have been cut off are still able to operate. The hospitals have had to cancel elective surgery, unless it is particularly urgent, so that they can free up beds that are needed.

But the real challenge, I think, hospitals are having, according to my advice, is the staff there are incredibly overworked. They are doing an incredible job to deliver the services they need to, to Queenslanders. A lot of them in the Ipswich area I know, for example, west of Brisbane, are cut off from their own homes. So, in many cases, it's things like ensuring that there are—there is accommodation for hospital workers and other health workers who are cut off from their own homes and things like that. But the situation we're told at the moment is that hospitals are coping, but we're certainly monitoring it very, very closely.

As for the issue of counseling, people who need counseling services right now have them available through either the Queensland Health Department, or also some of the organizations well-known to your listeners like Lifeline. The head of "Beyondblue"rang me a few hours ago to say that they're willing to do their bit.

But in the longer term, which is really as the recovery process starts and, in many cases, as the grieving process really settles in, we know that from previous natural disasters that we've suffered in Australia, there is the need to make available extra psychological counseling services. So we already made some changes recently to the existing programs to fund those services through Medicare, to ensure that more were available in the event of disaster.

But in addition to those recent changes, I've announced today that $1.3 million of funding, to fund additional services that we expect to be needed over coming weeks and months. And again, we'll monitor that pretty closely to see whether or not that money satisfies the need that is going to inevitably emerge from this disaster.

Thank you!

复述要点提示（主要信息逻辑点及层次）

讲话主题：简短总结澳大利亚政府在昆士兰洪灾中所做的工作，表达了政府对灾区人民的关心和政府救灾的决心。

内容概要：如何面对这次洪灾对澳大利亚人民所带来的沉重打击。

首先，政府和昆士兰州卫生机构密切合作，保证为所有需要帮助的医疗人员提供力所能及的帮助。从联邦政府的角度出发，因为洪灾导致当地人民丢失各种医疗证明，如处方、医疗卡、优惠卡等，而灾区的医疗工作者自己可能也是洪灾的受害者，所以政府采取应急措施，保证所有需要帮助的灾民在不需要凭证的情况下也可以获得必要的药物。

其次，政府充分认识到面对灾难人们除了物资上的帮助还需要心理上的关怀，而且这种关怀通常是长期性、持续性的，所以联邦政府专门拨付资金保证人们的心理健康。

另外，联邦政府认识到灾区的医院和医院工作人员处在援助工作的最前线，发挥最重要的作用。医院独立的供电系统保证了电力供应，确保了需要紧急治疗的病人都可以得到治疗。另外医院的工作人员在洪灾中超负荷工作，而他们中很多人的家庭在洪灾中受到伤害。政府要为这些人员提供必要的帮助。

此外，政府还调动社会组织参与为人们提供心理帮助的工作。人们可以通过昆士兰州的卫生部门，通过一些社会团体如生命线和“超越忧郁”等，获得必要的援助。

最后，政府从这次洪灾中吸取的经验教训让联邦政府开始对现有的卫生制度进行必要的改变，让遭受灾害的人们能够得到更多。

五、英译汉练习

Text 3

“Are We Ready?”—The Need for Deep Preparation

The Ambassador Extraordinary and Plenipotentiary of the United States of America, Peter A. Prahar’s Speech at the Third Annual Public Health and Hospital Emergency Preparedness Summit

26 March 2012

As you can see, a large number of people with a wide range of expertise have come to this beautiful location to participate in this 3rd Annual Public Health and Hospital Emergency Preparedness Summit.

This of course underscores both the importance and the complexity of this subject. The agenda covers the topic thoroughly, but I would like to draw special attention to the presentations on the Yap Dengue Outbreak and the Murilo Turtle Event. These emergencies severely tested the capacity of the Yap and Chuuk State medical services, the first with an emergency which lasted for months and affected over a thousand people, the other with an unexpected, severe event on a remote island that resulted in six deaths. I believe interesting lessons can be learned from both events—lessons that can help you mitigate the effects of future public health emergencies.

Unlike you, I am not an expert in the public health and hospital emergency preparedness field. But my long career in the US Air Force and in the US Foreign Service certainly has given me some considerable experience in dealing with emergencies of various sorts. So please let me offer a few observations to consider as you ask yourselves: Are we ready?

First, as previous speakers have noted, we can and should plan and practice for dealing with emergency situations of all sorts. But as you know, no emergency ever unfolds in the precise way it was envisioned. For this reason, I think an effective response to an emergency goes well beyond plans and specific skill sets. An effective response requires what I call "deep preparation."

Let me suggest four elements of "deep preparation".

First, "deep preparation" requires responders to not only have the skills but also clearly understand—and accept—their responsibilities and authority.

Second, "deep preparation" requires sound public infrastructure. In this area I am proud to draw attention to the role the US through the Compact of Free Association and other US federal grants, programs, and services is playing in establishing the infrastructure the FSM needs to respond not only to the daily needs of its citizens, but also to their needs in emergencies.

Over the last three years, Aircraft Rescue and Firefighting buildings have been built at the international airports in Kosrae, Yap, and Chuuk and another is nearing completion in Pohnpei. These facilities are equipped with advanced fire-fighting equipment and staffed by personnel trained to the highest standards in order to deal with what we hope never happens: an emergency involving an aircraft.

Also, a major renovation project is now underway at the Yap State Hospital. I am pleased to report that just last week the U.S.-FSM Joint Economic Management Committee directed that Compact funds be used to construct a new hospital in Kosrae, which has never had a proper hospital facility.

Finally, deep preparation requires that the public have confidence in its law enforcement officers, medical personnel, and government leaders. Law enforcement officers must have a reputation for integrity and skill in dealing with difficult situations. Medical personnel must have a reputation for offering authentic medical information and reliable care. Government leaders must have the reputation of putting the public's interest foremost and for being able to lead a stricken citizenry through an emergency.

They are what I think worth considering when answering the Summit's question: "Are we ready?"

I wish you all the best as you work together over the next three days and in the future to serve and protect the people of this region we love and serve.

Text 4

UN Secretary-General Ban Ki-moon Briefs to the General Assembly on the Emergency in Haiti

13 January 2010

Mr. President, Excellencies, Ladies and gentlemen,

Our hearts and minds today are with the people of Haiti. We are still struggling to learn the full extent of the devastation from yesterday's earthquake, but you have all seen the images on television—collapsed hospitals and schools, public buildings in ruins, including the parliament, presidential palace, cathedral, the ministry of justice and many government offices. Tens of thousands of people are in the streets, without shelter. Uncounted numbers remain trapped in the rubble.

Large portions of the capital, Port-au-Prince, have been badly damaged. Basic services such as water and electricity have collapsed almost entirely. Some major transportation routes have been severely disrupted by surface cracks or blocked by rocks, fallen trees or collapsed buildings. Medical facilities are besieged; many are simply not functioning.

To take control of the situation and direct our immediate emergency response efforts, I am dispatching Assistant Secretary General Edmond Mulet, our former SRSG for MINUSTAH, to Haiti this evening. He will be on the ground tomorrow morning to assume full command of the United Nations mission at this juncture. He will begin his work by seeking a meeting with the top leadership of the country.

MINUSTAH troops worked through the night to reach those under the debris. So far, several badly injured people have been retrieved and transported to the MINUSTAH logistics base, which remains largely operational.

MINUSTAH has approximately 3,000 troops and police in and around Port-au-Prince to help maintain order and assist in relief efforts. MINUSTAH engineers have also begun clearing some of the main roads in Port-au-Prince which will allow assistance and rescuers to reach those in need.

The most urgent need is emergency search and rescue. A Chinese team has arrived in Port-au-Prince; at least two US teams will arrive by this evening, and two more tomorrow morning. Additional search and rescue teams are reported to be arriving from Guadeloupe and the Dominican Republic, and still others are on their way from many countries that have sprung to action.

Let me say that I am very grateful, on behalf of the United Nations and on Haiti's behalf, for these urgent efforts. Clearly, a major relief effort will be required. In any emergency like this, the early hours and days are critical. That is why I have directed the United Nation's humanitarian agencies to mobilize swiftly and in close coordination with the international community.

In the next few days, we will issue a flash appeal for Haiti. I expect my humanitarian coordinators to perform the necessary assessment of needs and funding as quickly as possible and report back to me at once. In the meantime, I have ordered $10 million to be released from the Central Emergency Response Fund, or CERF, to kick-start our response.

Ladies and gentlemen, to the people of Haiti, I say this: we are with you.

We are working quickly—as fast as humanly possible.

On behalf of the people of Haiti, I thank you for your support, and I urge you to work closely with us at the United Nations and the MINUSTAH mission, so that we may deliver for those so in need.

Thank you very much.

六、汉译英练习

Text 5

卫生部应急办主任梁万年在国务院青海玉树地震新闻发布会上的开场白

2010年4月23日

各位媒体朋友们，女士们、先生们：

下面我代表卫生部就青海玉树地震灾区医疗卫生救援工作的有关情况给大家做一个简要的介绍。

一、工作进展

（一）医疗救治工作成效显著

一是紧急调援，全力抢救伤员。地震发生后，我们迅速调动全国军地医疗和卫生应急救援队伍，多方配合、齐心协力抢救伤员。共组织军地医疗救治队伍35支3 346人，配备急救车近400辆，携带大量医疗器械和保障物资在灾区开展紧急医疗救援工作。截至4月22日，累计接诊灾区伤病人员4万余人次，累计收治伤员9 145人次。目前，灾区医疗救治工作逐步由紧急救援向提供基本医疗服务转变。

二是果断决策，实施伤员转运，提高救治效果。于震后3天完成了1 434例重症伤员的大规模转运。转运重伤员至西宁、海南州、格尔木、兰州、成都、西安、昌都等5省7市38所医疗条件和技术较好的综合医院和专科医院并进行有效救治。

三是集中优势，全力救治危重伤员。调整整合医疗资源，重点加强西宁和格尔木等地医疗救治力量。卫生部组建联合专家组，为每一位伤员实施个体化治疗。截至22日，已全部完成非择期手术544例，累计治愈出院伤员154例。

（二）卫生防疫工作全面展开

一是灾区卫生防疫工作扎实有序推进。全面展开环境消杀、帐篷消毒、供水点监测、传染病和鼠疫疫情监测、健康宣教等工作。目前，灾区已开展环境消杀121.5万平方米，消毒帐篷6 600顶；对68个供水点进行了水体监测；在27个医疗点开展了传染病监测，动物鼠疫疫情监测面积累计达470万平方米。卫生防疫组还组建了250余人的卫生防疫预备队，可按需求随时赶赴灾区开展工作。

二是大力开展健康宣传教育和心理干预活动。编印鼠疫和高原病等防治知识要点以及环境、食品饮水卫生宣传要点，由青海卫生部门翻译成当地语言。灾区卫生救援人员开展健康教育咨询2.8万人次。同时，快速组织国家专家赶赴西宁市，对通晓当地民族语言和风俗的186名地震灾后心理援助人员进行师资培训，指导做好伤员转运和灾区群众的心理疏导服务。

二、下一步工作安排

1. 对前一阶段卫生救援工作进行认真总结梳理，继续强化与灾区卫生部门的沟通，加强与军队及中央派遣单位的协调配合，确保各方卫生救援力量形成合力，共同推进灾区各项医疗卫生工作。

2. 继续全力做好转出伤员的救治工作，加强对重症伤员医疗救治工作的指导。按照“四集中”（集中伤员、集中专家、集中资源、集中救治）原则，努力提高治愈率和康复率，最大限度地降低死亡率和致残率。

3. 全面落实卫生防疫，确保大灾之后无大疫。帮助灾区卫生部门尽快实现防疫工作“四个全覆盖”（即监测报告、环境消杀、饮食饮水卫生、健康教育工作全覆盖），加快动物尸体无害化处理，加大灾区人畜牧共患病和重大动物疫病的防控工作力度。谢谢大家。

Text 6

李斌向世卫组织通报H7N9进展情况

瑞士日内瓦

2013年5月21日

尊敬的主持人卡琳女士，

尊敬的世界卫生组织总干事陈冯富珍女士、西太平洋区域主任申英秀博士、助理总干事福田敬二博士，

尊敬的世界动物卫生组织总干事贝尔纳博士、联合国粮农组织首席兽医官胡安博士，

女士们、先生们：

在这次世界卫生大会期间，中国和世界卫生组织联合召开人感染H7N9禽流感防控工作边会，邀请来自世界卫生组织、联合国粮农组织、世界动物卫生组织以及各国的卫生官员和专家，沟通疫情防控信息，共谋防控之计。这种畅通的沟通和交流非常必要，这体现了对全球卫生安全和人类健康的高度负责。

今年3月末，中国卫生计生部门在接到地方报告3例不明原因肺炎病例后，用很短时间就确认病例为H7N9禽流感病毒感染。截至5月20日，中国大陆累计报告确诊病例130例，病例呈散发，分布于浙江、上海、江苏等10个省份。目前，治愈72人，死亡36人。

疫情发生以来，中国政府高度重视。国家主席习近平、国务院总理李克强第一时间要求各地、各有关部门要高度重视，把疫情防控工作作为关系国计民生的重要任务来抓。专门有一名副总理直接指挥防控工作，建立由卫生计生委牵头，农业部、林业局等16个部门组成的联防联控工作机制，指导各地采取了一系列有力、有序、有效、有度的措施，国家根据各省的疫情和需求，向各省提供不同的应对策略和指导，积极开展疫情防控工作。一是全力做好患者救治，及时制定下发诊疗方案，开展医务人员培训，做到早发现、早报告、早诊断、早治疗，并按照集中患者、集中专家、集中资源、集中救治的原则，加强重症病例救治，努力减少重症和死亡病例。保障患者救治费用，确保不因费用问题影响患者救治。二是加强监测。卫生部门强化了不明原因肺炎、流感样病例和病原学等监测，农业、林业部门加强了对动物、家禽和野鸟监测。及时开展风险评估，研判疫情形势。各地组织落实疫情溯源、现场流行病学调查、密切接触者追踪管理、卫生学处置等防控措施。三是地方政府根据当地疫情防控工作实际需要，有针对性地采取暂时或永久关闭城市活禽市场等措施，控制疫情源头，并采取规范活禽运输、强化健康教育等综合性措施，严防疫情扩散。四是中央财政安排6亿元人民币约9 700万美元扶持家禽产业健康

发展，统筹做好科学防控疫情，推动家禽产业转型升级。五是坚持公开透明，及时准确发布疫情和防控工作信息，广泛宣传防治知识，加强公众风险沟通。六是紧急组织实施诊断技术、疫苗、病原学及溯源、流行病学、临床救治、动物模型等应急科研专项，为疫情防控提供科技支撑。

在疫情防控过程中，中国与世界卫生组织沟通顺畅、配合默契。中国切实履行《国际卫生条例》，及时向世界卫生组织、有关国家和地区通报疫情信息。主动与世界卫生组织流感参比和研究合作中心以及指定的实验室共享毒株，保持定期交流及技术讨论。我与陈冯富珍总干事专门通电话，商谈防控合作。世界卫生组织专家接受邀请来华与中国专家组成联合考察组，考察疫情应对工作，对防控工作提出了很多宝贵的建设性意见。我们还举办了联合新闻发布会，向中外媒体通报疫情进展和防控措施。中国的疫情应对工作得到了来自世卫组织、粮农组织、世界动物卫生组织及有关国家和地区的支持与帮助。借此机会，我代表中国政府，向各方表示衷心的感谢!

女士们、先生们，人感染H7N9禽流感等新发传染病是人类面临的共同挑战。中国政府愿与各国一道在《国际卫生条例》框架下，支持世界卫生组织在全球卫生领域发挥积极作用，协同遏制各种新发传染病的传播，保障人类的生命安全和身体健康。

谢谢大家!

资料来源:

Text 1 www.flu.gov/blog/2010/02/blog20100216.html

Text 2 http://www.health.gov.au/internet/ministers/publishing.nsf/Content/tr-yr11-mb-mbtr130111b.htm

Text 3 http://kolonia.usembassy.gov/speech-2012-04.html

Text 4 http://www.un.org/apps/news/infocus/sgspeeches/statments_full.asp?statID=699#.UYEQd-2xFnY

Text 5 http://www.china.com.cn/zhibo/zhuanti/ch-xinwen/2009-01/23/content_19890589.htm

Text 6 http://field.10jqka.com.cn/20130523/c534886154.shtml

参考答案

四、摘要练习

Text 1

美国卫生及公共服务部第21任部长凯瑟林·西贝利瓦厄斯
在公共卫生危机应急峰会上的讲话

2010年2月16日

女士们、先生们：

今天的卫生应急工作比以前任何时候都艰巨。我们面临着前所未有的公共卫生挑战。这种挑战可能来自地铁上放置的炸弹，可能来自境外食物污染引发的危机，可能是一种威胁儿童的新的流感病毒，比如新的H1N1病毒。美国的家庭正在依靠我们应付所有这些威胁，哪怕我们面临的是一种从未见过的威胁。

2009年10月的H1N1流感是我们的公共卫生系统所经受的一次考验。我宣誓就职的时候正是我们发现第一波疾病的时候。在我成为秘书长的不到一个小时内，我就被招到白宫情报室并被告知疾病的情况。从上任的第一天我就开始应对H1N1流感。H1N1流感最严重的就是它并不朝着我们设计的方向发展。我们做了应对从远离美国的大陆传来的疾病的准备。然而H1N1这种疾病虽然杀伤力不大（感谢上帝），但是已经在好几个州出现。我们的做法证明了我们公共卫生防御的灵活的“全危险方法”的正确性。最危险的公共卫生威胁往往就是那些我们最没有意料到的，所以我们试图对任何东西都做好应对准备。

当H1N1流感4月袭来时，这些付出的努力终于取得了成效。在确认了这种流感后，我们做的第一件事就是从国家战略储备中发放了1 100万只抗流感剂，1 350万个手术面罩，和2 500万个防毒面具。这些措施保证了商业流通领域商品的短缺不会影响我们的应急反应。

我们的医院应急项目则是另外一个公共卫生应急成功的例子。自2002年起我们向各州、各地区和美国境内的公共卫生部门拨放了超过30亿美元用于加强我们的医疗急救能力。因为这项投资，许多医院实际上在流感来袭之前就已经进行了演练，它们知道在医院床位开始紧张时该做些什么。

像这样的举措使我们的公共卫生应急体系成功运作。和政府、产业以及全世界合作伙伴一起合作，我们快速确定了病毒的种类，开发了可用的疫苗，在确保疫苗的安全性后开始大量生产。通过快速反应，在病毒被确定后不到6个月时间内，就是10月份，我们就有了第一批流感疫苗。

同时我们开展了一项前所未有的多媒体的信息交流运动，首先教育美国人如何识别流感和预防流感的传播，接下来鼓励他们注射疫苗。我们教会孩子们如何打喷嚏，然后建立了一个无比强大的叫作flu.gov的一站式网站以供百万美国人使用。

所有这些成功都有一个相似点：都是通过统一的公共健康反应机制实现。在一些情况下，这意味着卫生部门之间的合作，如美国疾控中心、美国国家卫生研究院和美国食品及药物管理局（FDA）。在另外一些情况下，它意味着和联邦政府不同机构之间的合作。如我们和教育部合作，开发了一个危机时刻学校封闭计划，以实现健康风险和正常上课之间的平衡。

更多时候这意味着像你们这样的州、当地卫生官员、部落和地方卫生官员之间的合作。在任何公共健康应急情况下，你们就是我们的眼睛和耳朵，是我们的第一道防线。在H1N1流感应急中就是这样。我们从应对H1N1事件中可以看出这些合作的作用。如果我们用一个声音说话，我们要传达的信息就会更清楚明确，当我们一起响应时，我们的努力就更有效果。一个很好的例子就是flu.gov网站上的疫苗接种点搜索工具，通过收集当地的诊所信息，美国任何一个家庭都能够非常容易地找到离自己最近的接种点。

我们无法预测我们的公共卫生健康系统会在什么时候遭遇危机，而危机又会以何种形式出现。但是通过利用H1N1反应系统的成功以及对我们经验的成功应用，我们可以肯定下一次危机袭来时我们会准备地更加充分。感谢你们的参与。我期待着在未来几个月里和你们合作以确保全体美国人的安全和健康。

Text 2

澳大利亚工党代表人马克·巴特勒谈政府援助昆士兰洪灾灾民

2011年1月13日

这次灾难的程度是让人极为震惊的，这样的灾难带给我们的卫生方面的启示是非常深远的。灾难不仅带来严重的人员伤亡和损失，特别是在洛克耶谷（Lockyer Valley）地区，也给我们许多卫生工作方面的启示，这一点是我们联邦政府层次清楚认识到的。

所以昨天我们启动了国家重大事件室，这是一种应急措施，可保证我们能够提供力所能及的帮助，特别是和昆士兰卫生部门充分合作，保证对有需要的医疗人员（包括全科医生、专职卫生工作人员、药剂师等）提供必要的帮助。

在联邦政府层次上我们有自己特殊的责任。其中一件事可能是有些需要药物的群众遗失了处方、医疗卡，或者优惠卡。而平时为他们服务的药剂师可能自己也是洪灾的受害者。于是政府做出安排保证这些群众可以在任何一个药店，无论他们有没有医疗卡、处方，或者优惠卡，都可以得到他们需要应急的几天的药物。

我们从之前的灾难中学习到，遭受灾难的人们需要心理咨询，特别是那些在灾难中失去了亲人的人们。但是更广泛和长期的影响是人们需要的是长期的心理方面的帮助，这种帮助可能会持续数周，甚至数月。

所以今天我宣布了几项额外的资金安排，用以保证在需要的时候（也许这个时候很快就会到来），那些需要持续的心理帮助的人们能够得到帮助。我们已经和援助项目的协调机构，即全科医疗部门取得了联系以保证人们能够得到这样的帮助。

灾区的医院也面临着许多困难，但是他们都已经通过发电获得了独立的电力供应。因此断电地区的医院仍然能够运行。这些医院不得不取消那些非紧急的手术，所以它们还能够接收有需要的病人。

但是根据我的经验，我认为医院所面临的真正的挑战是超负荷的工作人员。他们正在从事着了不起的工作，为昆士兰的居民提供所需的服务。据我所知，伊普斯威奇地区的西布里斯班市的许多医务工作人员都和自己的家人失去了联系。所以我们需要为这些和家人失去联系的工作人员提供必要的帮助。但是我们现在被告知医院正在努力处理所有的问题，我们正在密切关注事情的进展。

至于为需要帮助的人们提供心理援助，人们可以通过昆士兰州卫生部门或者一些广为人知的组织，如“生命线”这样的组织获得必要的心理帮助。专门帮助抑郁人群的精神健康组织“超越忧郁”的负责人几个小时前刚给我打来电话表达了提供帮助的意愿。

但是从更长时间的角度来说，正如我们从澳大利亚以前所遭受的自然灾害中所了解到的，人们还需要额外的精神方面的咨询服务。所以我们最近已经对现有的项目做出了一些改变，通过全民医疗保险来提供必要的帮助，让遭受灾害的人们能够获得更多的帮助。

但是除了最近的一些变化外，我今天还宣布了一笔130万的资金，以满足未来几周或几个月内的额外需求。我想再次强调的是，我们会密切关注这笔资金，确保其用于这次灾难中可能出现的紧急情况。

谢谢大家。

五、英译汉练习

Text 3

“我们准备好了吗？”
——彼得·普拉哈在第三次年度公共卫生和医院应急准备峰会致词

美国特命全权大使波特·普拉哈
2012年3月26日

许多有着不同经验和知识背景的人们来到这个美丽的地方参加第三次公共卫生和医院应急准备峰会。

这当然彰显了这个题目的重要性和复杂性。这次会议将会详细地讨论这个题目，但是我还是希望能够提醒大家对雅浦岛（YAp）地区登革热疫情以及穆里洛（Murilo）毒龟事件的特别注意。这些危机事件严重考验着雅浦岛（Yap）和楚克州（Chuuk）（密克罗尼西亚群岛组成部分）卫生服务系统的应急能力。前一个危机持续数月，影响上千人，而后一个危机则属于荒岛上突发的严重事件，导致6人死亡。我相信通过这两次事件我们可以学到不少东西。它们可以帮助你们减轻未来公共卫生危机带来的危害。

和在座各位不同，我不是公共卫生和医院应急准备方面的专家。但是我长期在美国空军和驻外事务服务的经验给了我不少应对不同危机的经验。所以这里我想和大家分享几点观察所见。请大家考虑一下这个问题：我们准备好了吗？

首先，正如之前的发言人所说，我们能够而且应该为各种紧急情况进行安排和演习。但是正如大家所知，任何危机都不会严格按照预想的方式发展。出于这个原因，我认为对危机的有效反应是超出计划和特别技术的。有效的反应需要我所说的“深度准备”。

我所说的“深度准备”有四个要素：

首先，“深度准备”要求反应者不但要有技巧还需要明确理解并且接受他们的责任和权力。如果对自己的责任和权力不够了解，那么危机时刻的混乱必然会削弱反应力。

第二，“深度反应”要求完善的公共基础设施。在这方面我很自豪地提请大家注意，美国政府通过自由联系条约和其他美国联邦政府资金、项目和服务建立起严密的基础设施结构，不仅可以满足密克罗尼西亚公民的日常需求，同时也能满足他们在危机时刻的要求。

过去三年内，库赛埃岛、雅浦岛、楚克州已经完成了在其国际机场的飞行救援和消防建筑建设，而波纳佩州的项目也正在建设中。这些设施都配备了先进的防火设备和接受过严格训练的人员以应对与飞行器有关的紧急情况（当然我们希望危机最好不要发生）。

另外在雅浦州医院正在进行一项大型的改造工程。我很高兴地告诉大家，上周美国-密克罗尼西亚联合经济管理委员会将资金用于在楚克州地区修建一所新的医院。在此之前这个地区还从来没有一所像样的医疗机构。

最后，“深度准备”要求公众对执法官员、卫生工作者和政府领导人的充分信任。执法官员必须拥有良好的口碑，而且有应付困难处境的技能。卫生工作者必须能够提供正确的信息和可靠的服务。政府领导者必须能够把公众的利益放在首位，能够领导危难中的群众走出困境。

再次感谢大家给我这个发言机会。我祝大家在接下来的三天里工作愉快，在未来的日子里能够有效地服务和保护这个区域的人民。

Text 4

联合国秘书长潘基文在联合国大会上关于海地地震危机的讲话

2010年1月13日

主席先生，各位阁下，女士们、先生们：

今天，我们所思所念的都是海地人民。

我们仍在试图完全了解昨天地震破坏的严重程度，但是，大家都已看到了电视图像——医院和学校倒塌……公共建筑变成一片废墟，其中包括议会、总统府、大教堂、司法部和许多政府部门的建筑。数以万计的人流落街头，无处栖身。还有无数的人仍然被困在瓦砾之中。

首都太子港已大范围严重被毁。水和电力等基础服务几乎完全瘫痪。一些主要的运输线路遭到严重破坏，路面断裂或被岩石、倒塌的树木或建筑物阻断。医疗设施也被堵隔，许多根本无法运转。

为了充分控制局势并指导我们眼下的应急工作，我派遣我们联海稳定团的前秘书长特别代表，现任助理秘书长艾德蒙德·穆莱特今天晚上动身前往海地。他将于明天上午抵达当地，并在这一关键时刻完全接管联合国特派团的工作。他开展工作的第一件事就是寻求与该国最高领导人会晤。

联海稳定团的部队通宵达旦地抢救那些埋在废墟下的人。到目前为止，有几名受重伤的人已被救出，并运到联海稳定团的后勤基地，该基地基本上还在运转。

联海稳定团在太子港及其周围地区有大约3 000名士兵和警察，可协助维持秩序，并协助救援工作。联海稳定团的工程师们也已经开始清除太子港一些主要道路，这将使援助和救援人员可以抵达灾区救灾。

现在，最迫切需要的是紧急搜救。中国的一支分队已经抵达太子港，至少有两支美国的分队将于今晚到达，另有两支明天上午抵达。据报，更多的搜救分队将从瓜德罗普岛和多米尼加共和国抵达。另外，还有许多国家立即采取了行动，它们派出的搜救队正在进发途中。

请允许我代表联合国和代表海地说一声，非常感谢这些应急努力。显然，我们必须进行一场大规模的救援。在任何如此严重的紧急情况下，最初的数小时和数天都是生死攸关的。正因如此，我已指示联合国的人道主义机构迅速动员起来，并与国际社会密切协调。

在接下来的几天中，我们会为海地发出紧急呼吁。我希望我的各位人道主义协调员尽快做出需求和资金评估并立即向我报告。情况已经表明，在医疗保健、食品、洁净水和住房等方面将有巨大的需求。同时，我已命令从中央应急基金释放1 000万美元用于启动我们的应灾行动。

女士们、先生们，对海地人民，我要说：我们和你们在一起。

我们正分秒必争地工作——能多快就多快。

我要代表海地人民感谢你们的支持，而且我要敦促你们同我们在联合国和在联合国海地稳定特派团的人员密切合作，以便我们能够为灾民送去救助。

非常感谢大家。

六、汉译英练习

Text 5

The Opening Speech at the News Conference of the State Council on Yushu Earthquake

Liang Wannian,

Director of Public Health Emergency Response, Ministry of Health

23 April 2010

Media Friends, ladies and gentlemen:

On behalf of Ministry of Health, I would like to give a brief introduction of the medical rescue at Yushu, the earthquake stricken area of Qinghai Province.

1. Progress

1) The Medical rescue work has made great progress.

Firstly, we spared no efforts in rescuing the wounded people. After the earthquake, we quickly assembled the military and local health care and emergency rescue forces to participate in the earthquake rescue work. Altogether we organized 35 teams and 3, 346 people, equipped with almost 400 emergency vehicles, and a great amount of medical equipment and facilities. By April 22nd, we had treated over 40,000 sick and injured people, with 9, 145 persons being hospitalized. Till now, the medical work at the earthquake stricken area has changed from emergent rescue to basic medical service.

Secondly, we transferred the wounded to other places to receive better treatment. Facing the harsh natural conditions and the severely damaged medical equipment, our working team made resolute decision to transfer seriously injured people to other places to receive treatment. With the concerted efforts of the military and local forces, 1, 434 seriously injured patients were transferred in just three days. They were sent to 38 hospitals located respectively in Xi'ning, Hainanzhou, Ge'ermu, Lanzhou, Chengdu, Xi'an and Changdu and received effective treatment.

Thirdly, we pooled our strength in rescuing the severely injured patients. We adjusted the deployment of medical resources according to the geographical location of the hospitals that received these patients and reinforced the medical strength of hospitals in Xining and Ge'ermu. Ministry of Health set up the expert team to give personalized treatment to every patient. Each hospital is trying its best to give the patients treatment. Till 22nd, we had finished all non selective operations, which amounted to 544, and cured and released 154 patients from hospital.

2) The comprehensive conduction of disease control and prevention.

Firstly, we have promoted the disease prevention and control work at the earthquake stricken areas in an orderly way. We have already started to disinfect the surrounding environment, the tents, the monitoring of water supplies, the monitoring of infectious diseases and plague epidemic. Till now, we have disinfected an area of 1.215 million square meters and 6,600 tents, monitored 68 water supply sites, conducted infectious disease monitoring at 27 medical sites, and monitored 4.7 million square meters' plague epidemic situation. The disease prevention and control team have also organized a reserve team of over 250 people, ready to go to the stricken area at demand.

Secondly, we have put great efforts in health education and psychological intervention. We printed the pamphlet about plague and high attitude disease prevention and environmental, food and water safety, and the health department in Qin Hai province translated it into local language for local people. Rescue workers gave 28,000 times of health consultation to local people. Meanwhile, we organized national experts to Xi'ning to give training to 186 post-disaster psychological consultants who are proficient at local languages and customs and to guide the psychologicalcounseling for local people and the transfer of the wounded.

2. Next Phase

Firstly, in accordance with the central government and the State Council's deployment and requirement about the earthquake relief work for the following stage, we will give a thorough summary of our health relief work of the first stage, continue to strengthen the communication with health departments of the stricken areas and the coordination and cooperation with the army and the units dispatched by the central government so as to ensure the smooth and efficient work at the disaster areas.

Secondly, continue to devote to the treatment of the wounded, especially the severely wounded. According to the principles of Four Concentration, the concentration of the wounded, of experts, of resources, of treatment, we try our best to increase the cure rate, and minimize the death rate and disability rate.

Thirdly, fully implement disease prevention and control to make sure there is no big epidemic after the disaster. Reinforce the cooperation with the army, divide the 19 responsibility areas, make clear of the responsibility, the measures and the support, and guide local health departments to realize the four "coverage" of disease prevention and control: the monitoring and reporting, environmental disinfection, the safety of food and drinking water, the coverage of education. In addition, speed up in the harmless treatment of animal remains and reinforce the disease control and prevention of zoonoses and major animal epidemics.

Text 6

Li Bin Briefs WHO on the H7N9 Avian Flu

Geneva, Switzerland

21 May 2013

Respected Madame Chair Ms. Karin,

Honorable WHO Director-General Dr. Magaret Chan, Reginal Director for the Western Pacific Region Dr. Shin Young-Soo, Assistant Director-General Dr. Keiji Fukuda,

Honorable OIE Director General Dr. Bernard Vallet, FAO Chief Veterinarian Officer Dr. Jouan Lubrth,

Ladies and gentlemen:

During this World Health Assembly, China and WHO jointly convened this side event on Influenza A (H7N9) in order for officials and experts from WHO, FAO, OIE and relevant countries to communicate epidemic information and discuss common methods for prevention and control. This type of smooth communication and exchange is very necessary, and this demonstrates our commitment to global health security and human health.

At the end of March this year, after receiving reports of three cases of pneumonia with unknown cause, in a very short period of time, the health authorities of China confirmed that those cases were human infections with the H7N9 avian influenza virus. As of May 20, a total of 130 confirmed cases had been accumulatively reported in mainland China. The cases are of sporadic nature, scattering around 10 provinces such as Zhejiang, Shanghai, Jiangsu, etc. Currently, 72 cases recovered, and 36 cases died.

The Chinese government has taken the epidemic outbreak very seriously and has always put people's life and health in the first place. President Xi Jinping, Premier Li Keqiang immediately demanded that all relevant localities and departments pay high attention, and take the epidemic prevention and control as an important task of protecting national welfare and people's livelihood. A Vice Premier served as the commander for prevention and control of epidemic. We held many high-level meetings to study the prevention and control strategies. Multi-sectoral prevention and control mechanism is set up, led by the National Health and Family Planning Commission and participated by 16 ministries, such as the Ministry of Agriculture, the State Forestry Administration, etc. Adhering to the principle of legal and scientific response, prioritized work and differentiated guidance, these institutions are guiding the nation for taking strong, orderly, effective, and appropriate prevention and control measures. According to their different epidemic situation and needs, the central government provided each province with distinctive response strategy and guidance.

Firstly, patients have been given utmost care. Health institutions have efficiently worked out treatment plans and carried out medical personnel training. Early detection, early reporting, early diagnosis and early treatment have been followed. Hospitals have been pooling experts and resources for focused treatment of patients, so as to reducing the number of severe cases and deaths. At the same time, no patient is left untreated due to lack of payment.

Secondly, surveillance has been intensified. Health institutions at all levels have strengthened the surveillance of pneumonia with unknown causes, influenza-like illnesses and pathologies. The agriculture and forestry authorities have strengthened the monitoring of animals, poultry and wild birds. We promptly carried out risk assessment and situation analysis. Local authorities have organized epidemic tracing, on-site epidemiology investigations, tracing of close contacts to poultry, and hygienic disposal, etc.

Thirdly, local governments have shut down live poultry markets temporarily or permanently as needed to control the source of outbreak. They have also taken integrated measures to standardize live poultry transports and strengthen health education to curb the epidemic from spreading.

Fourthly, the central government has allocated RMB￥600 million, around 97 million USD to support healthy development of the poultry industry. Scientific prevention and control of the epidemic can go hand in hand with the poultry industry restructuring and upgrading.

Fifthly, information has been open and transparent. Epidemic updates have been timely and accurately released. Prevention and control knowledge has been widely disseminated. Risk communication with the public has been strengthened.

Sixthly, we have organized focused research programs on diagnostic techniques, vaccines, etiology, epidemiology, clinical treatment, and animal models, etc. These researches provide scientific and technological support for the epidemic prevention and control.

In the process of epidemic prevention and control, China and WHO had smooth channels of communication and good collaboration. The Chinese government has effectively implemented the International Health Regulations and timely notified the World Health Organization and relevant countries and regions of the epidemic. We have taken the initiative to share the virus strains with the WHO Influenza Reference and Research Collaborating Centers as well as their designated laboratories, and conducted extensive international exchange and cooperation. I had a phone conversation with Dr. Margaret Chan on the epidemic cooperation. Upon our invitation, WHO experts came to China and joined Chinese experts in assessing China's response to the epidemic. They gave us a lot of valuable constructive suggestions. We held a joint press conference with WHO to inform domestic and international media of the epidemic updates and our prevention and control progress. China's response efforts have been supported by WHO, FAO, OIE and relevant countries and regions. On behalf of the Chinese government, I would like to take this opportunity to express our heartfelt gratitude to you all!

Ladies and gentlemen, emerging infectious diseases, such as avian influenza A (H7N9), are common challenges to humanity. The international community needs to work actively to strengthen the institutional capacity building of public health, facilitate epidemic communications, exchange experiences in prevention, control and treatment, share scientific findings, and jointly cope with epidemic threat. Under the framework of International Health Regulations, the Chinese government is ready to join hands with all countries to support WHO's role in coordinating global efforts to curb any emerging infectious disease and protect life and health.

Thank you!

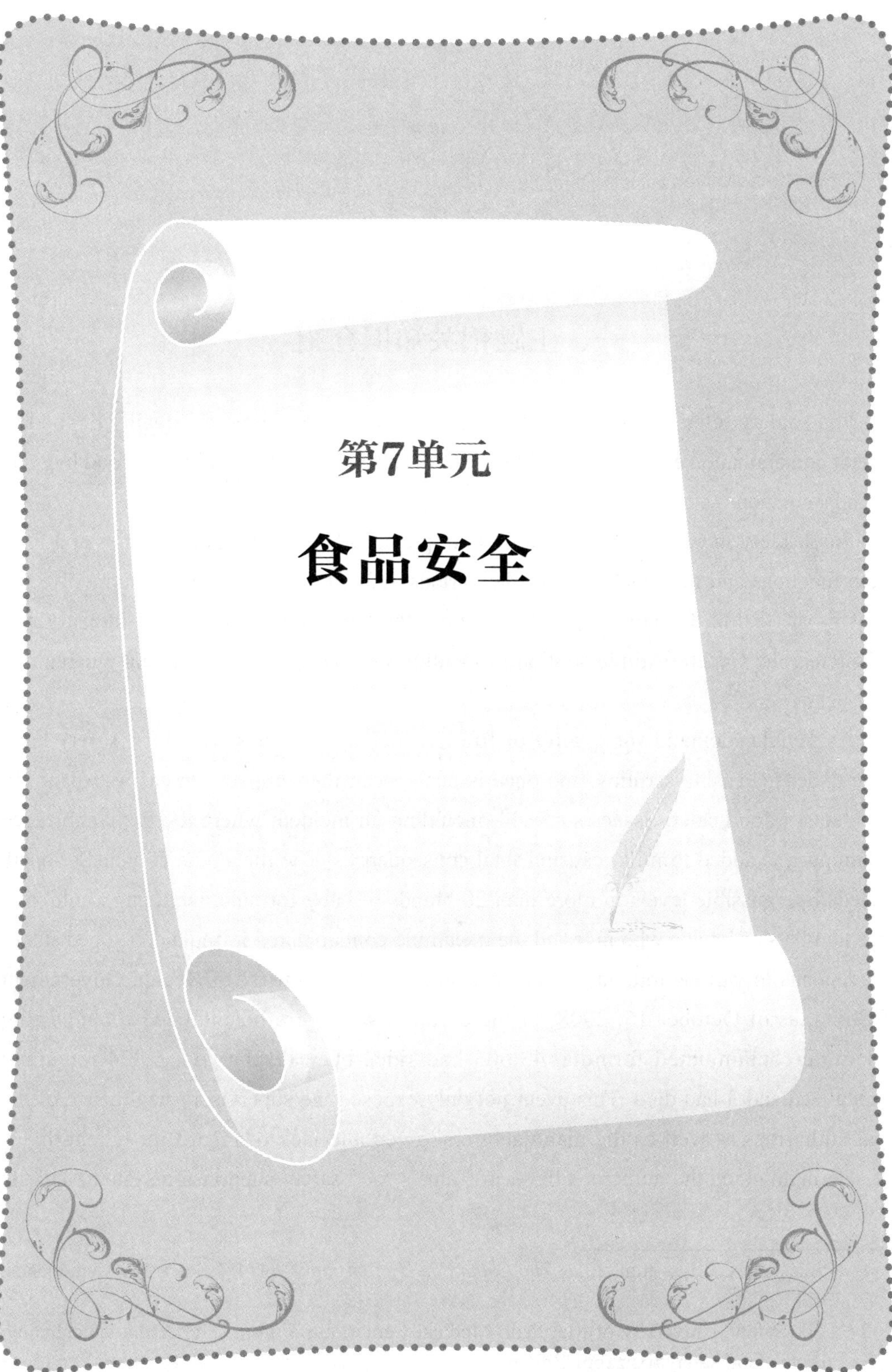

第7单元

食品安全

一、主题相关知识介绍[1]

Food safety refers to the conditions and practices that preserve the quality of food to prevent contamination and foodborne illnesses. It is also alternatively known as food hygiene or food sanitation.[2]

Food safety in China is regulated by multiple agencies, creating ambiguities and gaps in the functions and responsibilities of the various authorities concerned. These involve the Ministry of Health, the Ministry of Agriculture, the State Administration of Industry and Commerce, the General Administration of Quality Supervision, Inspection and Quarantine, etc.

As popular demand for quality of life has increased, issues with food safety have come under increasing scrutiny, and once issues appear, their impact can easily expand. In 2008, severe food safety issues surfaced, including an incident where the toxic substance melamine was added to milk, causing fatal consequences. The melamine content seriously exceeded permissible levels in more than 20 brands of baby formula, including Sanlu, and large numbers of infants who ingested the melamine-contaminated formula developed stone-like deposits in various internal organs. According to the Ministry of Health, Government of China, as of October 15, 2008, of the children who were hospitalized for ingesting melamine-contaminated formula, 43,603 had since been discharged, 5,824 remained hospitalized and 3 had died. This event not only exposed the supervisory negligence of the local authorities as well as the manufacturers' greed and lack of regard for human lives, but also highlighted the numerous flaws in China's food safety supervision system, and the

1 Ru X., Lu X., Li P., et al. 2011. *The China Society Yearbook*. Vol. 4. Leiden, The Netherlands: Brill.

2 Food safety. University of Maryland Medical Center. http://umm.edu/health/medical/ency/articles/food-safety#ixzz2bpUZN6od.

issues exposed by the formula event have since received a great deal of attention from the government. On July 27, 2008, the State Council issued *Special Provisions on Strengthening Food Safety Supervision*[1]. On October 9, the Stated Council announced *Regulations on the Supervision and Administration of the Quality and Safety of Dairy Products*[2]. On September 18, the General Office of the State Council issued Notice on the Abolition of Food Quality Inspection-Exempt Provisions[3]. In October, the National People's Congress conducted its third review of the Food Safety Act (Draft)[4], which was promulgated in April, 2008. The third review resulted in the addition of new items governing food safety supervision, including the abolition of food quality inspection exemptions, state-unified food safety standards, the requirement for food additives to receive Ministry of Health authorization, a requirement for businesses to recall their food products when an issue with these problems arise, lacking which, the government is authorized to enforce a product recall. It is clear that 2008 would become a year of symbolic significance in China's history of food safety.

"The Chinese Food Safety Act" was passed after the fourth review by the Standing Committee of the National People's Congress in early 2009. After some revisions, the Food Safety Act puts greater emphasis on the accountability of both the central government (relevant competent authorities) and local governments and the responsibility of food businesses.

Chinese food standards consist of state standards, local standards, industry standards and enterprise standards. The multi-level standards sometimes conflict with each other, and most of these standards are outdated or lower than the international ones. To systematize these food standards, China has committed to unify national food safety standards by conferring standard-making powers on the Ministry of Health. Furthermore, given situations such as the production and marketing of substandard food and food products, the conflicting standards set by different bodies, the regulation based on outdated standards or without established standards, it is also necessary to set up the general principles and requirements with regard to the standards setting procedures in order to ensure uniformity and consistence. To this end, Article 23 has provided that the national food safety standards should be approved by a national review committee of standards which consists of experts with food related background and government officials. In addition to this, before decisions are taken,

1 《加强食品安全监管特别规定》。
2 《乳品质量安全监督管理条例》。
3 《关于废除食品质量免检制度的通知》。
4 《食品安全法草案》。

the committee should consider the comments of different stakeholders and the results of risk assessment as the basis for setting standards.

二、技巧指导：缩写、符号及口译笔记本的空间结构

业内很多人都知道实战口译笔记“少字多义，少写多划，少横多竖”的原则，因此在学习笔记记法的时候，可以了解某些缩写和符号，比如中、英文缩写词，中英文符号和速记符号等，以达到快速记录的效果。英文缩写词中，有的缩写词已经被广泛应用。例如：

技术性缩写词：

H	氢
Pb	铅
Na	钠
Si	硅
Atm	大气压
IU	国际单位
LF	低频，低频率，低生长率
DNACVI	儿童免疫创议
AVG	平均
FW	淡水
SG	比重
Ibid	the same with above 同上
3D	3-Dimensional 三维
4WD	Four Wheel Drive 四轮驱动
AI	Artificial Intelligence 人工智能

普通词汇缩写：

cf	compare, comparative 相比较，比较的
e.g.	example 例如
s	sum 总计
f	frequent, frequency 频繁，频度
cap	capitalism, capitalist 资本的，资本主义，资金的

bio	biology, biological, biologist 生物学，生物学的，生物学家
Info	information, informative 信息，提供信息的
max	maximum，maximize 最大值，最大化，增至最大限度
min	minimum，minimize 最小值，最小化，减至最低限度
w/	with 与
w/o	without 无
co	company 公司
asap	as soon as possible 尽快

国名缩写：

br巴西，ca 加拿大，cn中国，eg埃及，fr法国，gb英国，hk香港，jm牙买加，mx墨西哥，no挪威

机构名称：

WHO	United Nations Health Organization 世界卫生组织
UNDP	United Nations Development Program 联合国开发计划署
WWF	World Wildlife Fund 世界野生动植物基金会
NIH	National Institutes of Health 美国国家卫生机构
BMA	British Medical Association 英国医学学会
HC	Health Canada 加拿大卫生部
NHFPC PRC	National Health and Family Planning Commission of People's Republic of China 中华人民共和国国家卫生和计划生育委员会
CDC	Chinese Center of Disease Control and Prevention 中国疾病防控中心
FAO	Food and Agriculture Organization of the United Nations 联合国粮食及农业组织
UNFPA	United Nations Population Fund（旧称United Nations Fund for Population Activities联合国人口活动基金会）联合国人口基金
UNICEF	The United Nations Children's Fund（旧称United Nations International Children's Emergency Fund 联合国国际儿童紧急救援基金会）联合国儿童基金会
EPI	Expanded Programme on Immunization 扩大免疫规划，来自《发展和坚持免疫方法与流行病监督计划，防止天花、白喉、百日咳、

	破伤风、麻疹、脊髓灰质炎、结核病等传染病》。
USFDA	US Food and Drug Administration 美国食品药品监督管理局
FFIB	Frozen Food Information Bureau (Australia)（澳大利亚）冷冻食品信息局
FSA	Food Standards Agency（英国）食品标准局

上述例子只是海量缩写词中的几例。由于缩写词量大，除了在平时学习中不断地参考英文缩写大全之外，另一个方法是在接受口译作业或任务之后，有范围、有针对性地选择记忆。

缩写英文单词的另一个方式是省去单词中的一个或多个元音，省去一个或多个辅音，或使用省略符号。这种方法有一定的规律，但口译笔记不是速记，目的不是记下以后慢慢回看，而是辅助即时回忆，所以要以能够有效提示自己回忆为主。在这种情况下，无须严格遵循缩写规律，可以有个人的偏好。例如：

problems可以缩写成prblms, probs, pros, 或prlmsd等。
government可以缩写成goven, govmt, gov, gov't或gmt等。
background可以缩写成bkrnd, bcrnd, bac, 或brnd等。
educational可以缩写成eductnl, educat'l, edu'nl, edunl, edu等。

中文表达中也有固定的缩写。例如：

中华人民共和国国家发展和改革委员会	发改委
新型农业合作医疗	新农合

口译笔记虽然不是速记，但仍然可以使用某些速记符号。下面的速记符号比较常用：

>	大于、多于、比……要好
<	小于、少于、比……差
≤	小于或等于
≥	大于或等于
=	等于、是、两者一样、意味着、也就是
≠	不等于、两者不一样
≈	大概、大致、约等于

:<	遗憾、悲哀
:)	高兴、荣幸
×	错误、否、不、否定
√	正确、对、好、肯定
N	不同意
Y	同意
↑	上升、增加
↓	下降、减少
+	强、好
+ +	更强、更好
−	弱、差
——	更弱、更差
∵	因为
∴	所以
∈	属于
V	胜利
?	问题、疑问
&	和、与
=>	结论是
↗	促进、发展
□	国家
□/□	国与国
←	原因
→	导致、结果
><	对立、冲突
< <	波折
∩	进入
∞	接触、交往
⊥	分歧
**	非常、十分重要
≡	坚持
!	关键，奇观
@	有关
∽	替换为

|| 但是
// 口译段分隔符
○ 轮子、空洞
△ 代表
vs 比
\ 因此、那么
& 和、并且

笔记中，短的单词一般不缩写，例如is，are，but，as，big等。笔记记的是主、谓、宾、定、状语，或名词、动词、形容词、副词、数字。只有语法功能的词，例如a，an，the，where等不记。

本科阶段，在A4大小的纸张上写的时候，有不少学生为了节省纸，笔记记得密密麻麻，从左至右横向写满页，翻译的时候到处找。这种写法难以分清层次，所以看不清楚。还有的同学喜欢在纸上竖着画一条中线，将空间一分为二，先左后右，从上往下写字。其实这样既不利于快速书写，看的时候也有干扰。好的笔记要便于自己回看，要考虑以意群为单位分区或排列。比较顺手的一是以方块形式，横向按意群段排列，在一方块之中，一个层次一短行。每个意群段完成之后，画一条斜线表示与下一段隔离开来，防止自己看错内容。另外也有阶梯式排列，一个意群段为一个阶梯，更加一目了然。

例一：

新年的钟声即将敲响。我们要继续努力，把人民的期待变成我们的行动，把人民的希望变成生活的现实。我们要继续全面深化改革，开弓没有回头箭，改革关头勇者胜。我们要全面推进依法治国，用法治保障人民权益、维护社会公平正义、促进国家发展。我们要让全面深化改革、全面推进依法治国如鸟之两翼、车之双轮，推动全面建成小康社会的目标如期实现。（习近平）

Bell
    Conti, exp→ act, hope→现
        Conti 全→深g, ∵弓X←, 改g t y√
            全 → fa□、fa: 权yi、≡社g，促□发
                Let全深g、全→fa□ be 2 wings, 2○s, →estb康 as

例二：

世界卫生组织2003年的调查结果显示，北京复发性脑中风的比例为27%，居世

界各国主要城市之首。我国学者对临床资料的分析也表明，门诊的脑中风患者中约40%为复发病例，25%～33%的脑中风患者将在3～5年内再次发作……我国缺血性卒中的比例快速上升，缺血性和出血性脑卒中的比例从1984年的1.25：1上升到2004年的6.06。

WHO 03 : re str 比 27%，no 1 worl

Clinic ana: op 40% re， 25-33% re 3-5y

I S↑! IS & ha：1984 1.25 →2004 6.6

（recurrent stroke 复发性脑中风，ischemic stroke 缺血性卒中，hemorrhagic apoplexy 出血性脑卒中）

做这种笔记，即便在学习阶段，最好还是用一个巴掌能握住的线圈本来做记录。线圈本的好处是容易拿在手中，并且容易翻页，尤其在写了几页后，可以一把翻回来正好翻到一段的开头，并立即开始翻译。这样养成习惯之后，实战的时候会更顺手。

三、词汇准备

Text 1

Codex Alimentarius Commission 国际食品法典委员会
Codex Alimentarius 国际食品法典
Director-General 总干事
Food and Agriculture Organization (FAO) 联合国粮食及农业组织
credibility 可靠性，可信度
standard-setting body 制订标准的机构
codes of practice 操作规范，实践准则
organic vegetable 有机蔬菜
vaccination 疫苗接种
distribute 经销
mandate 委任，授予权限
eradicating hunger and malnutrition 彻底消灭饥饿和营养不良
be food secure 得到足够食物的保障
improve access to 增多获取途径

World Trade Organization (WTO) 世界贸易组织

Agreement on Sanitary and Phytosanitary Measures 《食品安全卫生与植物卫生措施协定》

block competitors unfairly 不公正地阻碍竞争

translate into 转化

safe-maximum levels for pesticide residue 农药残留的最高安全水平

veterinary drug 兽药

contaminant 污染物

food additive 食品添加剂

harmonize 使协调、和谐

Hazard Analysis and Critical Control Point (HACCP) 危害分析与关键控制点

food-borne disease 食源性疾病

be recognized and embraced by 得到……认可和接受

Text 2

institutional 制度上的，机构的

joint venture 联合、合作事业

collaborative 合作性的

undertakings 事业

profoundly 极深的，深厚的，深远的

glaring 显眼的；突出的

sound scientific foundation 合理的科学依据

rigour 严谨性

consistency 一致性，一贯性

step in 插手干预；介入

safety net 安全网

World Health Assembly 世界卫生大会

hazard 危险，危害

toxin 毒素

processed, semi-processed, and raw food commodities 加工、半加工、原料食品商品

benchmark 标准，尺度

benchmark standards 参照基准，参考标准

level the playing field 创造公平竞争的环境

on an equal footing 在平等的基础上，平等地

consumer confidence 消费者的信心
rigorous scientific methodology 严谨的科学方法
inclusive 内容丰富的，范围广的
be in a better position to... 处于更好的位置，更容易做到
outbreak 疫情，疾病暴发，突然发生，发作（尤指疾病或暴力行为）
take the heaviest toll on... 对……造成巨大危害
enduring concern 引起长期关注的问题
distinct seasons 四季分明
on a grand scale 大规模
recall 产品召回
obesity 肥胖

Text 3

FDA (Food and Drug Administration) Commissioner 美国食品与药品监督管理局局长
bear on 对……造成影响
consumption 消耗，食用
caffeine 咖啡因
dietary supplement 膳食补充
diet cola 健怡可乐
ingest 咽下，摄取
pharmacologically active substance 具有药理学活性
central nervous system 中枢神经系统
stimulant 兴奋剂
coffee beans 咖啡豆
kola nut 可乐坚果
soft drinks 不含酒精的饮料
cocoa pods 可可豆荚
barrage 倾泻，接二连三
moderate consumption 适度食用、使用
adverse effect 不良影响
supersized 超大号，超大杯（饮料）
food additive 食品添加剂
inundate 淹没，泛滥
consumer advocates 消费者权益倡议人士

energy drinks 能量饮料
be loaded with 装载大量的，含有大量的
waffle 奶蛋格子饼，华夫饼
syrup 枫糖浆
breakfast oatmeal 早餐燕麦片
jelly beans 彩色软糖豆，豆状胶质糖果
marshmallow 棉花糖
sunflower seeds 葵花籽
caffeinated 含有咖啡因的
regulatory agency 监管机构
medical professional 医务人员
be at increased risk for 存在更高风险
dosage 剂量
cumulative 累积的
relevant literature 相关文献
vulnerable population 弱势人群
data gap 数据缺口
deliberation 熟思，商议

Text 4

deputy commissioner 副局长
bottom line 底线，最重要的因素
dynamic 动态的
incredibly 不可思议地，惊人
obsolete 已不用的，陈旧的
political alignment 政治联盟
bipartisan 两党的，代表两党的，得到两党支持的
overhaul 彻底检查
Department of Health and Human Services 美国卫生及公共服务部
Secretary Sebelius 西贝利厄斯部长
prevention-oriented 以预防为主
from farm to table 从农业生产到餐桌食用的各个方面
tenure 任期
silver bullet 奇迹般的解决方法

magic wand 魔法杖

Text 5

监测 monitoring
评估 assessment
食品安全风险评估 risk assessment for food safety
有害因素 harmful substance
试行 trial
食源性疾病 foodborne disease
隐患 potential problem
重点领域 key area, priority area
监管部门 supervisory body
化学污染物和食品中非法添加物以及食源性致病微生物监测点 monitoring sites of chemical contaminants, illegal food additives, and foodborne pathogenic microorganisms
食源性异常病例或健康事件 abnormal cases of or health events caused by foodborne diseases
应急和常规食品安全风险评估项目 emergency and routine food safety risk assessment project
三聚氰胺 melamine
丙烯酰胺 acrylamide
苏丹红 Sudan red dye, magdala red, naphthalene red
氯丙醇 chloropropanol
溴酸盐 bromate
二噁英 dioxin
风险监测评估制度规范 risk monitoring and assessment system regulations
工作机制和程序 working mechanisms and procedures
参比实验室 reference laboratory
放射性物质 radioactive substance
检测 testing
风险评估模型 risk assessment model
技术支撑体系 technical support system

Text 6

切身利益 concern the vital interests of

执行力 execution capacity

中国共产党总书记 CPC General Secretary

指示 give instructions on

重点工作任务 prioritized tasks

有关部门 the departments concerned

贯彻落实 implement, carry out

专项整治 rectification activities targeted at specific issues

高发态势 high incidence

非法添加和滥用添加剂 illegal use and overuse of food additives

制售假冒伪劣食品 manufacturing and selling of counterfeit and shoddy food commodities

道德缺失、自律缺失 fail to follow vocational ethics and lack self-discipline

监管 supervision, oversight

监管交叉和空白 regulatory overlaps and gaps

既要打好攻坚战，又要打好持久战 be ready to tackle the difficult issues on a long-term basis in the battle against food safety problems

综合整治 comprehensive rectification campaigns

综合治理 comprehensive management

专项整治 specific corrective activities

规范建设 setting up standards

使命 mission

四、摘要练习

请听下面英语语篇，第一篇用源语言复述此段主要信息逻辑点及层次，第二篇用译入语复述此段主要信息逻辑点及层次。注意信息点之间的逻辑联系。

Text 1

Address at the 36th Session of the Codex Alimentarius Commission[1]

José Graziano da Silva, Director-General of Food and Agriculture Organization, United Nations

Rome, Italy

2 July, 2013

Mr. Sanjay Dave, Chairperson of this Commission,

My sister Margaret Chan, Director-General of the World Health Organization,

Excellencies,

Fifty years ago, right here in Rome, the Codex Alimentarius Commission officially came into being.

In July 1963, the Commission held its first session as the principal organ of the Joint FAO/WHO Food Standards Program.

Since then, Codex has contributed to bringing about safer and more nutritious food around the world.

Codex began with 30 members. And has grown to include 185 Member governments, one Member organization and 220 observers.

The results that Codex delivers, its science based decision-making, its participatory nature and truly global membership contribute to Codex's credibility and high reputation as a standard-setting body.

Nowadays, it would be difficult to imagine what our food, our health, and even our economies would be like without Codex Alimentarius, and its international food standards, guidelines and codes of practice.

And yet, even today, many people are not aware of its vast influence on our everyday lives.

Whether you shop at a supermarket, produce organic vegetables, use vaccinations on livestock, or distribute seafood, your life is affected, or protected, in some way, by Codex. And these are just a few examples.

All of you are responsible for helping to make this happen, so I thank you.

---

1 国际食品法典委员会（Codex Alimentarius Commission，简称CAC）是联合国粮农组织、世界卫生组织于1962年共同创建的协调各成员国食品法规、技术标准的唯一政府间国际机构。CAC制定的标准致力于保护各国消费者的健康安全，维护国际公平的食品贸易，为各国食品标准的制订提供重要的科学参考依据。

Ladies and gentlemen,

Codex and standard setting are an important part of FAO's mandate, as recognized in our reviewed strategic framework and program of work.

Food safety is also important to FAO's global goal of eradicating hunger and malnutrition, since people cannot be food secure, if their food is not safe.

So FAO is proud to be part of the past, present and future of Codex.

And the Codex Alimentarius is as relevant today as when it was created.

Codex helps to improve access to healthy, nutritious food, and provides standards to guide people who depend directly on agriculture and the food system for their livelihoods.

Over the past 50 years, the Codex Alimentarius Commission has done much to strengthen national food safety systems and foster international food trade, which has grown from 22 billion dollars in 1963, to more than 1.3 trillion dollars.

Codex is an important reference for the work of the World Trade Organization.

The WTO refers to Codex as the ultimate standard setting body for food safety in its Agreement on Sanitary and Phytosanitary Measures.

The WTO agreement is designed to help countries protect their populations with food safety and health standards, while discouraging them from using those standards to block competitors unfairly.

Playing an active role in Codex has helped countries to compete in global food markets, while also improving food safety at home.

Much of the work done by Codex can translate directly into national legislation.

It includes thousands of safe-maximum levels for pesticide residues, veterinary drugs, contaminants, and food additives.

Also, Codex has helped to harmonize food labeling across the world, has helped to develop practices to help producers reduce and prevent contamination, and has helped to establish improved food hygiene through the Hazard Analysis and Critical Control Point system (HACCP).

Codex has also established and applied risk analysis for food safety decisions. Its food safety standards are firmly based on the solid scientific advice that FAO and WHO provide through independent expert bodies.

Where it has not directly set standards, Codex has given detailed advice to countries looking to set their own rules.

In sum, Codex has shown that without compromising its values and scientific approach, it can act quickly and set needed standards within a year.

This week, we can take a moment to celebrate the benefits of the work that we have done together—within countries and internationally. However, there is still a lot of work to be done.

New food-borne diseases are emerging, or being identified, new food products emerge and new production methods. This means that we need new standards.

Ladies and gentlemen,

Codex must keep pace with a changing world in which transportation, communications and scientific developments move at a much faster pace than before with direct and significant implications for food safety.

We also have several funding challenges. We are having a hard time finding the needed funding for the scientific advice on which Codex is based. We need to find a sustainable solution.

The Codex Trust Fund was formed with generous voluntary contributions from its Members and has helped make the Codex Commission truly global. But as the fund comes to an end in 2015, we will need to consider how we can continue offering support to those who need it.

Another issue is that Codex has created important links at all levels of the food chain but it has remained a mostly invisible player in the background.

One of the questions we will need to consider in the coming years is how to ensure that Codex is recognized and embraced by more actors outside its immediate circle.

We need more interaction with consumer associations and more participation at country level.

Above all, it is important to act together, to strive for even greater collaboration, across different sectors, across national borders, and among different jurisdictions.

FAO, WHO, Codex, the World Organization for Animal Health (OIE) and the International Plant Protection Convention (IPPC) are working closely on designing a framework of standards, guidelines and codes that can live up to this ideal.

This is in line with the "One Health"[1] approach to working across many disciplines, for the health of people, animals and the environment.

Let me add that, as FAO, we are not only celebrating 50 years of Codex but also, one of the longest standing collaborations in the UN system.

I would like to personally thank my counterpart from WHO for ensuring the success of

1 One Health（唯一健康）是一个针对人类、动物和环境卫生保健的各个方面的跨学科协作和交流的全球拓展战略。

this joint effort.

I also thank everyone who has supported us in the effort to guarantee safe, good food for everyone, and a healthy, sustainable future for us all.

Thank you for your attention.

复述要点提示（主要信息逻辑点及层次）

Purpose of the speech:

Giving congratulations on and commendation of the contribution of Codex Alimentarius Commission, or commonly referred to as Codex, to bringing about safer and more nutritious food around the world. Reflecting on the future challenges facing Codex.

Two keynotes of the speech:

1. Congratulations on the achievements made by Codex in the 50 years of its history. Codex sets up the standards used to regulate the production, processing and distribution of food commodities across the world. The influence of Codex standards pervades across the world, yet most people are not aware of it.

2. Codex plays multiple functions. Codex is closely involved in the work of other organizations and its member countries. Codex helps FAO realize its goal to eradicate global hunger and malnutrition. Codex helps WTO promote world trade. The member countries have integrated Codex standards into their national legislation for food safety, e.g., the safe-maximum levels for pesticide residues, veterinary drugs, contaminants, and food additives. Codex helps standardize food labeling. It helps food producers reduce risks for food safety problems and has helped improve overall food safety in the world. Codex funds research in order to obtain the needed scientific evidence for standards setting and Codex standards are based on solid scientific evidence.

3. Codex is faced with a lot of future tasks and challenges. First of all, the world is developing rapidly, resulting in the emergence of new food-borne diseases and new food products. Consequently, Codex has to keep pace with the changes and adapt itself accordingly. Secondly, Codex has funding challenges. The Codex Trust Fund provides funding for research on food safety standards or guidelines, but the fund ends in 2015. There has to be a new and sustainable plan to raise fund. Thirdly, Codex wants to become more visible in the future because the organization intends to play a more important role through increased interaction with consumer rights associations and participation at country level.

4. Codex will reinforce efforts in cross-institutional, cross-disciplinary, and cross-border cooperation.

Text 2

Statement Commemorating the 50th Anniversary of the Codex Alimentarius Commission

Dr. Margaret Chan, Director-General of the World Health Organization

Rome, Italy

2 July 2013

Excellencies, distinguished delegates, representatives of civil society, the private sector and scientific institutions, our sister agencies in the UN system, ladies and gentlemen,

Let me express my warm congratulations to the Codex Alimentarius Commission on its 50th anniversary. WHO can take some institutional pride in commemorating the many transformational changes introduced by Codex over these five decades.

Codex began as a joint venture between FAO and WHO, supported by countries. This is one of the longest-running collaborative undertakings in the UN family, and it has been profoundly effective.

Codex was established to meet a great and glaring need. In the early 1960s, legislation aimed at controlling the quality and safety of food varied greatly from country to country.

Laws were often enacted without a sound scientific foundation, and basic principles of nutrition were frequently overlooked. This confusion, variation, and lack of rigour and consistency was a significant barrier to trade.

Codex stepped in to reduce these barriers, to put science in the service of consumer protection and, in effect, to cast a safety net around the world's food supply.

WHO has always been a most willing partner in the work of Codex. In fact, this is part of our job. The establishment of international standards for food is a function mandated by the WHO Constitution.

In 1953, the World Health Assembly expressed concern about the increasing use of chemicals in the food industry as a new health problem that needed to be addressed.

Consumers were also showing concern. Most food that has gone bad looks bad and smells bad. But hazards arising from the presence of toxins, additives, pesticides, and veterinary residues in food were invisible and could be neither smelled nor tasted. Consumers wanted some assurance of safety. They wanted to be protected.

Codex addressed these and many other concerns.

Over the decades, Codex has produced standards for a wide range of food commodities, whether processed, semi-processed, or raw, from spices and dried fruits to fresh milk and meat, and foods for special dietary uses.

The output has been remarkable. Altogether, Codex has established more than 200 food standards and more than 100 guidelines and codes of practice for food production and processing.

Codex has also addressed those "invisible" hazards. Maximum permissible levels have been established for thousands of food additives, contaminants, pesticides, and veterinary drug residues.

Today, Codex standards are the benchmark standards for food safety. There is no competition. They are internationally recognized as the best, at every point along the food chain.

Food standards promote fair practices in food trade. Food that conforms to international standards moves more freely across borders. Food standards level the playing field. Developing countries producing food that meets international standards can enter international trade on an equal footing.

Codex has had an enormous impact on how food producers and processors operate and on consumer confidence in the safety and nutritional quality of food, whether consumed in the home country or when travelling abroad.

Today, consumers expect that a purchased food item conforms with what is stated on the label. This trust is thanks to decades of work by Codex.

Codex standards contribute to equity. Everyone in the world deserves the same assurance that the food they eat is safe and nutritious.

Rooted in a rigorous scientific methodology, Codex has also lifted the standards for assessing food quality by stimulating food-related scientific and technological research.

Today, Codex membership covers 99% of the world's population. Developing countries benefit from Codex standards once they have been adopted. But participation needs to be more inclusive.

As you have heard, WHO and FAO established the Codex Trust Fund in 2003. In its ten year history, the Fund has been used to support more than 2000 participants from 134 countries to attend Codex meetings and working groups. Countries that understand the process by which standards are set are in a better position to interpret and implement them effectively.

Ladies and gentlemen,

Safe and nutritious food sustains human life, ideally in good health. Unsafe food can cause disease, sometimes in very large outbreaks. Contaminated food can be deadly, usually taking its heaviest toll on the very young and the very old.

Hunger and undernutrition, and all the adverse consequences for health, continue to be priority issues of international concern. Talk about food security[1] is on the table in discussions about sustainable development and the post-2015 development agenda.

In the midst of these enduring concerns, the world food supply has changed dramatically. Food production is increasingly industrialized. Distribution networks now span the globe. The notion that fresh fruits and vegetables have distinct seasons has all but vanished.

This has brought some advantages. Hunger has receded in many parts of the world, and dietary diversity can introduce significant health benefits.

But there is a negative side. Economic integration and the globalization of food trade mean that a single meal can contain ingredients from all around the world. The complexity of the food chain has increased, introducing more critical points where something can go wrong.

And when something does go wrong, it often does so on a grand scale. Investigations of outbreaks can involve multiple countries on multiple continents. Recalls can be massive, with huge economic losses. Consumer confidence can be shattered, and take a very long time to recover.

And there are other problems. Today, the cheapest, most convenient, most accessible, and best-tasting foods are often energy rich, yet nutrient poor.

Today, obesity and diet-related noncommunicable diseases often exist side-by-side with undernutrition in the same country, even in the same community or household. It is good to know that Codex is now addressing this issue through its nutrition and food labeling committees.

This may be one of the next great challenges for Codex: to introduce greater balance in the world's food supply.

This is what we all want to see: safe, nutritious, and health-promoting food for all, whether home grown or a product of international trade.

Thank you.

---

1 Food security指食物保障，即所有人在任何时候都能在物质上和经济上获得足够、安全和富有营养的食物以满足其健康而积极生活的膳食需要（世界粮食首脑会议行动计划第一段）。这涉及四个条件：充足的粮食供应或可获得量、不因季节或年份而产生波动或不足的稳定供应、具有可获得的并负担得起的粮食、优质安全的食物。

复述要点提示（主要信息逻辑点及层次）

讲话包括五项内容：

1. 祝贺国际食品法典委员会（CAC）成立50周年。代表世卫组织祝贺50周年庆。简述CAC建立背景和发展历史：50年前各国的食品质量和安全的法律存在非常大的差异，已有的法律没有健全的科学基础，这些都构成贸易堡垒；粮农组织和世卫组织联合建立CAC以消除贸易堡垒、保护消费者；世卫组织和CAC是长期合作伙伴，建立食品标准是世卫组织的职责之一，1953年世卫大会对食品工业中使用的化学品提出担忧；消费者担忧食品工业中化学品的使用，希望得到安全保障。

2. 总结CAC的工作和产生的影响。CAC在50年间制订了各种各样的食品标准，对世界产生巨大影响。建立了200多个食品标准和100多个食品生产和加工实践指南及守则。为数以千计的食品添加剂、污染物、农药和兽药残留建立了最高允许水平。CAC的食品标准是世界各国的参照标准。CAC的食品标准促进了公平竞争，提高了消费者对食品安全和营养质量的信心。CAC的食品标准促进了公平性，每个人都享有安全且富有营养的食物。标准制订基于严谨的科学方法，促进食品质量评估标准的提高。成员国覆盖世界人口的99%，但不足之处是发展中国家参与不足。CAC信托基金支持134个国家的2 000多人参加食品法典委员会的会议和工作组，帮助各成员国更好地诠释和实施标准。

3. 食品和健康的关系。安全和有营养的食物维持人类的生命，有助于维持良好的健康状况。反之，不安全的食品可能导致疾病，甚至是严重的疾病暴发。粮食安全对健康的影响是人们持续关注的问题。

4. 世界的变化、发展和全球化对食品安全带来新的挑战。食品生产的工业化水平提高，蔬菜水果季节性特征不再明显，带来的好处是消除饥饿，饮食多样性促进改善健康；不好的方面是食品成分和食物链的复杂性提高，出问题的可能性增高，容易造成严重问题、巨大经济损失、消费者信心丧失。食品还存在热量高、营养低的问题，造成肥胖、饮食相关的非传染性疾病、营养不良共存的问题。食品法典委员会的营养和食品标签委员会正在努力解决这个问题。

5. 对CAC未来工作的展望。引入更加平衡的世界食品供应，促进健康。

五、英译汉练习

Text 3

Caffeine in Food and Dietary Supplements: Examining Safety

Remarks by Dr. Margaret Hamburg, FDA Commissioner to a Meeting of the Institute of Medicine, Food and Nutrition Board and Board on Health Sciences Policy National Academy of Sciences

Washington, D. C.
5 August 2013

Thank you, Dr. Goldman, for that generous introduction, and for taking on the responsibility of chairing this important committee. I also want to thank the members of the committee for their service and for bringing their knowledge, expertise and insights to bear on the issues surrounding the potential health hazards associated with the consumption of caffeine in food and dietary supplements.

As a brief glance around the room this morning confirms, many of us begin our days with some caffeine, in the form of a cup of coffee, tea and, for some, diet cola.

That's not surprising. Caffeine is probably the most frequently ingested pharmacologically active substance in the world. A central nervous system stimulant, it occurs naturally in more than 60 plants, including coffee beans, tea leaves, kola nuts used to flavor soft drinks and cocoa pods used in making chocolates.

But if the barrage of coffee cups across the room is not surprising, neither should it be seen as alarming. Years of research and study have shown that moderate consumption by adults of products with naturally occurring sources of caffeine is not associated with adverse effects.

Of course, the traditional cup of coffee or tea—even when it's "supersized," as is so often the case today—is not the concern or focus of your important work here today. For the Food and Drug Administration, caffeine is both a drug and a food additive. And your mission is to take a closer look at the many new and novel products that are inundating the marketplace today that have added sources of caffeine.

Some of these products have already begun to be publicly examined and challenged—by consumer advocates, scientists and the medical profession. For instance, we've seen a good deal in the news recently about some of the energy drinks that are loaded with caffeine. But the assortment of products being created with caffeine added to them is much more extensive. It includes everything from waffles and syrup to chewing gum, breakfast oatmeal to jelly beans, marshmallow to sunflower seeds. It even includes caffeinated water.

This new marketplace raises many questions and concerns, both for us as the public health regulatory agency responsible for overseeing these products, and also for the food industry whose responsibility it is to ensure the safety of its products. And we're asking you to take a close look at these products. Surely a key question—one already identified by numerous consumer advocates, medical professionals and scientists—concerns the safety, availability and marketing of many of these products primarily to target populations that we might not ordinarily associated with caffeinated products, primarily children and adolescents.

Studies have demonstrated that, compared to adults, children are at increased risk for possible health effects from ingestion of even naturally occurring dosages of caffeine. And, with caffeine now appearing in so many different product types, it's possible that a young child may be at risk of ingesting caffeine from many sources in a given day without even having any sense of the exposure they are having from what they are eating and drinking. The consequences of this cumulative exposure are deserving of greater analysis, attention and understanding.

All of which is why we have asked the Institute of Medicine to undertake this workshop.

Specifically, we have requested that this workshop review the relevant literature, describe the vulnerable populations of concern and the health risks from dietary supplements and foods to which caffeine is being added, and, importantly, to identify data gaps.

The meetings today and tomorrow will allow us to take a close and thorough look at what is happening in the marketplace, how industry is proceeding with so-called innovation, what the science reveals about this area, and what actions, if any, might be necessary. It occurs at a critical time and offers a critical opportunity to evaluate the data and to reach some informed conclusions. Your deliberations will help guide us as we consider the right steps forward to protect public health.

Thank you.

Text 4

Remarks Presented by Michael Taylor, Deputy Commissioner for Foods, Food and Drug Administration on Global Food Safety Summit

Washington, D.C.
4 February 2010

I really do appreciate the chance to be here today and join so many people who are colleagues and partners in food safety. Today, I want to talk about how we—and I do mean all of us—are going to make food safer. And I have one very simple message, which is that I really do believe we are all in it together and that together, we can succeed in making food safer.

I'm going to talk about FDA's role in making food safer. But I really think it's critical to put FDA's role in a much broader food system context because the bottom line is that food safety is a food system challenge.

I don't need to review what the challenges are for this audience. You know the dynamic nature of the food system and the challenges we face. We do have a persistent burden of food-borne illness in this country. And recently, in particular, we've had some very visible, very large-scale outbreaks that have resulted in declining consumer confidence in the food safety system itself and big economic impacts for the industry.

And we at FDA encounter this situation in a time where it has been a very long time since our laws have been modernized. We do operate under obsolete food safety laws and it has been a struggle to create the capacity to keep up with new scientific developments and the incredibly dynamic nature of the food system.

But the opportunity for progress has also never really been greater. And I think all of us who have been watching the political alignment around food safety in the United States are keenly aware of this. We really do have an opportunity to make some interesting changes. The White House has made food safety a priority. Congress is working on bipartisan food safety legislation that really would overhaul FDA's food safety laws. Within the Department of Health and Human Services, Secretary Sebelius, and FDA Commissioner Hamburg have a really deep, personal commitment to building a stronger program at FDA.

It's clear that we need a system that is prevention-oriented. That's really the fundamental principle of public health. We also need a system that's science- and risk-based. Don Zink, who spoke before me, and his colleagues are certainly leaders in that enterprise. This is really essential if we're going to have a system that's both effective and efficient in reducing food-borne illness and preventing food safety problems and a system in which the public can have confidence. Also important is a system that addresses food safety comprehensively from farm to table—again, a very familiar principle to the people in this room. And we also need a system here in the United States—and I know this goal is shared by countries around the world—a system that holds imported foods to the same standards that we set for domestic facilities.

So we really look forward to working with all of you here at GFSI[1]. We look forward to working with the food industry more broadly. I was delighted to accept the invitation to speak here because this really is a great place for me to be, early in my tenure, as I express my desire to open up a dialogue.

You know, we're really clear at FDA that there are no silver bullets, there are no magic wands for food safety. We're in a long-term, system-building mode at FDA. And I think it's the same in the private sector.

But FDA is certainly in it for the long haul. We have more than a 100-year history. We'll have another 100-year history. We want to get on with building a program and a food safety system we can all be proud of. And so we look forward to working with all of you and to future opportunities to get together.

六、汉译英练习

Text 5

新华网权威访谈：食品安全风险监测网络逐步覆盖全国
——卫生部部长陈竺谈食品安全风险监测与评估（节选）

食品安全风险监测评估制度建立实施

问：我国2009年颁布的食品安全法规定，要建立实施食品安全风险监测评估制

1 GFSI，即Global Food Safety Initiative，“全球食品安全倡议”，是由主要来自欧洲的国际性食品零售商于2000年5月创立的非营利性组织，其主要目标在于加强全球食品安全，切实保护消费者，增强消费者的信任度，建立必要的食品安全计划，通过食品供应链改进效能。

度。这项制度包括哪些内容？对促进食品安全管理有什么作用？

答：风险监测评估制度是食品安全法确立的一项重要制度。国内外实践证明，食品安全不存在“零风险”。为应对不断暴露的食品安全问题，国际社会普遍采用食品安全风险评估的方法评估食品中有害因素可能对人体健康造成的风险，并被世界贸易组织（WTO）和国际食品法典委员会（CAC）作为制定食品安全监管控制措施和标准的科学手段。

按照食品安全法及其实施条例的有关规定，卫生部于2009年组建成立了国家食品安全风险评估专家委员会，建立了专家委员会相关规章制度。先后出台《食品安全风险评估管理规定（试行）》《食品安全风险监测管理规定（试行）》等系列管理制度。牵头组织制定实施年度国家食品安全风险监测计划，各地根据国家计划组织制定实施本区域的风险监测方案。进一步扩大医疗机构等对食源性疾病隐患的监测布点，完善网络体系，及时组织开展隐患评估工作。

通过食品安全风险监测和评估可以为制定或者修订食品安全国家标准提供科学依据、确定监督管理的重点领域、发现食品安全隐患。同时，通过将风险监测和评估结果及时通报各食品安全监管部门，可以预防控制食品安全事故的发生，提高监督执法的针对性。

食品安全风险监测网络逐步覆盖全国

问：食品安全风险监测评估工作进展如何？

答：我们逐步建立了覆盖全国的食品安全风险监测网络。食品安全法公布实施以来，食品安全风险监测体系初步建立，国家食品安全风险监测计划已连续实施两年，对全面掌握全国食品安全状况和开展针对性监管执法提供了重要依据。目前，全国共设置化学污染物和食品中非法添加物以及食源性致病微生物监测点1 196个，覆盖了100%的省份、73%的市和25%的县，在416个医疗机构主动监测食源性异常病例或健康事件。此外，我们还开展了一系列应急和常规食品安全风险评估项目，完成了三聚氰胺、丙烯酰胺、苏丹红、氯丙醇、溴酸盐、二噁英污染等风险评估基础性工作。

在构建食品安全风险监测网的同时，我们努力提高我国食品安全风险监测评估工作水平。建立健全风险监测评估制度规范，完善相应工作机制和程序；建设国家食品安全风险监测参比实验室、食品中非法添加物和放射性物质检测等实验室；建立监测数据共享平台，研究设立风险评估模型，不断提高食品安全风险监测评估能力。特别是在党中央、国务院的高度重视下，在有关部门的支持下，国家食品安全风险评估中心于去年10月正式挂牌组建，我相信评估中心的成立将对完善食品安全技术支撑体系、进一步提高风险监测评估水平发挥重要作用。

Text 6

李克强副总理在国务院食品安全委员会第四次全体会议上的讲话（节选）

2012年2月8日

食品安全事关人民群众切身利益，事关经济发展与社会和谐稳定，事关政府形象及其执行力，也事关我国国际形象。党中央、国务院对食品安全工作高度重视，胡锦涛总书记、温家宝总理都对此做出重要指示。今天的会议，主要是总结2011年工作，分析研究当前形势，安排部署2012年食品安全重点工作任务。刚才，回良玉、王岐山副总理发表了重要意见，有关部门负责同志也提出了很好的建议，我都赞成。下面，我讲几点意见。

一、充分肯定成绩，全面认识食品安全工作的重要性、长期性和艰巨性

2011年，各地区、各有关部门认真贯彻落实党中央、国务院关于食品安全工作的各项决策部署，加大力度，创新方式，完善机制，依法开展重点专项整治，统筹推进各项任务，有效遏制了食品安全事件高发态势，维护了人民群众利益，得到社会各界肯定。

在肯定成绩的同时，我们也要清醒地看到，食品安全面临的形势依然严峻。

一是食品安全事件仍然频发，在食品中非法添加和滥用添加剂、制售假冒伪劣食品以及环境污染造成的食品安全等问题凸显。二是食品产业基础仍然薄弱，食品生产经营单位多、小、散特点突出，带来大量食品安全风险隐患。三是食品安全诚信环境有待改善，一些食品生产经营者道德缺失、自律缺失，一些不法分子见利忘义、以身试法。四是食品安全监管仍然薄弱，人员装备和技术手段相对落后，监管交叉和空白并存，长效机制亟待建立。这些都表明了保障食品安全的复杂性、长期性和艰巨性，各地区、各有关部门一定要进一步提高认识，以对党和国家、对人民群众高度负责的态度，把食品安全工作摆在更加突出的位置，须臾不可放松，既要打好攻坚战，又要打好持久战，切实提高我国食品安全水平。

二、深入开展综合整治，打好食品安全攻坚战

从去年的工作经验看，在当前食品安全问题集中多发、矛盾复杂叠加的阶段，集中力量进行综合治理和专项整治是行之有效的必要手段，必须打好食品安全综合治理和专项整治攻坚战，向人民群众昭示政府坚定不移地抓好食品安全的决心和信心。

三、着力构建长效机制，打好食品安全持久战

在打好治理整顿攻坚战的同时，必须牢固树立打持久战的思想。保障食品安

全，既要抓当前，更要管长远，狠抓基础工作和规范建设，标本兼治，形成食品安全工作的长效机制。

四、真抓实干、全力以赴，做好2012年食品安全工作

做好食品安全工作，是党和人民赋予我们光荣而艰巨的使命，是民心工程[1]、德政工程[2]。各地区、各有关部门一定要进一步增强责任感和使命感，全力以赴、开拓创新、真抓实干，努力做好今年食品安全工作。

资料来源：

Text 1 http://www.fao.org/fileadmin/user_upload/newsroom/docs/2013-07-02-36th-session-codex-alimentarius-statement-DG-speech-en.pdf

Text 2 http://www.who.int/dg/speeches/2013/codex_alimentarius_20130702/en/

Text 3 http://www.fda.gov/NewsEvents/Speeches/ucm363925.htm

Text 4 http://www.fda.gov/AboutFDA/CentersOffices/OfficeofFoods/ucm206457.htm

Text 5 http://www.jdzx.net.cn/article/40288ce4062bb60401062bb60cef0014/2012/2/2c909e8c33151ad001357a7dafe51192.html

Text 6 http://views.ce.cn/main/qy/xzgl/201106/15/t20110615_22480356.shtml

1 政府为解决老百姓的困难，改善老百姓的生活而采取的措施和实施的项目。

2 有益于人民的政治措施和工作。

参考答案

四、摘要练习

Text 1

国际食品法典委员会第36届会议发言

联合国粮食及农业组织总干事何塞·格拉齐亚诺·达席尔瓦
意大利罗马
2013年7月2日

国际食品法典委员会主席，桑杰·戴维先生，
我的姐妹，世界卫生组织总干事陈冯富珍，
各位尊敬的阁下：

国际食品法典委员会50年前在罗马正式成立。

1963年7月，作为FAO/WHO联合食品标准计划的主要机构，国际食品法典委员会举行了第一次会议。

从那时起，食品法典委员会已给世界各地带来更安全、更有营养的食品。

自创建开始，食品法典委员会有30名成员，现已发展到成员包括185个国家政府、一个会员组织和220名观察员。

食品法典委员会提供的结果、以科学为基础的决策过程、参与性和真正意义上的全球会员制度促成了食品法典委员会的信誉和作为标准制定机构较高的声誉。

如今，很难想象如果没有食品法典委员会及其国际食品标准、指南和实践标准，我们的食物、身体健康甚至经济会是什么样的情况。

然而，即使在今天，很多人都没有意识到食品法典委员会对我们日常生活的巨大影响。

无论是在超市购物、生产有机蔬菜、为家畜接种疫苗或经销海鲜，在某种程度上，你的生活都会受到食品法典委员会的影响或保护，以上只是其中的几个例子。

在座的各位负责帮助实现这一点，因此我要感谢你们。

女士们、先生们，

食品法典委员会标准的制定是粮农组织的重要职责，在我们评审通过的战略框架和工作方案中也得到确认。

对于粮农组织彻底消除饥饿和营养不良的全球目标而言，食品安全也非常重

要，因为如果人们的食物不安全，就无法实现得到足够粮食的保障。

因此，粮农组织感到非常自豪，能够参与食品法典委员会的过去、现在和未来。

此外，食品法典在其创建之时具有重大意义，今天依旧如此。

食品法典委员会使健康、营养丰富的食物更易获取，为直接依赖于农业和食品体系谋取生计的人提供标准和指导。

在过去的50年，食品法典委员会已经做了很多工作来加强各国的食品安全系统和促进国际食品贸易，国际食品贸易的总额已经从1963年的220亿美元增长为超过1.3万亿美元。

食品法典是世界贸易组织的工作的重要参考。

世界贸易组织将食品法典委员会作为其《食品安全卫生与植物卫生措施协定》的最终标准制定机构。

制订世界贸易组织协议的目的是通过食品安全和卫生标准帮助各国保护本国人民，同时防止他们使用这些标准对竞争对手进行不公平的阻碍。

成员国在食品法典委员会中积极发挥作用，协助各国在全球食品市场竞争，同时还可以提高本国的食品安全。

食品法典委员会所做的大部分工作可以直接转化为国家立法。

它包括数以千计的农药残留、兽药、污染物、食品添加剂的最高安全水平。

此外，食品法典委员会还帮助各国协调统一世界各地的食品标签，开发操作方法以帮助生产者减少和防止污染，通过危害分析与关键控制点体系（HACCP）建立和改善食品卫生。

食品法典委员会还建立并应用了食品安全决策的风险分析。粮农组织和世卫组织通过独立专家机构提供了切实的科学依据，为食品法典委员会建立食品安全标准提供了坚实基础。

对于未直接设置标准的领域，食品法典委员会给出详细的建议，以帮助成员国建立自己的规定。

总之，食品法典委员会已表明，在不影响其宗旨和科学方法的前提下，它可以迅速采取行动，并在一年之内设置急需的标准。

本周，我们可以花点时间来庆祝我们一起工作所取得的成效——在各国国内以及国际范围的成效。当然，我们仍然有大量的工作要做。

新的食源性疾病不断涌现，或者被发现，新的食品产品和生产方法也不断出现。这意味着我们需要新的标准。

女士们、先生们，

食品法典委员会必须跟上不断变化的世界，因为当前世界的交通、通讯和科学发展均已飞速提升，对食品安全直接产生重大影响。

我们也有一些资金方面的挑战。在筹集资金进行研究并为建立食品法典提供科学依据方面，我们经历了重大困难。我们需要找到一个可持续的解决方案。

法典信托基金通过食品法典委员会成员大量自愿捐款形成，使食品法典委员会成为真正的全球性组织。但是，基金将于2015年结束，我们需要考虑如何继续提供必需的支持。

另一个问题是，食品法典委员会虽已创建各级食品链的重要环节，但它仍然是一个置身幕后几乎隐形的参与者。

我们在未来几年将需要考虑的问题之一是如何确保食品法典委员会在直接影响圈外得到更多认可和接受。

我们需要增加与消费者协会的互动和国家层面的参与。

首先，重要的是要一起行动，争取实现更大的跨越行业、跨越国界、跨越不同管辖范围的合作。

粮农组织、世卫组织、食品法典委员会、世界动物卫生组织（OIE）和国际植物保护公约（IPPC）组织密切合作，设计满足这个理想的框架、标准、指南和守则。

这也符合“唯一健康”的方式来进行跨学科工作，实现人、动物和环境的健康。

让我代表粮农组织再补充一句话，我们庆祝的不仅是食品法典委员会建立50年，法典委员会是历史最悠久的联合国系统内的合作机构之一，这也非常值得庆祝。

我还想亲自感谢世卫组织总干事为确保联合工作成功做出的努力。

我也感谢大家支持我们的工作，以保证每个人享有安全、优质的食物，并保证我们所有人拥有健康、可持续发展的未来。

感谢您的关注。

Text 2

庆祝食品法典委员会成立50周年发言

世界卫生组织总干事陈冯富珍博士

意大利罗马

2013年7月2日

各位尊敬的阁下，尊敬的代表，来自民间组织、私有部门、科研机构、联合国系统内我们姐妹机构的代表，女士们、先生们：

请允许我对国际食品法典委员会成立50周年表示热烈的祝贺。食品法典委员会这50年来带来了许多转变，世界卫生组织非常自豪地参与庆祝活动。

起初，食品法典委员会是粮农组织和世界卫生组织之间的合作事业，得到了各国的支持。它是联合国大家庭中运行时间最长的合作事业，也已产生深远的影响。

成立食品法典委员会是为了满足一个巨大而且突出的需要。在20世纪60年代初，各个国家涉及控制食品质量和安全的法律存在非常大的差异。

制订法律往往没有健全的科学基础，也总是忽视营养学的基本原则。混乱、差异、缺乏严谨性或一致性的情况对贸易构成重大壁垒。

食品法典委员开始介入，目的是消除这些贸易壁垒，以科学的方式提供保护消费者的服务，围绕世界食品供应建立实质性的安全网。

世界卫生组织一直是食品法典委员会工作上最热心的合作伙伴。事实上，这也是我们工作的一部分。国际食品标准的建立，是世界卫生组织宪法规定的世界卫生组织的职责。

1953年，世界卫生大会对食品工业中化学药品的使用越来越多表示关注，认为这是一个需要加以解决的新的健康问题。

消费者也表达了担忧。大多数坏了的食品看起来很糟糕，味道也不好闻。但食品中毒素、添加剂、农药和兽药残留的存在造成的危害是眼睛看不到、鼻子闻不到、嘴巴尝不出来的。消费者想要一些安全保障。他们希望得到保护。

食品法典委员会解决了这些问题和许多其他问题。

在过去的几十年中，食品法典委员会制订了适用于广泛范围的食品标准，包括加工、半加工、原料食品商品，例如香料和干果、新鲜牛奶和肉类、特殊膳食用食品。

产生的效果令人瞩目。食品法典委员会一共建立了200多个食品标准和100多个食品生产和加工实践指南及守则。

食品法典委员会还讨论了那些“隐形”危害，为数以千计的食品添加剂、污染物、农药和兽药残留建立了最高容许水平。

如今，食品法典委员会的标准是食品安全标准的参照基准。没有其他机构能和他们竞争。他们是国际上公认最好的，食物链上的每一个环节都能做到最好。

食品标准促进食品贸易中的公平做法。符合国际标准的食品能更自由地实现跨越国界的移动。食品标准提供了公平的竞争环境。发展中国家生产的符合国际标准的食品可以在平等的基础上进入国际贸易。

食品法典委员会已经对食品生产者和加工者的经营方式、消费者对食品安全和营养质量的信心产生了巨大影响，无论是在本国或国外销售的食品都是如此。

如今，消费者会期望他们购买的食品与标签上注明的信息相符。这种信任来自于食品法典委员会几十年的工作。

食品法典委员会的标准促进公平性。世界上的每个人都应当得到同样的保障，吃到既安全又富有营养的食物。

食品法典委员会以严谨的科学方法为基础，通过激励食物相关的科学技术研究，提高了食品质量评估标准。

如今，食品法典委员会的成员涵盖了世界人口的99%。发展中国家一旦采用法典标准，也会受益匪浅。但食品法典委员会需要更加广泛的参与。

正如你们已经听到过的，世界卫生组织和联合国粮农组织于2003年成立了法典信托基金。在其10年的历史中，法典信托基金已被用于支持来自134个国家的2 000多人参加食品法典委员会的会议和工作组。一个国家如果非常了解食品标准设立的过程，将能够更好地诠释和实施标准。

女士们、先生们，

安全和有营养的食物维持人类的生命，在理想状态下还可以维持良好的健康状况。不安全的食品可能导致疾病，有时甚至导致非常严重的疫情。被污染的食物有可能致命，通常会对非常年幼或年老的人造成最严重的危害。

饥饿、营养不良及其对健康造成的不良后果始终是引起国际关注的首要问题。关于粮食安全的谈话是可持续发展的讨论内容，也是2015年之后发展计划的讨论内容。

在这些引起长期关注的问题之中，世界食品供应有了很大的改变。食品生产工业化程度越来越高。现在，销售网络也遍布全球。新鲜水果和蔬菜有明显的季节性这一概念几乎已经完全消失了。

这带来了一些好处。饥饿在全世界许多地方已经减少，饮食的多样性可以带来显著的健康效益。

但也有不好的一面。经济一体化和食品贸易的全球化意味着一顿饭可能包含来自世界各地的成分和原料。食物链的复杂性也有所增加，形成了更多可能出问题的关键点。

而且一旦出问题，往往就是非常大的问题。疫情的调查可能涉及多个洲的许多国家。可能需要大面积的召回，造成巨大的经济损失。消费者的信心一旦破灭，将需要很长的时间来恢复。

还有其他问题。如今，最便宜、最方便、最容易获得、最好吃的食物通常都热量高，但营养价值低。

今天，肥胖和饮食相关的非传染性疾病常常和营养不良并存于同一个国家，甚至同一个社区或家庭。好消息是现在食品法典委员会正在通过营养和食品标签委员会解决这个问题。

食品法典委员会的下一个巨大挑战可能是：引入更加平衡的世界食品供应。

我们希望看到的是：每个人都享有安全、营养、促进健康的食品，无论是本地生产或是国际贸易的产品。

谢谢。

五、英译汉练习

Text 3

食品和膳食补充剂中的咖啡因：安全检查

——美国食品药品监督管理局局长玛格丽特·汉伯格博士在美国国家科学院食品和营养董事会及健康科学政策董事会医学研究所会议上的讲话

美国华盛顿特区

2013年8月5日

感谢戈尔德曼博士介绍中的美言，也感谢你承担委员会主席的重要责任。我还想感谢委员会成员的工作，他们用自己的知识、专业能力和见解来影响食品和膳食补充剂中的咖啡因摄入带来的潜在健康危害问题。

今早我在会议厅里四周打量了一下，看到我们中的许多人以咖啡因开始我们的一天，咖啡因可能来自一杯咖啡或茶，也有些人喝健怡可乐。

这并不奇怪，咖啡因可能是世界上最经常被人们摄入的具有药理学活性的物质。咖啡因是中枢神经系统兴奋剂，天然存在于60多种植物中，包括咖啡豆、茶叶、用于给汽水调味的可乐坚果和用于制作巧克力的可可豆荚。

然而，如果房间里摆满咖啡杯并不奇怪，也就不应该引起人们的警惕。多年的调查和研究表明，成人适度使用含有自然产生的咖啡因的产品和不良影响无关。

当然，传统的一杯咖啡或茶——即便是现在人们常常喜欢要的“加大杯”——并不是你们今天工作的核心关注问题。对于美国食品和药品监督管理局，咖啡因既是药物也是食品添加剂。而你们的任务是仔细检查许多最新和新颖的产品，这些添加咖啡因的产品如今已在市场上泛滥。

其中一些产品已经开始接受公开审查和挑战——由消费者权益倡导人士、科学家和医学界进行。例如，我们在最近的新闻中看到大量关于某些添加咖啡因的能量饮料的报道。但添加了咖啡因的产品琳琅满目，种类非常广泛，包括蛋奶饼、糖浆、口香糖、早餐燕麦片、彩色胶质糖豆、棉花糖、葵花籽等各种食品，甚至还包括含咖啡因的水。

这个新的市场引发了许多疑问和担忧。我们作为公共卫生监管机构关注这个问题，因为我们负责监督这些产品；食品行业也对这一问题加以关注，因为它们的职责是确保产品的安全。请你们务必仔细检查这些产品。当然，众多消费者权益倡导者、医务人员和科学家都发现了一个关键问题，即许多以儿童和青少年为主要目标人群的产品的安全性、可获得性和销售方式，虽然我们通常不会将儿童、青少年和含咖啡因的产品联系起来。

有研究表明，与成人相比，即使摄入自然产生剂量的咖啡因也可能增加给儿童健康造成危害的风险。咖啡因现在存在于这么多不同类型的产品中，可能造成一个年幼的儿童对自己的饮食中存在的咖啡因没有任何了解的情况下，在任意一天中从许多来源摄入咖啡因。对这种累积摄入的后果应当进行更深入的分析、关注和了解。

所有这一切，就是我们要求美国医学研究所开展本次研讨会的原因。

具体而言，我们请本次研讨会回顾相关文献，描述引起关注的弱势群体，描述添加咖啡因的膳食补充剂和食品可能造成的健康危害，并完成一项非常重要的任务——找出数据的缺口。

今天以及明天的会议将帮助我们深入并全面地了解市场上发生的活动、行业如何进行所谓的创新、科学在这个领域中揭示了什么内容，以及如果要采取行动，应当采取什么样的行动。本次会议举办的时间是一个关键时刻，提供了一个重要的机会来评估数据，并在了解情况的基础上形成一些结论。你们的讨论将有助于引导我们找到正确的步骤来保障公众健康。

谢谢。

Text 4

食品药品监督管理局分管食品副局长迈克尔·泰勒在全球粮食安全峰会上的讲话

美国华盛顿特区

2010年2月4日

非常感谢有机会来到这里，见到这么多食品安全的工作同僚和合作伙伴。今天，我想谈谈我们——我是说所有人一起——如何使食品更安全。我想传达一个非常简单的信息，就是我深信食品卫生与我们所有人都息息相关，而且通过一起努力我们一定可以成功地使食品更安全。

我要谈谈食品药品监督管理局（FDA）在食品安全方面的职责。我认为有必要让FDA在更广泛的粮食系统范围内发挥作用，因为说到底，食品安全是整个食品系统的挑战。

我不需要为大家回顾食品安全挑战包括哪些内容。大家都知道粮食系统的动态性质和我们面临着哪些挑战。美国一直有食源性疾病的负担尤其是在近日，我们经历了一些非常突出的大规模食源性疾病疫情，已导致消费者对食品安全系统信心下降，对食品行业造成巨大经济影响。

FDA面对这些情况，而我们的法律已经很长一段时间没有进行现代化的更新了。我们工作的基础是过时的食品安全法律，要跟上新的科学发展和食物系统惊人的动态性，并培养相应的工作能力，非常困难。

但FDA也面对了最大的发展机遇。而且我认为，我们这些人一直关注着美国各地涉及食品安全的政治取向，我们都敏锐地意识到了这个机遇。我们真的有机会做出一些有意义的改变。白宫已将食品安全列为一个优先事项。国会正在制定两党共同支持的食品安全立法，将对FDA的食品安全法律进行彻底检查。美国卫生及公共服务部的西贝利厄斯部长和FDA汉伯格局长都非常重视建立FDA更强大的食品卫生部门，他们对此做出了个人承诺。

很明显，我们需要一个以预防为主的系统，这也的确是公共卫生的基本原则。我们还需要一个以科学和风险为基础的系统。我前面的发言人是唐纳德·辛克，他是FDA食品安全和应用营养中心高级科学顾问，他和他的同事们肯定是这项事业的领导者。我们还必须建立一个系统，能够有效且高效地减少食源性疾病和预防食品安全问题，使公众拥有信心。同样重要的是这个系统能够全面解决从农业生产到餐桌食用的各个方面的全部食品安全问题——再次强调，这也是参加这次会议的所有人都清楚的一项原则。此外，我们在美国也需要食品安全系统能够对进口食品实施和国内食品生产设施一致的标准，我知道这不仅是美国的目标，也是全世界各国共同的目标。

所以，我们非常期待与在座的各位通过全球食品安全倡议一起合作。我们期待与食品行业进行更广泛的合作。我非常高兴能得到邀请，在这里发言，因为这次会议满足了我在任职初期表达的对创建对话的愿望。

其实，FDA的人都很清楚我们没有什么撒手锏，或是彻底解决问题的魔杖。FDA正处在一个长期的、系统建设的模式之中。而且我认为私有部门也处于同样的状态。

但FDA将长期参与这项工作。FDA有超过100年的历史，我们将有另一个100年的历史。我们希望能建立引以为豪的食品卫生部门和食品安全系统。因此，我们期待和你们合作，期待未来团聚的机会。

六、汉译英练习

Text 5

Interview with Xinhua News Agency on Food Safety Risk Monitoring and Assessment: Food Safety Risk Monitoring Netwook to Gradually Cover China (Excerpt)

Chen Zhu

Minister of Health, Government of China

The establishment and implementation of the food safety risk monitoring and assessment system

Q: According to the Food Safety Act issued in 2009, a food safety risk monitoring and assessment system was to be established and implemented in China. What is included in this system? What kind of role does the system play in the promotion of food safety administration?

A: Risk monitoring and assessment system is an important system established by the Food Safety Act. Domestic and overseas practice has shown that "zero risk" in food safety does not exist. In response to the constant emergence of food safety problems, the international community generally adopts risk assessment for food safety to assess the potential health risk of harmful substances contained in food. In addition, the World Trade Organization (WTO) and the Codex Alimentarius Commission (CAC) use risk assessment for food safety as the scientific method for formulating food safety related guidelines, standards and codes.

In accordance with the Food Safety Act and the relevant provisions in its implementation regulations, the Ministry of Health founded the national expert committee for food safety risk assessment and established rules and regulations for the committee in 2009. Then, Food Safety Risk Assessment Regulations (Trial), Food Safety Risk Monitoring Regulations (Trial) and a series of other policies were introduced. The leadership organizations develop the annual national plans for the implementation of national food safety risk monitoring and assessment program, the institutions concerned at the local level develop and implement their local risk monitoring and assessment programs on the basis of the national plan. Medical institutions will further expand and improve the monitoring network of potential risks for foodborne diseases. Risk assessment activities will be conducted whenever they are needed.

Food safety risk monitoring and assessment helps provide solid evidence for the formulation or revision of national food safety standards, determine key areas of supervision and management, and identify potential food safety problems. Meanwhile, findings from risk monitoring and assessment activities will be reported to the food safety supervision department promptly, which will help prevent and control food safety problems. In addition, specific supervision and law enforcement actions will be adopted for specific problems.

Food safety risk monitoring network will gradually cover the whole country.

Q: What progress has been made for food safety risk monitoring and assessment?

A: We are gradually setting up a nationwide food safety risk monitoring network. Since the promulgation and implementation of the Food Safety Act, a food safety risk monitoring system has been gradually established and the national food safety risk monitoring plan has been implemented for two years, providing solid evidence for a thorough understanding of the food safety issues across the country and facilitating targeted regulatory and law enforcement actions. Currently, the government has set up 1,196 monitoring sites of chemical contaminants, illegal food additives, as well as foodborne pathogenic microorganisms, covering all the provinces, 73% of the cities, and 25% of the counties in China. 416 medical service facilities have provider-initiated monitoring program for abnormal cases of foodborne diseases or health problems. In addition, we also carried out a series of emergency and routine food safety risk assessment projects and successfully completed the risk assessment of melamine, acrylamide, Sudan red dye, chloropropanol, bromate, and dioxin contamination.

In addition to building a food safety risk monitoring network, we are striving to improve the competence of food safety risk monitoring and assessment in China. We have established and improved the risk monitoring and assessment system regulations and improved the relevant working mechanisms and procedures. We have built national food safety risk monitoring reference laboratories and labs to test illegal food additives and radioactive substances. We have also established a platform to share monitoring data. We are conducting research into risk assessment models because we intend to continuously improve our capacity in food safety risk monitoring and assessment. Thanks to the special attention from the Central Committee of the Communist Party of China (CPC) and the State Council and the support from the departments concerned, the National Center for Food Safety Risk Assessment was established and opened in October last year. I believe that the risk assessment centers will help improve the technical support system for food safety, and that they will play an important role in improving China's capacity of risk monitoring and assessment.

Text 6

Speech at the Fourth Plenary Session of Food Safety Commission of the State Council by Li Keqiang, Vice Premier of the State Council (Excerpt)

8 February 2012

Food safety concerns the vital interests of the people. It is also closely associated with economic development, social harmony and social stability. It bears on not only the image of the government and its execution capacity, but also China's international image. CPC Central Committee and the State Council attach great importance to food safety. Both CPC General Secretary Hu Jintao and Premier Wen Jiabao have given important instructions on food safety. At today's meeting, we will sum up the work done in 2011, analyze the current situation, and make arrangements for the prioritized tasks for food safety in 2012. Just now, Vice Premier Hui Liangyu and Vice Premier Wang Qishan made some important comments and officials from the departments concerned made some good suggestions. I completely agree with what they have said. Now, I'd like to make a few comments.

First of all, I'd like to fully affirm the achievements, but we must also be aware that our work in food safety is not only very important, but also protracted and difficult.

In 2011, the local governments and the departments concerned implemented the food safety decisions and plans made by the CPC Central Committee and the State Council. They intensified their efforts, adopted innovative methods and improved mechanisms. In accordance with relevant laws and regulations, they have carried out rectification activities targeted at specific issues and made an effort to coordinate the implementation of various activities. As a result, they were able to effectively curb the high incidence of food safety problems, safeguard people's interests, and win the approval of various circles of the society.

While it is important to recognize achievements, we must also be acutely aware of the gravity of the situation in food safety.

A) Food safety incidents are still constantly emerging. Some of them deserve special attention, for example, illegal use and overuse of food additives, manufacturing and selling of counterfeit and shoddy food commodities, and food safety problems caused by environmental pollution. B) The food industry does not have a strong basis.

Food manufacturers and businesses are large in number and small in size, and are widely dispersed, causing a lot of potential risks for food safety hazards. C) The overall environment of vocational ethics for food safety still has to be improved. A number of food producers and businesses fail to follow vocational ethics and lack self-discipline. What's more, some unscrupulous criminals are happy to defy the law if they will make profits by doing so. D) Food safety supervision remains very weak. Human resources, equipment and technical means are all relatively backward and obsolete. Regulatory overlaps and gaps co-exist and there is an urgent need to establish long-term mechanisms. All these problems indicate that food safety is a complicated, protracted and arduous journey. The local governments and departments concerned must raise their awareness, keep a responsible attitude to CPC, the nation and the people, and give high priority to food safety. We will take the problem very seriously. We'll be ready to tackle the difficult issues on a long-term basis in the battle against food safety problems and eventually, we will effectively improve food safety in China.

Secondly, we will carry out comprehensive rectification campaigns to deal with food safety problems in the long run.

Based on the experience from last year, current food safety issues are characterized by multiple and concentrated incidence and a contradictory, complicated and overlapping nature. Therefore, the answer to the problem and a necessary step to take is to pool our forces and implement comprehensive management and specific corrective activities in response to specific problems. By so doing, we are showing the government's determination, commitment and confidence in resolving the food safety problems.

Thirdly, we will work hard to build long-term mechanisms and get ready to fight food safety problems in the long run.

When we start the campaign to tackle challenging food safety problems, we must be mentally prepared that this is going to be a protracted battle. When we look at the food safety issues, we have to think about not only the present moment, but also the future. It is important that we pay close attention to the basic work, set up standards, deal with the problem not only on the surface, but also at the root, and form a long-term mechanism for food safety.

Fourthly, we should make solid effort and go all out to do a great job to improve food safety in 2012.

It is certainly a great honor that the CPC and the people handed us the arduous mission of improving food safety, which will benefit the people and help improve their confidence in the government. The local governments and departments concerned will further enhance their sense of responsibility and mission, and dedicate themselves to the improvement of food safety.

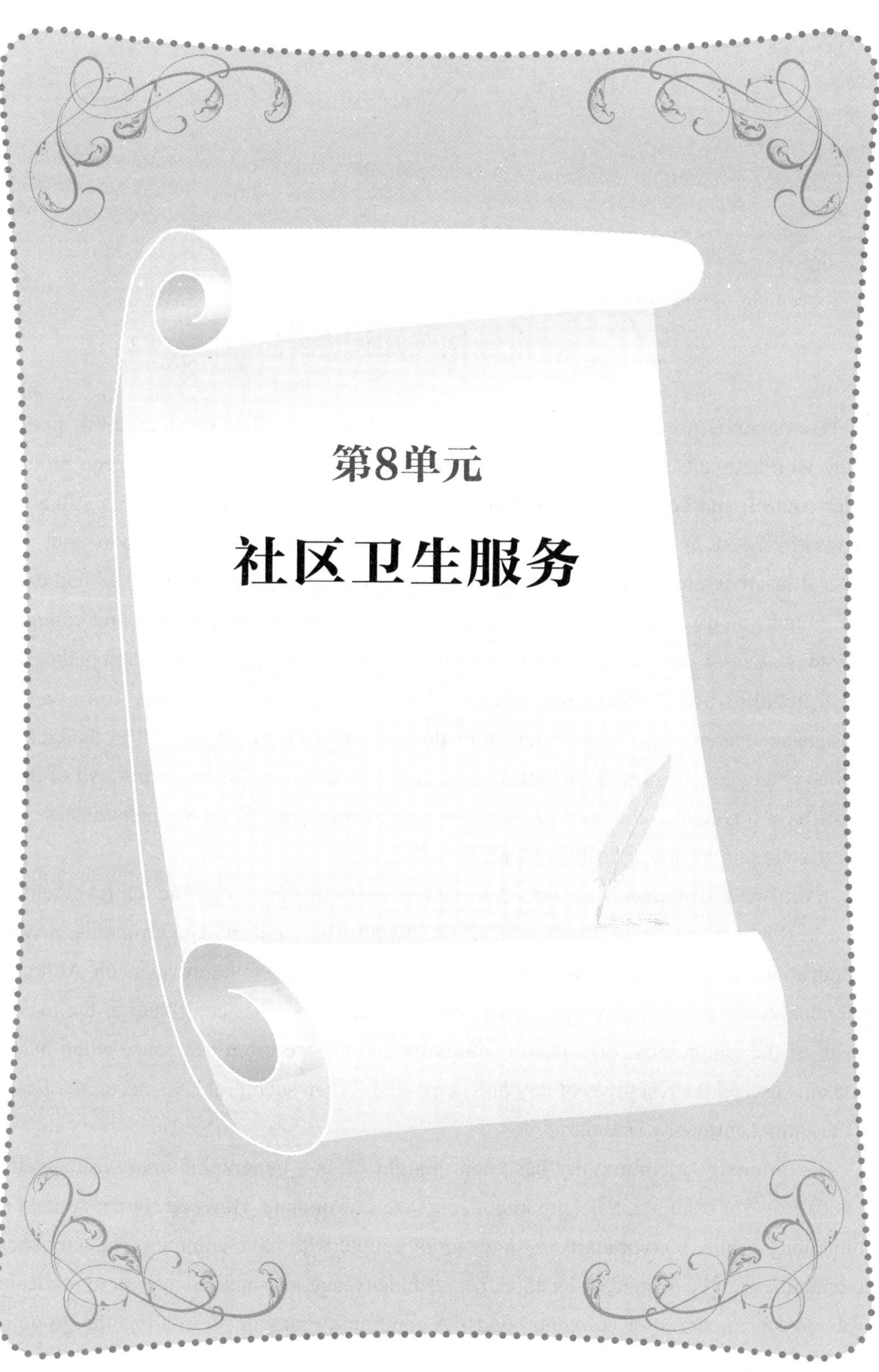

第8单元

社区卫生服务

一、主题相关知识介绍

Tremendous progress has been made in the health and life expectancy of people of the world. Infant mortality dropped, any of the infectious diseases have been brought under control, and better family planning became available. However, there is still room for improvement! Individual health behaviors, such as the use of tobacco, poor diet, and physical inactivity, have given rise to an unacceptable number of cases of illness and death from noninfectious diseases such as cancer, diabetes, and heart disease. New and emerging infectious diseases, such as the 2009 H1N1 flu and those caused by drug-resistant pathogens, are stretching resources available to control them. And events stemming from natural disasters such as earthquakes and human-made disasters such as the oil spill in the Gulf of Mexico and terrorism around the world have caused us to refocus our priorities. All of these events have highlighted the need for improvement in emergency response preparedness and infrastructure of the public health system.

Even with all that has happened in recent years in the world, the achievement of good health remains a worldwide goal of the twenty-first century. Governments, private organizations, and individuals throughout the world are working to improve health. Although individual actions to improve one's own personal health certainly contribute to the overall health of the community, organized community actions are often necessary when health problems exceed the resources of any one individual. When such problems occur, the health of the entire community is at risk.

Traditionally, a community has been thought of as a geographic area with specific boundaries—for example, a neighborhood, city, county, or state. However, in the context of community health, a community is "a group of people who have common characteristics; communities can be defined by location, race, ethnicity, age, occupation, interest in particular problems or outcomes, or common bonds."A community may be as small as the group of people who live on a residence hall floor at a university or as large as all of the individuals who make up a nation. "A healthy community is a place where people provide leadership in assessing their own resources and needs, where public health and social infrastructure and policies support health, and where essential public health services, including quality health care, are available."

Community health refers to the health status of a defined group of people and the actions and conditions to promote, protect and preserve their health. For example, the health status of the people of Muncie, Indiana, and the private and public actions taken to promote, protect and preserve the health of these people would constitute community health.

Community health activities are activities that are aimed at protecting or improving the health of a population or community. Maintenance of accurate birth and death records, protection of the food and water supply, and participating in fund drives for voluntary health organizations such as the American Lung Association are examples of community health activities.

There are a great many factors that affect the health of a community. As a result, the health status of each community is different. These factors may be physical, social, and/or cultural. They also include the ability of the community to organize and work together as a whole as well as the individual behaviors of those in the community.

二、技巧指导：目的语信息重组的几个方法（Ⅰ）

译员工作时，要执行多重任务（multitasking）：耳听信息片段，分辨信息片段，记录信息片段，然后回忆信息片段，语言转换信息片段，产出信息片段。整个阶段包含了解析信息、逻辑整理、综合信息和信息重组的过程。语言转换和信息产出阶段包含了信息重组概念。为了使产出的信息符合译入语的习惯和表达方式，满足听众理解的要求，我们总结了几种能够有效完成信息重组的方法，包括顺句驱动与适当调整法、重组法、拆句法、合并法、增译法、简译法、倒置法、包孕法、插入法等。要注意的是，教科书中分成多种方法来写，是为了讲清每一种方法，但在口译实践中，这些方法不是截然分开而是相辅相成的，需要在实践中融会贯通，配合使用。

●顺句翻译与适当调整（syntactic linearity and appropriate adjustment）

顺句翻译是指对照源语言的语序将需要翻译的内容译成译入语，换句话说，翻译之后，译入语的语序与源语言的语序大致相同。是否用这个方法，首先要判断原语言句型是否适合顺句对译，其次这个过程经常伴随着适当调整。适当调整是指在顺句对译的过程中，不完全按照源语言的语序，而根据需要在局部做微小调整，例如增补、删减、换位、合并等。一般综合使用两个方法，先听到的内容先处理，后听到的内容后处理，在个别信息单位上稍作调整。调整实际上融合了多种方法。由于此法便捷，在信息重组的时候能够减轻负担，因此是首选之良策。

英译中例句：

1. A standard may be *mandatory* (required by law), *voluntary* (established by professional organizations and available for use), or *de facto* (generally accepted by custom or convention way of dress, manners or behavior). It can be measured and enforced in a wide variety of ways.

标准可以是强制性的（法律要求），也可以是自愿性的（由专业机构制定，方便使用），还可以是实际存在的（习俗和惯例接受的，如穿着方式、行为方式）。标准可以用各式各样的办法来衡量和执行。

2. The role of PHAC is to: Promote health; Prevent and control chronic diseases and injuries; Prevent and control infectious diseases; Prepare for and respond to public health emergencies; Serve as a central point for sharing Canada's expertise with the rest of the world; Apply international research and development to Canada's public health programs; and Strengthen intergovernmental collaboration on public health and facilitate national approaches to public health policy and planning.

PHAC的作用是：促进健康，预防并控制慢性疾病和外伤；预防并控制传染病；准备并应对突发公共卫生事件；承当中心点，与世界其他地区分享加拿大的专业知识；申请国际研究和开发，为加拿大的公共卫生项目申请国际研究和开发项目；加强公众健康方面的政府间合作，并协助国家手段在公共卫生政策和规划方面的应用。

中译英例句：

1. 站在新的起点上，卫生系统要进一步统一思想，明确任务，充分发挥行业组织优势和专业优势，认真贯彻李克强副总理重要讲话和本次会议精神，全面落实"十二五"医改规划和2012年医改主要工作安排确定的各项任务，坚定不移地将医改推向深入。

Standing now on a new starting point, we in the health system must further unify our thoughts, clarify our tasks, and give full play to our organizational and professional advantages. We must earnestly implement the guidance of Vice Premier Li Keqiang's important speech and of this meeting, fully implement the "12th Five-Year" medicare reform plan and tasks identified by 2012 healthcare reform, and unswervingly deepen medicare reform.

2. 新医改提出“保基本，强基层，建机制”的基本原则，明确了医疗卫生事业的公益性质，突出了政府在医疗卫生事业中的主导作用，有效弥补了医疗卫生领域“市场失灵”的问题，切实维护了基本医疗卫生的公益性，促进了社会公平公正。

The new healthcare reform has put forward the basic principles of "insuring essentials, strengthening services for the grass-roots, and establishing mechanism", clarified that medical and health enterprises are public services, highlighted the dominant role of government in medical and health enterprises, effectively repaired "market failure" in medicine and healthcare, practically maintained the commonweal nature of the essential medicare service, and promoted social fairness and justice.

●重组法（reorganization）

当两种语言句法结构完全不同时，使用顺句翻译便会难以操作，这时就要尽快抓住原文的主要信息点，放弃原文的表达顺序，按照译入语的表达习惯重新组织原句的信息，翻译出原文所要表达的意思。

英译中例句：

This is important for two reasons. First, when uninsured people who can afford coverage get sick and show up at the emergency room for care, the rest of us end up paying for their care in the form of higher premiums.

之所以说这个重要，有两个原因。首先，有些人能够承受医疗费用但又没有买保险，当这些人生了病并到急诊室求医的时候，我们其余的人实际上在为这部分人支付医疗费，付款的方式是支付更高的保费。

中译英例句（既有重组也有顺译）：

近几年，我国专家在脑中风筛查及干预试点中发现，许多病人由于颈动脉狭窄引致的中风体征，如肢体活动障碍、失语、听力减退甚至丧失、视网膜或黄斑病变以及视力明显下降等，在颈动脉狭窄解除后，均得到了明显改善或恢复。甚至在核磁共振影像上已显示脑功能区部分坏死的病人，在解除颈动脉狭窄后，其已丧失的功能又出现恢复的奇迹。

In recent years' stroke screening and intervention pilot project, our experts finds that many patients with carotid artery stenosis have developed stroke signs, such as limb movement disorder, aphasia, hearing loss, retina macular degeneration, and decreased vision. These symptoms have obviously mitigated or disappeared after carotid artery stenosis was treated. Patients with partial necrosis in functional areas of brain reflected in magnetic resonance imaging have miraculous recovery of their lost function after carotid stenosis is treated.

三、词汇准备

Text 1

Secretary of the Department of Health and Human Services （美国）卫生及公共服务部部长

community health centers 社区卫生服务中心

uninsured 没有保险的

coverage （保险）覆盖

expansion of health coverage 扩大医保覆盖面积

outreach workers 外展工作人员

create bilingual education material 编写、制作双语宣传教育材料

boost technological capacity 增强、提高技术能力

get the word out 把消息传开去，发布信息

health center award recipient 社区卫生中心拨款获得者

shine a light on 使明了、了解

business community 商业界，商界

Blue Cross Blue Shield 蓝十字蓝盾协会

frustrated 沮丧的，挫败的，失意的

gouge 敲（某人）的竹杠，漫天要价

turn away 拒绝接待，不加理睬

affordable 负担得起的，实惠的

undertaking 任务，工作

pale 相形失色

stand to gain 一定获利，一定受益

a robust plan 强有力的计划

Text 2

wellness 健康，幸福
objectives 目标（与goal相比，goal的目标更长远）
vision, envision 愿景
commitment 承诺，承担
Nurse Practitioners 执业护士
FASD fetal alcohol spectrum disorder 胎儿酒精谱系障碍
substance abuse 滥用药物
Yukon 加拿大育空地区
cost-effective 最具成本效益的
Client-oriented care 以客户为中心的关怀
evidence-based interventions 询证干预
community inclusion 社区接纳
performance measurement 绩效评估
Patient/Client-centred service delivery 提供以患者/客户为中心的服务
live fully 充实地生活
empower 赋能

Text 3

initiatives 倡议，新方案
Secretary of Health and Human Services (HHS) （美国）卫生及公共服务部部长
Administrator of the Health Resources and Services Administration （美国）卫生资源和服务局局长
Deputy Secretary of HHS （美国）卫生及公共服务部副部长
quality care 优质医疗卫生服务
promoting wellness 促进良好状态
unmet 未满足的
critical 严重的，不稳定的，可能有危险的
medical needs 医疗需求
reduce ethnic and racial disparities in care 减少、缩小医疗中的民族和种族差异
accessing primary health care 使用初级医疗保健服务
underserved areas 缺医少药的，缺乏医疗资源的
regular checkup 定期体检
routine screenings 常规疾病筛查

tough it out 忍耐过去，咬紧牙关挺过去
hope for the best 做最好的打算；抱乐观的态度
complications 并发症
chronic conditions 慢性疾病
have no place in 不应发生或存在
where on the political spectrum we fall 在政治光谱上的位置，每个人的政治立场
defend 为……辩护
health insurance reform 医疗保险改革
Recovery Act 经济复苏法案
recession 经济衰退
be well on one's way to 顺利进行
Congressional Budget Office （美国）国会预算办公室
renewable energy 可再生能源容量
chicken coop 养鸡场
cramped 拥挤的
fire station 消防站
double-book 重复预订（将同一房间、座位、餐桌等同时预订给不同的人）
standing room 立足之地，空间只容站立的地方
skyrocketing 飞涨的，猛涨的
economic downturn 经济衰退
health information technology system 医疗信息技术系统
manage administrative and financial matters 管理行政和财务事物
paper file 纸质版档案
electronic medical record 电子病历
providers （医疗卫生服务）提供机构
demonstration project 示范项目
"medical home" model of care "医疗之家"医疗保健服务模型
keep track of 追踪，记录，密切注意……的动向
referral 转诊
plan of care 医疗保健计划
peace of mind 内心的宁静，平静，安心
be there for 愿随时提供帮助，在那里
take up a cause 承担这一事业
pave the way for 为……创造条件，为……做好准备

with so much at stake 利益攸关
memo 备忘录

Text 4

health center sites 社区卫生服务中心服务点
cornerstone 基石，基础，奠基石
Powering Healthier Communities 增强健康社区
private insurance 私营保险
proven 得到证实的，已证明有效的
ripple through 传播到，波及
dental checkup 检查牙齿，齿科检查
fill one’s prescription 按处方配药、取药
make... a top priority 把……列为头等大事，对……予以优先考虑
Affordable Care Act 平价医疗法案
add new locations 开设新的服务点
vulnerable population 脆弱人群
immunizations 免疫接种，疫苗接种
manage conditions 管理疾病
miss work 误工
bolster local economies 加强当地经济

Text 5

深化医药卫生体制改革 deepen reform in the medical and health care system
践行科学发展观 adopt the scientific concept of development
实施方案 implementation plan
全面部署 make comprehensive arrangements for
加强 reinforce, strengthen
基本公共卫生服务均等化 equitable basic public health services
城市化 urbanization
老龄化 population aging
疾病谱 disease spectrum
医疗卫生事业 health care industry
覆盖城乡居民的基本医疗卫生制度 a basic health care system that covers urban and rural residents

安全、有效、方便、价廉的医疗卫生服务 safe, effective, convenient and affordable health care services

健康教育 health education

传染病防治 prevention of infectious diseases

慢性病管理 chronic disease management

妇幼保健 maternal and child health care

普及医疗卫生知识 popularize information on health care

预防为主的 prevention-based, prevention-oriented

主动服务 take an initiative to provide services

上门服务 deliver services to homes

弱势人群 vulnerable populations

获得基本医疗卫生服务 access basic health care services

采取适宜的医疗技术 appropriate use of medical technology

常见病、多发病和诊断明确的慢性病 commonly-encountered diseases, frequently-occurring diseases and diagnosed chronic conditions

诊疗服务 diagnosis and treatment

医疗保障 health insurance

夯实 reinforce

缓解"看病难、看病贵"问题 alleviate the problem of "difficult access to and expensive cost of health care"

医疗救助 medical aide

就近就医 get health care services from the nearest provider

载体 carrier

国家基本药物制度 National Essential Drugs System

收支两条线管理 the separate management of the income and expenditure

试点 pilot

公益性 public service, serving public welfare

基本药品目录 inventory of essential drugs

Text 6

电视电话会议 teleconference

健康档案 health records

电子健康档案 electronic health records

健康管理 health management

慢性病人 patients suffering from chronic conditions

重点人群 key populations

家庭或个人健康档案 family or individual health records

有针对性地提供服务 provide targeted services

城市社区卫生服务机构基本服务内容 Urban Community Health Institutions' Essential Services

居民健康信息管理 residents' health information management

规范记录 standardized documentation

双向转诊 two-way referral

医药费用 medical costs

制定卫生政策 formulate health care policies

管理粗放 be not carefully managed

造假行为 fabricate unreal health records

档案管理与服务提供"两张皮" the complete separation between record management and service delivery

死档 dead records

基础设施 infrastructure

四、摘要练习

请听下面英语语篇，第一篇用源语言复述此段主要信息逻辑点及层次，第二篇用译入语复述此段主要信息逻辑点及层次。注意信息点之间的逻辑联系。

Text 1

Community Health Centers Outreach and Enrollment

Kathleen Sebelius, Secretary of the Department of Health and Human Services (HHS)

Washington, D. C.

10 July 2013

Good morning. I'm pleased to be joined by Mary and Jim to announce the latest steps we're taking to help millions of Americans get ready to enroll in quality, affordable health insurance plans this fall.

Today, we're announcing that we've awarded $150 million to nearly 1,200 community health centers across the country. This funding—which was made possible by the Affordable Care Act—will help health centers reach uninsured Americans and get them signed up for coverage in the new Marketplace this fall.

Our national network of health centers serves more than 21 million patients each year, many of whom are uninsured. They are trusted resources—not only of care, but of information—in some of the neighborhoods that stand to benefit most from the expansion of health coverage. They have the ear of so many of the Americans we're trying to educate about the Marketplace this summer and fall. And these awards will help them do just that.

All told, this funding will allow those nearly 1,200 community health centers to assist up to an estimated 3.7 million Americans with enrollment. The awards will go towards things like hiring almost 3,000 new outreach workers, training staff, creating bilingual education materials, and boosting technological capacity.

As you know, the next few months represent an unprecedented opportunity for millions of Americans to get connected with the security that quality, affordable health coverage provides—in some cases for the first time ever. Education and outreach will be a critical part of seizing that opportunity. And because of the role they play in thousands of communities across the country, health centers are uniquely positioned to contribute to our educational and outreach efforts.

Of course, today's announcement is just one piece of our progress when it comes to getting ready for October 1st. We recently announced an initiative with America's libraries—which, like health centers, are another trusted institution in countless communities nationwide. And we're pleased that many libraries will serve as convenient locations for families to get information about the Marketplace this summer and to enroll for coverage this fall.

In addition, I'll be traveling to communities across the country between now and October to help get the word out about enrollment. Today I'll be visiting one of our health center award recipients, the Mountain Park Health Center in Phoenix, Arizona. And after that I'll be in different cities nearly every week, helping to shine a light on our education and outreach efforts, and speaking to people from all corners of our country about the enormous opportunity we have ahead of us.

Additionally, we're pleased that members of the business community are joining in the effort to get Americans enrolled. Just this morning, Walgreens announced that they'll be partnering with Blue Cross Blue Shield to help educate people about the law so that they'll be ready for October.

Over the summer, we'll continue to build on the incredible momentum we've seen so far. We know it won't be easy. So many Americans have spent their whole lives being frustrated, gouged, or turned away by our health care system—and connecting them with the information they need to finally get quality, affordable coverage is a huge undertaking. But the challenge of enrollment pales in comparison to the benefits that millions of American families stand to gain. That's why we're doing this. And we have a robust plan to get the job done.

Thank you again for joining us.

And now, I'd like to turn things over to Mary.

复述要点提示（主要信息逻辑点及层次）

Theme of the speech:

The US government will award $150 million, raised through the Affordable Care Act, to approximately 1,200 community health centers (CHC) across the country. Then, the CHCs will use the money to provide education and outreach services to help Americans get ready to enroll in Health Insurance Marketplace when it starts operation in the Fall.

Three keynotes of the speech:

1. Why is the money awarded to CHCs and what will CHCs do with the money?

Enrollment in Health Care Marketplace will start in the Fall, 2014 and education and outreach services will be provided before that to prepare Americans who do not have health insurance to enroll in Marketplace and gain access to health coverage through the Marketplace. The CHCs are in a very good position to undertake the task. Firstly, they are providing health service to more than 21 million patients each year, many of who are uninsured. Therefore, they have already got the access to reaching uninsured Americans. Secondly, CHCs are trusted institutions in communities. Community members are willing to listen to them. Therefore, the education about enrollment in Marketplace will be more effective if it is offered by the CHCs.

2. An overview of education and outreach service for enrollment

- The CHCs will use the awarded funding to help an estimated 3.7 million people enroll in the Marketplace.
- Those who enroll in Marketplace will have quality, affordable health coverage.
- An initiative with America's libraries will be launched and the libraries will serve as convenient locations for families to get information about the Marketplace to enroll for

coverage.

● Secretary Sebelius herself will be travelling around the country to speak to people about enrollment.

● Businesses, e.g., Walgreens and Blue Cross Blue Shield are also involved in carrying out education activities for enrollment.

3. The challenges

People have had a lot of frustrating experience with the health care system. As a result, it is not going to be easy to convince them of the benefits. However, the benefits outweigh the challenges of enrollment. Therefore, education activities still have to be carried out.

Text 2

Healthy Communities—Wellness for All

It is my pleasure to present the 2014-2019 five year strategic plan for Health & Social Services. This plan describes our objectives and outlines the key strategies the department will be implementing over the next five years, in pursuit of its identified goals and ultimately the vision of healthy communities and wellness for all.

Over the past few years, much work has been done towards fulfilling many of the commitments made by our government in 2011. Support of nongovernmental organizations in addressing needs of various populations; increased emergency shelter options for vulnerable youth and adults; new legislation regulating Nurse Practitioners; establishment and strengthening of partnerships aimed at supporting persons with FASD—these are just a few examples of progress we've made towards the commitments relevant to this department and are all part of a strategic focus on our vision.

The goals and strategies outlined in this plan will further the progress being made towards improving access, quality, and sustainability. We can expect to see continued work on mental health and substance abuse; improved integration of delivered services; ongoing work on recruitment and retention; integration of a wider range of health professionals and programs, and more.

Accompanying this work is an increased focus on accountability and an ongoing need to manage cost escalation. Ensuring that Yukon residents have appropriate access to a continuum of social supports and health services requires a significant investment, resulting in the budget for Health and Social Services being the largest of any Yukon government department. This price tag and the importance of the work that we and our partners carry out necessitate good governance, accountability, and effective planning processes, to maximize resources while ensuring the best possible outcomes for our population. Health and Social Services staff are committed to using best evidence to guide practice and evaluate outcomes, ensuring that the services we offer are meeting the needs of our population in the best and most cost-effective way possible.

Meaningful improvements in health and well-being across the population will require the Department of Health and Social Services to move to Client/Patient-centred delivery; to work with our system partners in new ways; and to lead in cross-ministry collaboration to address both immediate needs, and as much as possible, those factors that impact our well-being from infancy to our older years. We, collectively, need to explore a new model of service and support delivery that works to build a new, unified identity of coordinated service and Client-oriented care.

As outlined in this plan, over the next five years we envision making progress towards our vision of healthy communities and wellness for all by focusing on three departmental goals. The gains realized in this five year period will mark the first stage of a long journey—a journey towards system transformation that began with the Needs Assessment for Watson Lake and Dawson City; followed by the information and evidence gathering phase of the Clinical Services Plan; and that will continue to be shaped by evidence, our values and our vision in the years to come.

1. Optimal physical and mental wellbeing

We will place focus on areas of health promotion and risk reduction, child development, mental wellness, chronic condition management, and environmental health risks.

2. Safety and well-being for vulnerable and "hard-to-serve" populations and those with complex conditions

We will expand service options for persons with addictions and mental health issues; collaborate with system partners in addressing service gaps for "hard-to-serve" persons; implement evidence-based interventions for vulnerable populations and improve identification and understanding of those with complex needs through integrated case-management. We will support vulnerable and hard-to-serve persons in achieving and maintaining optimal independence and community inclusion.

3. Access to integrated, quality services

Both within Whitehorse and the smaller communities, we will change how and where residents are accessing service in order to improve their access and experience. We will do this by ensuring a variety of health and allied professionals work together to provide quality care in our smaller communities. We will use innovative ways to deliver services, such as through expanded use of Telehealth. We will support residents in accessing care locally, outside of a hospital setting (where appropriate), reducing the burden on our hospital system with the result being improved care experiences for Patients and Clients.

Beyond our focus areas, we will improve and expand upon performance measurement across the department, so we can ensure that our work is having the intended impact, and so we can examine factors and make appropriate adjustments when outcomes are not what we expect.

Progress on these goals, most importantly, will lead to improved outcomes in the population. Improvements in those factors that impact health, while vital at all ages, will have particular impact for our youngest residents, in leading to reduced risk of chronic conditions throughout life.

I am confident that the 5-year plan laid out in the following pages will support progress towards our aim of healthy, vibrant communities and populations; maximized use of limited resources; innovative approaches to increase access and quality; Patient/Client-centred service delivery; appropriate resource use; and Yukon services, designed and structured based on needs and aligned with best practices.

Through reduced risks of injury and disease; improvements in wellness for those with health challenges; and effective and appropriate changes to our services, we will see a population better able to live fully and a system better able to handle new issues and opportunities that may arise.

Achieving this will require working together with partner organizations and empowered, informed residents, and we hope you will join us in accepting this challenge.

Sincerely,
Minister
Health and Social Services

复述要点提示（主要信息逻辑点及层次）

今天展示2014至2019年社区和社会服务五年战略计划。阐明该计划的目标，未来五年的战略重点、追求的目标。

政府已完成2011年的承诺。例如在解决各种人群需要方面，支持非政府组织、为弱势青少年和成人增加应急避难场所、规范执业护士的新立法、在支持有胎儿酒精谱系障碍的人方面建立和加强合作伙伴关系等。

今后的大目标：将继续改善可获得率、质量与可持续性。将继续改善精神健康和难以戒除的瘾，改进服务一体化，继续形成卫生专业人员的一体化等。

途径是更加注重责任感与成本管理。投资应该与良好的政府管理、问责、有效规划相结合，才能最大限度地利用资源，使人民得到优质服务。

具体目标：1. 民众拥有最佳的身体与心理健康。2. 弱势群体、难以服务人群、情况复杂者获得安全与健康。3. 获得综合优质服务。

与之对应的工作方法：1. 服务方式转变成以客户/病人为中心，以统一的身份给予关怀。2. 对成瘾族和精神问题族扩大服务选项；为难以服务的人群解决服务空白，对弱势群体实施询证干预，改善社区管理，改善对有复杂需要的人群的识别和理解。为弱势人群和难以服务的人群实现并维持最佳独立状态和社区的接纳。3. 改变居民获得服务的方式和地点，改善获得服务的途径和经验。

将改进跨部门绩效评估，在未能达到预期结果时检验各种因素，做出适当调整。

将支持最大限度地利用有限的资源。

五、英译汉练习

Text 3

Remarks on Community Health Centers

US President Barack Obama

9 December 2009

Good afternoon, everybody. I am pleased that you could all join us today as we announce three new initiatives to help our community health centers provide better care to people in need all across America.

I want to thank our Secretary of Health and Human Services, Kathleen Sebelius; our Surgeon General, Dr. Regina Benjamin; our Administrator of the Health Resources and Services Administration, Dr. Mary Wakefield; and our Deputy Secretary of HHS, Bill Corr, for being here today and for their outstanding work to support community health centers. There they are. By the way, Regina, it's good to see you in your uniform. We had been waiting for that.

I also want to thank the many members of Congress who are with us today both in the audience and up on the stage, particularly Bernie Sanders and Representative Jim Clyburn. We are grateful for all that you've done.

And I especially want to recognize the leaders here today from health centers across the country for what all of you are doing in your communities every day—working long hours to provide quality care at prices that people can afford, with the dignity and respect they deserve, and in a way that takes into account the challenges that they face in their lives.

For you folks, health care isn't just about diagnosing patients and treating illness—it's about caring for people and promoting wellness. It's about emphasizing education and prevention, and helping people lead healthier lives so they don't get sick in the first place.

And it works. Studies show that people living near a health center are less likely to go to the emergency room and less likely to have unmet critical medical needs. CHCs are proven to reduce ethnic and racial disparities in care. And the medical expenses of regular CHC patients are nearly 25 percent lower than those folks who get their care elsewhere—25 percent lower.

So you can see why, in a speech marking the first anniversary of the first community health centers in America, Senator Ted Kennedy declared, "You have not only assured the best in health care for your families and neighbors, but you've also begun a minor revolution in American medicine."

Now, unfortunately, today, nearly 45 years later, that care has yet to reach many of the folks in this country who need it most. Today, millions of Americans still have difficulty accessing primary health care, and many of them are uninsured. Many have insurance, but live in underserved areas, whether in urban or rural communities. So they don't get regular checkups, they don't get routine screenings. When they get sick or hurt, they tough it out and hope for the best, and when things get bad enough they head to the emergency room.

So we end up treating complications, crises and chronic conditions that could have been prevented in the first place. And the cost is measured not just in dollars spent on health care, or in lost workplace absences and lower productivity, but in the kind of raw human suffering that has no place in the United States of America in the year 2009.

No matter what party we belong to, or where on the political spectrum we fall, none of us thinks this is acceptable. None of us would defend this system. And that's why we've taken up the cause of health insurance reform this year. It's why many of the folks in this room fought so hard to ensure that the Recovery Act included unprecedented investments—a total of $2 billion—to upgrade and expand our health centers—investments that embody the act's core mission: to help folks hardest hit by this recession, to put people back to work, and to leave a legacy of improvements that will continue to lift up communities for generations to come.

Today, we're well on our way to meeting these goals. We've created or saved up to 1.6 million jobs, according to the CBO—the Congressional Budget Office—through the Recovery Act. Our economy is growing again. We're doubling our capacity in renewable energy and rebuilding schools and laboratories, railways, and highways. Yesterday, the Kaiser Family Foundation issued a new report showing the Recovery Act has helped many states keep and improve access to health insurance for families in need.

And so far, we've allocated nearly $1.4 billion to health centers across America so they can get to work building and renovating and hiring new staff this year. And today, I'm pleased to announce that we're awarding more than $500 million to 85 centers in more than 30 states and Puerto Rico that are providing critical care for so many folks with nowhere else to turn.

We're investing in places like Canyonlands Community Health Care in Arizona, that has one facility operating in a building originally constructed as a chicken coop and another in a cramped fire station. We're investing in places like Avis Goodwin Community Health Center in Dover, New Hampshire, that's become so overcrowded—you must be from there. It's become so overcrowded the doctors are using bathrooms and closets as offices. We're investing in Bucksport Regional Health Center in Maine, where doctors are double-booked and the waiting rooms are often standing room only. We're giving places like these the funding they need to upgrade and expand their facilities so they can meet the skyrocketing demand for services that's come with this economic downturn. But we won't just want our health centers to provide more care for more patients; we want them to provide better care as well. So starting today, we're making $88 million in funding available for centers to adopt new health information technology systems to manage their administrative and financial matters and transfer old paper files to electronic medical records. These investments won't just increase efficiency and lower costs, they'll improve the quality of care as well—preventing countless medical errors, and allowing providers to spend less time with paperwork and more time with patients.

That's the purpose of the final initiative I'm announcing today as well—a demonstration project to evaluate the benefits of the "medical home" model of care that many of our health centers aspire to. The idea here is very simple: that in order for care to be effective, it needs to be coordinated. It's a model where the center that serves as your medical home might help you keep track of your prescriptions, or get the referrals you need, or work with you to develop a plan of care that ensures your providers are working together to keep you healthy.

So taken together, these three initiatives—funding for construction, technology, and a medical home demonstration—they won't just save money over the long term and create more jobs, they're also going to give more people the peace of mind of knowing that health care will be there for them and their families when they need it.

And ultimately, that's what health insurance reform is really about. That's what the members of Congress here today will be voting on in the coming weeks.

Now, let me just end by saying a little bit about this broader effort. I know it's been a long road. I know it's been a tough fight. But I also know the reason we've taken up this cause is the very same reason why so many members from both parties are here today—because no matter what our politics are, we know that when it comes to health care, the people we serve deserve better.

The legislation in Congress today contains both Democratic ideas and Republican ideas, and plenty of compromises in between. The Senate made critical progress last night with a creative new framework that I believe will help pave the way for final passage and a historic achievement on behalf of the American people. I support this effort, especially since it's aimed at increasing choice and competition and lowering cost. So I want to thank all of you for sticking with it, for all those late nights, all the long weekends that you guys have put in. With so much at stake, this is well worth all of our efforts.

It is now my pleasure to sign the memo that will direct Secretary Sebelius to get started on that medical home demonstration. So let's do that.

Text 4

Statement from HHS Secretary Kathleen Sebelius on Community Health Center Week

6 August 2012

There are 8,500 health center sites across the country, treating more than 20 million people each year. They are the cornerstones of stronger communities. They also boost local economies, adding more than 25,000 jobs in the last three years. This year, as we celebrate Community Health Center Week and its theme of "Powering Healthier Communities", we keep in mind that for 45 years, community health centers have served individuals and families whether they have private insurance, insurance through a public program like CHIP or Medicaid, or no insurance at all.

They are a proven health care model. When a community health center opens up or adds new services, the benefits can ripple through an entire community. They are a place where mothers can take their children for dental checkups, where seniors can fill their prescriptions, where families turn when they need help finding a job or access to child care services, and so much more.

Community health centers are one of the best investments our country can make in its future. This Administration has made expanding our nation's network of community health centers a top priority.

Through the Affordable Care Act, we're making an historic $11 billion investment in our nation's community health centers. Health centers are already using some of these funds to add new locations, hire more providers and offer additional services to our nation's most vulnerable populations. The law has also added thousands to the ranks of the National Health Service Corps to place doctors and nurses where they're needed most.

These investments and the work of community health centers mean more people are getting primary care and staying out of the emergency room, which can lower health care costs for the whole community. They mean kids are getting the immunizations they need to thrive in school, which can raise educational achievement. They mean adults can fill prescriptions and manage conditions so they don't miss work, meaning productivity can rise. And they can mean more jobs to bolster local economies.

We are building a stronger, healthier nation, one community at a time.

六、汉译英练习

Text 5

抓住机遇，迎接挑战——加快推进社区卫生服务健康发展

卫生部部长陈竺在2009年全国社区卫生工作会议上的讲话

2009年8月13日

今天，卫生部召开2009年全国社区卫生工作会议。这是在推进深化医药卫生体制改革关键时期召开的一次重要会议。本次会议的主题是，践行科学发展观，贯彻落实中央关于深化医药卫生体制改革意见和重点实施方案精神，全面部署加强社区

卫生服务体系建设、促进基本公共卫生服务逐步均等化、深化运行机制改革等社区卫生重点工作任务，统一思想，交流经验，推进全国社区卫生服务健康、持续发展。下面，我想谈谈社区卫生工作在深化医药卫生体制改革中的重要作用。

我国人口众多，将长期处于社会主义初级阶段，随着城市化、老龄化进程的加快以及疾病谱、医学模式的转变和人民生活水平的改善，我国城市医疗卫生服务体系面临着新的挑战。发展社区卫生服务，是我国在深入总结多年医疗卫生体制改革与发展经验的基础上，从医疗卫生事业发展规律和广大人民群众的要求出发，采取的有效促进群众健康的服务方式。

第一，发展社区卫生服务是建立基本医疗卫生制度的重要内容。深化医药卫生体制改革的总体目标是建立健全覆盖城乡居民的基本医疗卫生制度，为群众提供安全、有效、方便、价廉的医疗卫生服务。这是与我国社会主义初级阶段经济社会发展水平相适应，国家、社会、个人能够负担得起的医疗卫生制度。社区卫生服务机构通过开展健康教育、传染病防治、慢性病管理、妇幼保健等公共卫生服务，普及医疗卫生知识，提高群众自我保健水平，改变不良生活习惯，尽可能不生病、少生病、晚生病，真正落实预防为主的卫生工作方针，有利于节约卫生资源。社区卫生服务机构植根于居民生活区，提供主动服务、上门服务，方便社区居民尤其是老年人、残疾人等弱势人群获得基本医疗卫生服务。社区卫生服务采取适宜的医疗技术、使用基本药物为社区居民提供最基本的医疗服务，广泛开展常见病、多发病和诊断明确的慢性病的诊疗服务，满足群众基本健康需求，减轻个人、家庭和社会的负担。社区卫生服务发展好了，对于建立基本医疗卫生制度将起到至关重要的作用。

第二，社区卫生服务是医药卫生四大体系的重要交汇点。中央深化医药卫生体制改革的意见明确提出，建设覆盖城乡居民的公共卫生服务、医疗服务、医疗保障、药品供应保障四大体系。社区卫生服务机构主要提供公共卫生和基本医疗服务，是公共卫生和基本医疗服务体系的双重网底，构建以社区卫生服务中心为主体的社区卫生服务网络，有利于夯实城市公共卫生和医疗服务体系的基础。加强社区卫生服务体系建设和提高社区卫生服务水平，也是缓解“看病难、看病贵”问题的重要手段。社区卫生服务机构也是城市医疗保障体系的重要支撑，充分发挥社区卫生服务在城镇职工、居民基本医疗保险以及医疗救助中的作用，有利于方便参保人群就近就医，同时也可以有效节约医疗保险费用。

社区卫生服务机构是城市实行国家基本药物制度的重要载体，社区卫生服务机构将全部配备和使用基本药物，实行零差率销售，保障群众基本用药，这不仅大大减轻居民的医药费用负担，而且必将促进社区卫生服务机构公益性的回归。因此，社区卫生服务是医药卫生体制改革的一个重要交汇点和突破口，必须予以重点加强。

第三，社区卫生服务发展为医药卫生体制改革积累了宝贵的经验。近几年来，各地积极探索社区卫生服务管理体制和运行机制改革。一些地区开展社区卫生服务机构收支两条线管理试点，强化政府责任，切断医务人员个人收入与医疗服务收入之间的联系，加强了公共卫生服务、降低了医疗费用，有效维护了社区卫生服务的公益性质。一些地区制定社区卫生服务机构基本药品目录，探索实行社区基本药物政府招标、统一配送、零差率销售，有效减轻了群众的药品费用负担，为建立国家基本药物制度提供了基础。

一些地区制定社区公共卫生服务项目，建立经费保障机制，规范服务内容，并免费为社区居民提供，为促进基本公共卫生服务逐步均等化积累了经验。这些实践探索对于完善深化医药卫生体制改革政策措施提供了重要的实践基础。

Text 6

陈竺部长在加快推进健康档案工作电视电话会上的讲话（节选）

2011年9月16日

今天卫生部专题召开电视电话会议，主要目的是，通报居民健康档案工作进展情况，交流经验，进一步动员和部署推进建立城乡居民健康档案工作，确保完成2011年电子健康档案建档率达到50%左右的目标任务。刚才，江苏、湖北、贵州、陕西4个省卫生厅的负责同志介绍了经验和做法，值得大家学习借鉴。下面我讲三点意见。

一、充分认识建立居民健康档案的重要意义

我国的居民健康档案始于20世纪90年代，社区卫生服务机构为方便对居民的健康管理，在服务过程中为慢性病人、老年人等重点人群建立家庭或个人健康档案。通过建立健康档案，社区卫生服务机构一方面可以了解服务对象及其家庭的健康状况，有针对性地提供服务，同时也是加强自身建设的一条路径。2000年卫生部印发了《城市社区卫生服务机构基本服务内容》，把居民健康信息管理纳入服务范围，建立健康档案成为各地区社区卫生服务机构普遍开展的一项工作。2009年，党中央国务院关于深化医药卫生体制改革的意见和医改近期重点实施方案，将建立统一规范的居民健康档案作为一项重要实施内容提出，并将建立居民健康档案工作纳入国家基本公共卫生服务项目。

健康档案是医疗卫生机构为城乡居民提供医疗卫生服务过程中的规范记录，是以居民个人健康为核心、贯穿整个生命过程、涵盖各种健康相关因素的系统化文件记录。规范的健康档案，有利于医疗卫生机构更好地了解居民整体健康状况，提供连续性、综合性健康管理服务。建立电子健康档案，通过信息化手段，可实现不同医疗卫生机构之间健康信息资源共享，促进公立医院与基层医疗卫生机构的双向转诊和分工协作，有利于提高卫生服务效率，改善服务质量，节约医药费用。随着健康档案建立范围的不断扩大，居民群体健康信息可作为各级政府制定卫生政策的重要参考依据。完整的健康档案记录，也是卫生行政部门对医疗卫生机构进行考核、评价的重要工具。

二、健康档案工作面临的主要问题

免费为城乡居民建立健康档案是一项新的工作，各地在开展工作过程中，也遇到一些困难和问题。一是健康档案管理不规范。一些地区未能按照统一规范和要求建档，存在档案信息不完整、管理粗放等问题，甚至存在部分造假行为。一些地方宣传不到位，不仅医务人员缺乏积极性，也得不到居民的普遍认可。一些地方对健康档案疏于管理，健康信息泄漏等安全隐患问题逐步暴露出来。二是健康档案使用效率较低。很多基层医疗卫生机构在健康档案建立过程中没有与其所开展的医疗卫生服务相结合，形成档案管理与服务提供“两张皮”，“死档”问题比较突出。三是以电子健康档案为基础的区域信息化进程缓慢。目前，基层医疗卫生机构尤其是农村地区的基础设施薄弱，多数地区尚未建立起电子化的信息系统，严重影响了健康档案的使用效率。

三、加快推进落实2011年健康档案工作任务

根据卫生部医改工作进展监测，截至2011年6月，全国城乡居民健康档案累计建档率达到50.2%，规范化电子健康档案建档率达为27.2%，其中城市地区为37.6%，农村地区为21.8%。北京、黑龙江、江苏、浙江、山东、湖北、陕西、青海8个省（区、市）规范化电子健康档案建档率超过40%。河北、山西、辽宁、吉林、安徽、福建、江西、四川、贵州、云南、西藏、宁夏、新疆13个省（区）低于20%。很多地区工作进展依然比较缓慢，如果不采取有力措施，将难以完成医改任务目标。为此，各地应做好以下几方面工作：

第一，以服务为切入点，努力提高健康档案建档率；第二，规范健康档案管理，努力提高使用率；第三，加快信息化建设，提高电子化建档率；第四，互相促进，着力推动居民健康卡建设；第五，加强人员培训，动员社会各方参与；第六，加强督导考核，落实经费保障措施。

2011年医改任务中，电子健康档案建档率要达到50%，现在到明年2月底还有5个多月时间。各地要积极采取措施，广泛动员各方力量，抓紧时间，查找薄弱环节，有针对性地开展工作，力争到年底前，各省（区、市）电子健康档案建档率达到40%以上。从2011年10月开始，各地要建立健康档案月报制度，每月月底前要将电子化健康档案进展情况报卫生部。对于进展明显缓慢的地区，卫生部将采取约谈、通

报等形式进行督促，确保完成医改任务目标。

为城乡居民建立健康档案是卫生系统建设的一项重要的基础性工作，各级卫生行政部门要高度重视，集中人力物力，加强信息系统建设，进一步提高电子健康档案建档率，规范健康档案管理，为推进医改整体工作贡献力量。

资料来源：

Text 1 http://www.hhs.gov/about/leadership/secretary/speeches/2013/index.html

Text 2 http://www.hss.gov.yk.ca/pdf/Health_and_Social_Services_Strategic_Plan_2014_-_2019.pdf

Text 3 https://www.whitehouse.gov/briefing-room/speeches-and-remarks

Text 4 http://www.hhs.gov/about/leadership/secretary/speeches/2013/index.html

Text 5 http://www.gov.cn/gzdt/2009-08/31/content_1405362.htm

Text 6 http://www.moh.gov.cn/mohzcfgs/s7857/201110/53190.shtml

参考答案

四、摘要练习

Text 1

社区卫生服务中心的外展服务和报名

美国卫生及公共服务部（HHS）部长凯瑟琳·西贝利厄斯

美国华盛顿特区

2013年7月10日

早晨好。我很高兴和玛丽、吉姆一起公布我们正在采取的最新的步骤，以帮助数百万美国人做好准备在今年秋天参加优质、支付得起的医疗保险计划。

今天，我们宣布，我们已经给全国各地的近1 200个社区卫生服务中心拨款1.5亿美元。这笔资金通过平价医疗法案筹募，将用于帮助社区卫生服务中心为没有医疗保险的美国人提供服务，让他们在今年秋天通过新的“医疗保险市场”签订保险合约，获取保险覆盖。

我们全国的社区卫生服务中心网络每年给2 100万名病人提供服务，其中很多人是没有保险的。在从医疗保险覆盖面扩大中获益最多的一些街区，这些社区卫生服务中心是值得信赖的资源，提供了可靠的服务和信息。我们将在今年夏天和秋天进行关于医疗保险市场的宣传教育，人们会更愿意接受卫生服务中心提供的信息，我们的这些拨款将帮助社区卫生服务中心完成医疗保险市场的宣传教育工作。

总而言之，据估计，通过这笔资金，约1 200个社区卫生服务中心将协助最多约370万美国人加入医疗保险。该项拨款将用于新增雇用近3 000名外展工作人员、开展人员培训、编写双语宣传教育材料、提高工作人员的技术能力等。

众所周知，随后的几个月将带来前所未有的机遇，帮助数以百万计的美国人获得高质量、可支付的医疗保险所提供的保障，对于某些美国人，这是有史以来第一次。宣传教育和外展服务是抓住这个机会的一个重要组成部分。因为社区卫生服务中心在全国各地数以千计的社区所发挥的作用，它们具备得天独厚的优势来协助我们的宣传教育和外展工作。

当然，“医疗保险市场”即将于10月1日开始投入使用，今天的公告只是准备工作的一部分。最近，我们宣布了一项和美国图书馆合作的倡议，图书馆和社区卫生服务中心一样，遍布在全国的无数个社区中，是受社区信赖的机构，是在全国无数社区中实施的一项举措。值得高兴的是，许多图书馆将作为方便的地点，在今年夏天给家庭提供“医疗保险市场”的相关信息，在今年秋天为他们报名参加“医疗保险市场”，从而获得医疗保险。

此外，从现在开始到10月为止，我将前往全国各地的社区，协助发布关于报名加入医疗保险市场的信息。今天，我将参观的社区卫生服务中心是亚利桑那州凤凰城的山园社区卫生服务中心，他们也获得了拨款。之后，我每周会去不同的城市，让更多人了解医疗保险市场的宣传教育和外展服务，我会不断告诉美国各地的人，这个巨大的机会就在我们面前。

此外，我们很高兴看到商业界成员加入进来，和我们一起努力让美国人报名加入医疗保险市场。就在今天早上，沃尔格林公司宣布，他们将与蓝十字蓝盾协会合作，帮助进行相关法律的宣传教育，帮助人们做好准备10月加入医疗保险市场。

今年夏天，我们将维持并加强惊人的发展势头。我们知道这不是一件容易的事情。所以，许多美国人一辈子都在卫生保健系统中不断经历挫折、勒索、拒绝，要让他们了解获取优质、可支付的医疗保险所需信息是一项非常艰巨的任务。但报名的挑战性远远低于数以百万的美国家庭加入医疗保险市场后一定会得到的收益。这就是我们要这样做的原因。我们有一个强有力的计划，一定能把工作做好。

再次感谢您加入我们的行列。

接下来由玛丽讲话。

Text 2

健康社区——健康为大家

我很高兴向大家介绍2014至2019年卫生和社会服务五年战略计划。这个计划描述了我们的目标，概述了我们部门在未来五年为实现既定目标并最终实现健康社区与健康为大家的最终愿景将实施的重点战略。

在过去的几年中，我们在完成政府2011年所做的承诺方面，已经做了大量工作。例如在解决各种人群需要方面支持非政府组织、为弱势青少年和成人增加应急避难场所、规范执业护士的新立法、在支持有胎儿酒精谱系障碍的人方面建立和加强合作伙伴关系……这些例子表明，与我们部门相关的、我们做出过的相应承诺已经取得进展，都是我们的愿景中战略重点的一部分。

这一计划中列出的目标和策略，将使我们在改善可获得率、质量与可持续性方面取得进一步的进展。我们将在精神健康和滥用药物方面继续努力工作，服务一体化将得到改进，招聘和留职的工作正在进行，各种卫生专业人员的整合工作也在进行。

伴随着这项工作的还有更加注重责任感以及眼下突显的成本管理的需求。要确保育空[1]居民有适当的途径获得连续的社会支持和健康服务，需要大量资金，这导致卫生和社会服务预算是所有育空政府部门中最高的。巨大的开支以及我和我们的合作伙伴工作的重要性使得我们需要良好的政府管理、问责与有效的规划过程，这样才能最大限度地利用资源，为人民带来尽可能好的结果。卫生和社会服务人员正在以充分的依据来指导实践和评估结果，确保我们所提供的服务能够以最优质、最具成本效益的方式满足人民的需要。

要得到人口健康和幸福方面最有意义的改善，就要求卫生与社会服务部的服务方式转变成以客户或病人为中心的方式上来，要求以新的方式与我们的系统伙伴合作，要求在跨部门协作当好领头人，尽可能多地解决眼前的问题，因为这些问题从婴儿到老年一直影响我们的幸福感。总的来说，我们需要探索新的服务模式与交付支持方式，这就是建立一个新的、统一的身份来协调以服务和客户为中心的关怀。

正如这个计划所描述的，在未来五年内，我们设想通过以三个部门的目标为重点，朝着我们设想的关于健康社区和全民身心健康的方向去取得进步。这五年期间实现的收益将是一个漫长旅程第一阶段的标志——这个旅程的目的是体制转型，以

1 育空（Yukon）是加拿大北部三个地区（Territory）之一，位于加拿大西北方，首府为怀特霍斯。

瓦森湖和道森市的需求评估为开始；其次是临床服务计划的信息和证据收集；我们将继续用证据、我们的价值观以及我们今后的理想打造该计划。

1. 身体与心理健康达到理想状态

我们将重点放在促进健康和减少风险上；儿童发展；心理健康；慢性疾病管理，环境健康风险。

2. 弱势群体和难以服务人口与情况复杂者的安全与健康

我们将对成瘾族和有精神问题的人群扩大我们的服务选项；在应对为难以服务的人群解决服务空白的问题上与系统伙伴合作；对弱势群体实施询证干预；通过综合案例管理，改善对那些有复杂需要的人群的识别和理解。我们将支持弱势人群和难以服务的人群实现和维持最佳独立状态，赢得社区的接纳。

3. 提供综合优质服务

在怀特霍斯社区和更小的社区，我们将改变那里的居民获得服务的方式和地点，以改善他们的获得服务的途径和体验。我们将确保各种健康专职人员和专业人员一起工作，给我们的小社区提供优质服务。我们将用创新的方法来提供服务，例如广泛使用远程医疗。我们将支持减轻医院系统的负担，使患者和客户获得良好的医护体验。

在我们的重点区域以外，我们将改进并扩大跨部门绩效评估，以便确保我们的工作达到预期的影响力，在未能达到我们预期的结果时，我们能够检验各种因素，做出适当调整。

最重要的是，在这些目标方面的进展将使人们更加健康。改善那些影响健康的因素在各个阶段都很关键，这在降低终身慢性疾病的风险方面，将给我们最年轻的居民带来特别重要的影响。

我相信，以下几页之中写下的五年计划将支持我们在建设健康、富有活力的社区与拥有健康、富有活力的居民方面取得进展；将支持最大限度地利用有限的资源；将支持用创新的方法增加获得服务，达到良好服务质量；将支持提供以患者或客户为中心的服务；将支持资源的合理使用，以及以需求为基础而设计和打造的育空地区服务。

通过降低损伤和疾病的风险，通过那些健康状况不佳人群健康状况的改善，以及我们服务的有效和适当的改变，我们将看到人民能够更好地生活，系统能够更好地处理可能出现的新问题和新机会。

要做到这一点，需要与合作机构以及被授予了权力、提供了相关信息的居民一同工作。我们希望你们能加入我们，接受这个挑战。

真诚的，

卫生和社会服务部部长

五、英译汉练习

Text 3

美国奥巴马总统关于社区卫生中心的讲话

2009年12月9日

下午好！欢迎大家的到来，今天我们将宣布三项新举措，帮助我们的社区卫生服务中心为全美国需要医疗保健的人提供更好的服务。

我要感谢美国卫生及公共服务部部长凯瑟琳·西贝利厄斯、美国公共卫生服务现役军团总医官丽贾娜·本杰明博士、卫生资源和服务局局长玛丽·韦克菲尔德博士和卫生及公共服务部副部长比尔·科尔出席今天的活动，感谢他们为支持社区卫生服务中心做出的出色工作。他们都在那儿。顺便说一下，丽贾娜，很高兴看到你穿着制服出席，我们一直在等待看到你穿着制服的身影。

我也想感谢许多国会议员出席今天的活动，他们有些在观众席上，有些在主席台上，尤其是参议员伯尼·桑德斯和众议员吉姆·克莱伯恩。我们非常感谢你们所做的一切工作。

我想特别感谢出席今天活动的来自全国各地的社区卫生服务中心的负责人，感谢你们每天在社区卫生服务中心所做的一切：每天长时间工作，为人们提供可以负担得起的优质医疗卫生服务，使他们能保有自己应有的尊严和尊重，在提供服务的过程中也充分考虑到服务对象在生活中面对的各种挑战。

对于你们而言，医疗保健不仅是诊断和治疗疾病，也是对人们的关怀和对健康的促进，强调宣传教育和预防，帮助人们过上健康的生活，这样他们就不会生病。

你们的工作已经产生了效果。研究表明，住在社区卫生服务中心附近的人去急诊室的可能性较低，出现危重医疗需求不能满足的情况的可能性也较低。已有证据表明，社区卫生服务中心减少了医疗中的民族和种族差异。和从其他医疗机构获取医疗服务的人相比，社区卫生服务中心普通患者的医疗费用少25%。

因此，你们也就了解为什么在美国首个社区卫生服务中心成立一周年之际，参议员特德·肯尼迪发布演说宣布："你们不但为家人和邻居获得最好的医疗保健服务提供了保障，而且也引导了美国医学的一场小小的革命。"

现在，不幸的是，在近45年后的今天，他提到的医疗保健服务仍未能覆盖到许多美国人，尤其是那些最需要这些医疗保健服务的人。今天，数以百万计的美国人仍然难以获得初级医疗保健服务，其中不少人没有保险。许多有保险的人生活在缺医少药的城市和农村社区，因此他们没有进行定期体检，没有接受常规疾病筛查。

当他们生病或受伤时，他们抱着乐观的态度坚持不看病，希望能咬紧牙关挺过去，当病情变得非常严重时，他们直接去急诊室看病。

结果导致我们最终要治疗本来可以避免的并发症、危重病和慢性疾病，产生的代价不仅是花在医疗保健上的金钱大大增加，或者工作场所缺勤和生产力降低，而且带来人类的原始苦难，在2009年的美利坚合众国不应该存在这样的苦难。

不管我们党派归属如何，或各自持有怎样不同的政治立场，所有人都同意这是无法接受的，谁都不愿意捍卫这样的系统。这就是今年我们已经开始进行医疗保险改革的原因。这就是今天在座的各位如此努力想要确保《经济复苏法案》投入前所未有的资金——总计20亿美元用于升级和扩展我们的社区卫生服务中心的原因。这笔投资体现了该法案的核心使命：帮助受这次经济衰退打击最沉重的人，帮助人们重新找到工作，留下一个改进的传统，从而世世代代不断提升社区的状态。

今天，我们在顺利地实现这些目标。根据美国国会预算办公室的说法，我们已经通过《经济复苏法案》创建或挽救了160万个就业岗位。我们的经济再次开始增长。可再生能源容量将翻倍，我们还在重建学校、实验室、铁路、公路。昨日，凯泽家庭基金会发表了一份新的报告，报告显示《经济复苏法案》已经帮助许多州有需要的家庭维持和改善医疗保险。

到目前为止，我们对美国各地的社区卫生服务中心的拨款已达到约14亿美元，这样他们今年就能够进行设施建设和改造、雇用新员工。今天，我很高兴地宣布，我们将为三十几个州和波多黎各的85个中心提供5亿多美元拨款，这些社区服务中心给很多人提供重要的医疗服务，这些人在其他地方无法得到这些服务。

我们投资的对象包括亚利桑那州的峡谷地社区卫生服务站，他们的一个分部运行的地点原本是用作养鸡场的，另一个分部在一个狭小的消防站设施里。我们投资的对象包括新罕布什尔州多佛市的安飞士·古德温社区卫生服务中心，这个中心已经拥挤不堪。您一定是从那里来的。这个中心拥挤的程度已经造成医生不得不把卫生间和壁橱用作办公室。我们投资的对象包括缅因州的巴克斯波特地区健康中心，那里的病人看病的预约经常排重，候诊室人太多，仅有立足之地。获得拨款的都是这类健康中心，他们需要资金来升级和扩展设施，这样才能满足经济衰退导致的迅速增长的患者需求。但我们的期望不是仅限于健康中心为更多的患者提供更多医疗保健服务，我们希望他们能提供更好的医疗保健服务。所以，从今天开始，我们将提供8 800万美元帮助健康中心采用新的医疗信息技术系统来管理他们的行政和财务事务，将旧的纸质文件转为电子病历。这些投资不仅能提高效率、降低成本，还能提高医疗保健服务质量，防止无数医疗失误的发生，并允许医疗卫生服务机构减少文书工作，节省出更多时间用在患者身上。

这是我今天宣布的最后一项举措的目的，这项举措是一个示范项目，用于评估许多社区医疗中心想要实现的“医疗之家”医疗保健服务模型。做这个项目的想法很简单，如果想要获得有效的医疗保健服务，必须要进行协调。在这个模型中，健康中心作为你的医疗之家可能会帮助你保持对自己处方药情况的了解，你能得到你所需要的转介，它能与你一起制定医疗保健计划，以确保为你提供医疗保健服务的不同机构一起合作来维持你的健康。

所以，这三项举措——建设用资金、技术和医疗之家示范，如果一起实施，将不只是在长远上省钱和创造更多的就业机会，它们也会使更多人心安，因为他们知道如果需要，他们和他们的家人随时可以获得医疗保健服务。

而最终，这就是医疗保险改革的真正核心，这就是今天在场的国会议员在未来几周内将要投票实现的事情。

现在，结束前我想稍微谈一下我们做得更广泛的工作。我知道这是一条漫长的道路。我知道这是一场艰苦的斗争。但我也知道，我们开始进行这项事业的原因也是今天有这么多两党的成员出席的原因：因为无论我们的政见如何，我们都清楚，当涉及医疗保健，我们所服务的人民应该得到更好的服务。

今天在国会的立法包含民主党思想和共和党的思想，以及大量的两党思想的妥协。昨晚参议院取得了至关重要的进展，代表美国人民通过了具有创造性的新的框架，相信这个新的框架将帮助我们做好准备，最终通过法案，并代表美国人民取得一项历史性的成就。我支持这项工作，特别是因为它的目的是增加选择和竞争，降低成本。所以，我要感谢你们所有人一直为医改坚持不懈，你们在无数深夜、节假日还坚持工作。因为利益攸关，我们所有的努力都是非常值得的。

下面，我很高兴能够签署这份备忘录，指示西贝利厄斯部长启动医疗之家示范项目。那么，让我们来做这件事吧。

Text 4

美国卫生及公共服务部部长凯瑟琳·西贝利厄斯关于社区卫生服务中心周的讲话

2012年8月6日

我们国家有8 500个社区卫生服务中心服务点遍布全国各地，每年治疗超过两千万病人，他们是形成强大社区的基础。他们还推动当地经济发展，在过去三年间增加了25 000个就业机会。今年，我们庆祝社区卫生服务中心周的主题为“增强健康社区”，我们必须牢记，在过去的45年中，社区卫生服务中心一直为个人和家庭提供服务，不论他们是否购买了私营性质的保险，是否通过公立性质的项目获取了保险，如儿童健康保险或联邦医疗补助，还是压根没有任何保险。

社区卫生服务中心这种医疗模式已被证实行之有效。当一个社区卫生服务中心开始营业或增加了新的服务，好处可以波及整个社区。在社区卫生服务中心，母亲能够带着孩子来检查牙齿，老年人可以按处方取药，当人们需要找工作或寻求托儿服务，也会来社区卫生服务中心寻求帮助，社区卫生服务中心还能提供很多其他服务。

社区卫生服务中心是我们的国家可以为未来进行的最佳投资之一。扩大我们国家的社区卫生服务中心网络是本届政府的工作重点。

通过《平价医疗法案》，我们正在将具有重大历史意义的11亿美元投资投入全国的社区卫生服务中心。社区卫生服务中心已经在使用这些资金用于开设新的服务点，聘请更多的医疗机构为最弱势的群体提供更多服务。该法案还促使成千上万人加入了国民卫生服务队的行列，将医生和护士送到最需要的地方。

对社区卫生服务中心进行这些投资和工作就意味着越来越多的人将获得初级医疗保健服务，这样他们就不用去急诊室看病，从而可以降低整个社区的医疗保健费用。这也意味着孩子们能获得免疫接种，在学校里能茁壮成长，从而可以提高教育成果。这也意味着成年人在不耽误工作的前提下就可以按处方取药和管理他们的疾病，带来生产力的提升。这也意味着更多的就业机会，从而可以巩固当地经济。

我们正在通过做一个个社区的工作建设一个更强大、更健康的国家。

六、汉译英练习

Text 5

Seizing Opportunities and Meeting Challenges
—Accelerating the Healthy Development of Community Health Care

Remarks by Chen Zhu, Minister of Health at the 2009 National Community Health Work Conference

13 August 2009

Today, the Ministry of Health held the 2009 National Community Health Work Conference. This is an important meeting held at a critical time of the campaign to deepen reform in the medical and health care system. The conference is focused on adopting the scientific concept of development, implementing the central government's suggestions and core ideas of the implementation plan for deepening health care system reform, making comprehensive arrangements for key areas of work of community health care, including reinforcing the construction of community health care system, promoting the gradual realization of equitable basic public health services, and deepening the reform of operation mechanism, uniting ideas, exchanging experiences, and promoting the healthy and sustainable development of the national community health care system. Now, I'd like to talk about the important role of community health care in deepening medical and health system reform.

China has an enormous population and will remain in the primary stage of socialism for a very long time to come. With the accelerating pace of urbanization and population aging, changes in the disease spectrum and medical model and the improvement of people's living standards, China's urban health care system is facing new challenges. After the government made in-depth review of the successful experience of the reform and development of the medical and health care system through the years and took into consideration the development principles of the health care industry and the demands of the people, the development of community health care was adopted as an effective service model to promote people's health.

First of all, developing community health care is an important component of establishing a basic health care system. The overall objective of deepening reform in the medical and health care system is to establish a basic health care system that covers urban and rural residents, and that provides people with safe, effective, convenient and affordable health care services. This is appropriate for the social development level of the primary stage of socialism in China, and this is also an affordable health care system for the whole country, the society, and individuals. Community health care institutions carry out such public health services as health education, prevention of infectious diseases, chronic disease management, and maternal and child health care, thus helping popularize information on health care, improve people's capability to take good care of their own health, and promote lifestyle changes so that people do not get sick, and even when they do get sick, it will happen only on very rare occasions or at a later time. The implementation of a prevention-based health policy is conducive to saving health resources. Community health care institutions are based in the residential areas. They always take an initiative to provide services and deliver services to homes, facilitating community members, especially senior citizens, people with disabilities, and other vulnerable groups to access basic health care services. Through the appropriate use of medical technology and basic drugs, community health care facilities provides basic medical services for community residents. They provide diagnostic and treatment service for an extensive range of commonly-encountered diseases, frequently-occurring diseases and diagnosed chronic conditions. Community health care helps communities meet the basic health needs of the people, and reduce the burden on individuals, families and the society. The development of community health care will play a crucial role in the establishment of a basic health care system.

Secondly, community health care is an important intersection point of the four major systems involved in medicine and health care. The Central Government proposed clearly in its suggestions for deepening health system reform that four systems covering urban and rural residents will be established. The four systems consist of public health services, medical services, health insurance, and drug supply system. Community health care institutions mainly provide public health and basic medical services. They serve as the bottom of the network of both public health system and basic medical service system. Building a community health care network based on community health care centers will help reinforce the foundation of public health and health care system in urban areas. Strengthening the construction of community health care system and improving the quality of community health care are importation measures to alleviate the problem of "difficult access to and expensive cost of health care". Community health care institutions also provide important support for the health insurance system in rural areas. Giving full play to the role of community health care in providing basic health insurance and medical aide for people working or living in urban areas will help promote people who have health care coverage to get health care services from the nearest provider, and effectively reduce the cost of health insurance.

Community health care institutions are an important carrier through which the government will implement the National Essential Drugs System in urban areas. All the community health care institutions will be fully equipped with all the essential drugs and they will be available at a reduced price so as to ensure that people have their basic medication. This measure not only greatly reduced the financial burden resulting from medical expenses, but also would definitely promote community health care institutions to resume their role in public service. Therefore, community health care is an important point of intersection and breakthroughs in medical and health system reform and deserves more efforts for reinforcement.

Thirdly, in the process of the development of community health care, we have accumulated invaluable experience for medical and health care system reform. In recent years, local governments have taken an initiative to experiment with the reformation of the management system and operation mechanism of community health care. Some areas piloted the separate management of the income and expenditure of community health care institutions, which helped strengthen government responsibility, sever the connection between the personal income of health workers and income of medical service, strengthen public health services, reduce medical costs, and effectively maintain the public service nature of community health care service. Some local governments formulated the inventory of essential drugs for community health care institutions, experimented with the implementation of government offering open bidding for the purchase order, unified distribution, and reduced price of essential drugs, effectively reducing people's burden of drug costs, and provided the foundation for the establishment of the national essential drug system.

Some local governments developed community public health programs, established mechanisms to ensure funding, standardized services, and provided free service for community residents. We have accumulated much experience for the gradual realization of equitable basic public health services. These practical experiments provide important foundation of practice for improving policies and measures for deepening the medical and health care system reform.

Text 6

Remarks by Chen Zhu, Minister of Health, China, at the Teleconference on Accelerating and Promoting the Implementation of the Health Records Program

16 September 2011

Today, the Ministry of Health called on a special teleconference for the main purpose of reporting information on the progress of the urban and rural resident health records program and exchange experiences so as to further mobilize forces, make arrangements for, and promote the establishment of health records for urban and rural residents, and ensure that the coverage of electronic health records reaches 50% of the target by 2011. Just now, the officials from the Departments of Health of Jiangsu, Hubei, Guizhou, and Shaanxi Provinces made introductions of their actual practice and experience and lessons. There's a lot we can learn from them. Now, I'd like to stress three things.

Ⅰ. Full recognition of the importance of establishing the health records

China's health records program started in the 1990s when community health institutions, in order to facilitate health management of the community residents, establish family or individual health records for patients suffering from chronic conditions, senior citizens and other key populations in the process of providing services. On one hand, through the establishment of health records, community health institutions learn more about the health condition of their clients and their families, and can provide targeted services subsequently. On the other hand, health records also help the community health institutions strengthen self-construction. In 2000, the Ministry of Health issued *Urban Community Health Institutions' Essential Services*, which incorporated the residents' health information management in the scope of services available. Consequently, establishing health records has become part of the responsibilities of the community health institutions across the country. In 2009, the CPC Central Committee and the State Council issued *Suggestions on Deepening Medical and Health Care System Reform and Key Short-Term Implementation Plans for Health Care Reform*, proposing that establishing standardized health records is an important task to be implemented, and incorporating the establishment of health records in the basic national public health service.

Health care institutions use health records to provide urban and rural residents with standardized documentation in the process of health services. They are centered on the health of individuals through the course of their entire life, systematically documenting a wide variety of health-related factors. Standardized health records help health care institutions gain a better understanding of the overall health condition of the individual so as to provide continued and comprehensive health management services. Creating electronic health records, by means of information technology, makes it possible for different health care institutions to share health information resources. It also promotes referrals, distribution of responsibilities, and collaboration between public hospitals and primary health care institutions. It will help improve the efficiency of health care services, improve service quality, and save medical costs. With the constantly expanding coverage of health records, governments at all levels can utilize the health information of different populations as important evidence and basis for formulating health care policies. Thorough health record keeping is also an important instrument for health administrative departments when they conduct evaluation and assessment on health care institutions.

Ⅱ. Main problems concerning the health records program

Establishing health records free of charge for urban and rural residents is a new task.

Therefore, in the process of implementation, the local governments have encountered some difficulties and problems. Firstly, health records management is not standardized. Some institutions have failed to follow the uniform standards and requirements for establishing health records. Some health records are incomplete. Some health records are not carefully managed. Some institutions even fabricated some unreal health records. Some institutions did not do much to inform and educate people of the health records, resulting in a lack of enthusiasm on the part of the health workers and lack of acceptance on the part of the community residents. Some institutions did not manage the health records well, causing potential risk of security breach such as leaking confidential health information. Secondly, the health records are not being used effectively. In the process of establishing health records, many primary health care institutions did not integrate health records in the health care services they provide, resulting in the complete separation between record management and service delivery. In addition, the problem of "dead records" is quite conspicuous. Thirdly, regional informationization based on electronic health records is progressing very slowly. Currently, primary health care institutions, especially those in rural areas, have a rather weak infrastructure. Consequently, most regions have not yet established electronic information system, which seriously impeded the effective use of health records.

Ⅲ. Accelerating and promoting the implementation of the tasks of the Health Record Program for 2011

According to the Ministry of Health's monitoring data on the progress of health care reform, as of June 2011, 50.2% of all urban and rural residents have established health records, and 27.2% of them are standardized electronic health records. The coverage of standardized electronic health records has reached 37.6% in urban areas and 21.8 % in rural areas. In eight provinces (or autonomous regions and municipalities under the direct administration of the Central Government of China), including Beijing, Heilongjiang, Jiangsu, Zhejiang, Shandong, Hubei, Shaanxi, and Qinghai, the coverage of standardized electronic health records has exceeded 40%. In 13 provinces (or autonomous regions), including Hebei, Shanxi, Liaoning, Jilin, Anhui, Fujian, Jiangxi, Sichuan, Guizhou, Yunnan, Tibet, Ningxia, and Xinjiang, the coverage is lower than 20%. Progress in many regions is still relatively slow. If we do not take effective measures, it will be difficult to accomplish the tasks of the health care reform. Therefore, all the local governments will carry out the following tasks: A. Use service as the entry point and make efforts to improve the health records coverage. B. Standardize the management of health records and strive to improve utilization. C. Accelerate informationization construction and raise the proportion of electronic health records. D. Promote mutual development and strive to promote the implementation of the health card program. E. Reinforce training and mobilize the involvement of people from all sectors of life. F. Reinforce supervision and evaluation and implement measures to ensure funding.

According to the defined tasks of health care reform for 2011, the coverage of electronic health records will reach 50% by the end of February next year. Now there is still a little over five months left. All local governments will have to take active measures to mobilize all forces available and make the most of the time left, find the weak links, carry out their work in a more targeted way, and strive to realize the target of reaching 40% or higher coverage of electronic health records in all the provinces (autonomous regions and municipalities). Beginning in October 2011, all local governments will make monthly reports on the progress of the health record program. The Ministry of Health will receive a report on the progress of electronic health records at the end of each month. For regions that are obviously making much less progress than the other regions, the Ministry of Health will supervise and urge on progress through interviews, reporting and other measures to ensure the accomplishment of all the targets of health care reform.

Establishing health records for urban and rural residents is an important basic task in the construction of the health care system. The health care administrative departments at all levels should give the program its due attention and pool all resources available to strengthen the construction of the information system, improve the coverage of electronic health records, standardize health records management, and contribute to the promotion of health care reform on the whole.

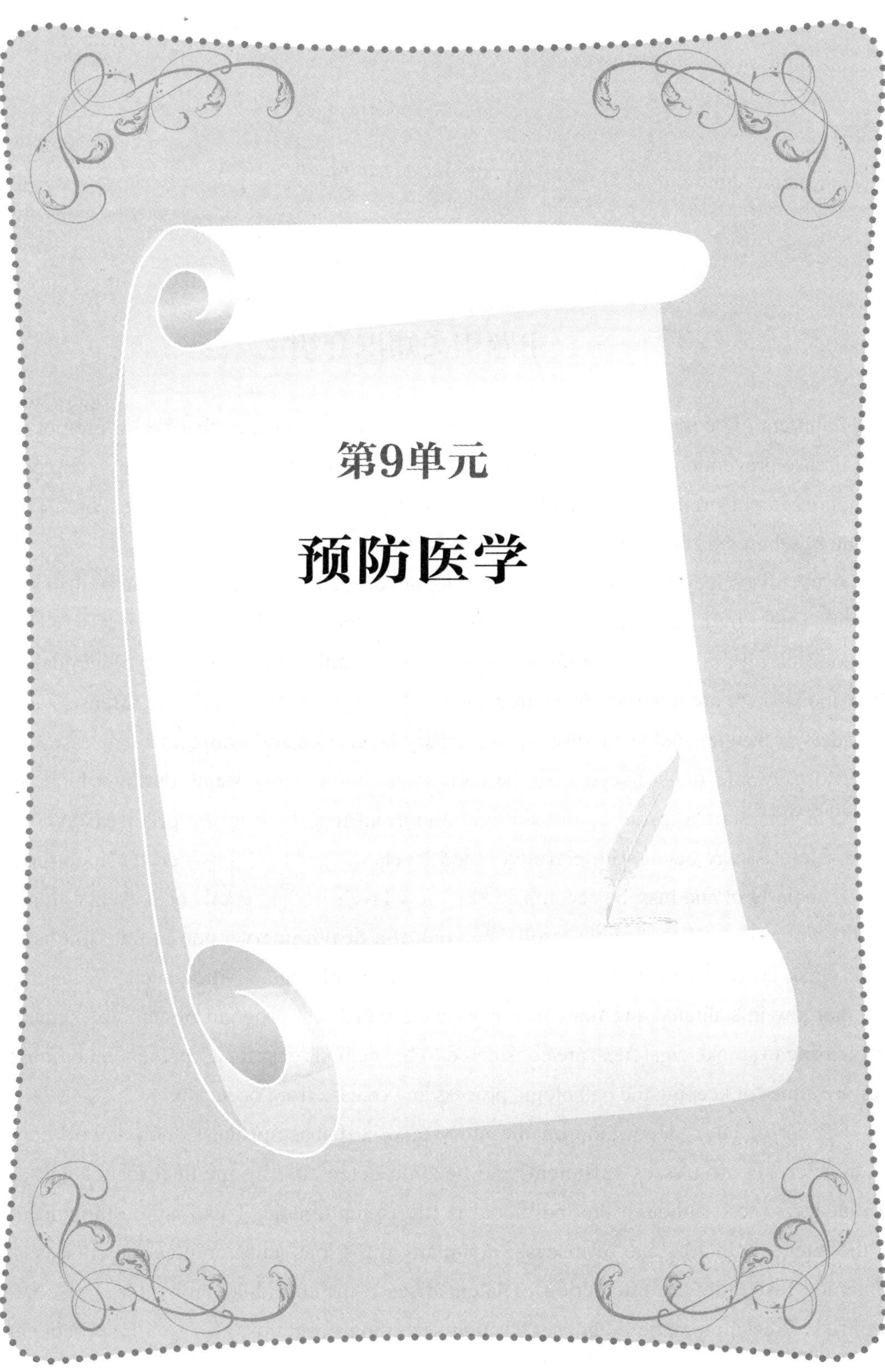

第9单元

预防医学

一、主题相关知识介绍

In an era of "cost consciousness", there are increasing demands that health promotion and disease prevention be proven economically worthwhile. Furthermore, many people in the political arena promote prevention as a means of controlling rising health care costs. This argument is based on the belief that prevention is always cost-saving.

A useful concept of prevention that was developed or at least popularized in the classic account by Leavell and Clark has come to be known as Leavell's levels. Based on this concept, all the activities of clinicians and other health professionals have the goal of prevention. There are three levels of prevention—primary prevention and pre-disease stage, secondary prevention and latent disease and tertiary prevention and symptomatic disease.

Most noninfectious diseases can be seen as having an early stage, during which the causal factors start to produce physiologic abnormalities. During the predisease stage, atherosclerosis may begin with elevated blood levels of the "bad" low-density lipoprotein (LDL) cholesterol and may be accompanied by low levels of the "good" or scavenger high-density lipoprotein (HDL) cholesterol. The goal of a health intervention at this time is to modify risk factors in a favorable direction. Lifestyle modifying activities, such as changing to a diet low in saturated and trans fats, pursuing a consistent program of aerobic exercise, and ceasing to smoke cigarettes, are considered to be methods of primary prevention because they are aimed at keeping the pathologic process and disease from occurring.

Sooner or later, depending on the individual, a disease process such as coronary atherosclerosis progresses sufficiently to become detectable by medical tests, such as cardiac stress test, although the individual is till asymptomatic. This may be thought of as the latent (hidden) stage of disease. For many infectious and noninfectious diseases, screening tests allow the detection of latent disease in individuals considered to be at high risk. Presymptomatic diagnosis through screening programs, along with subsequent treatment when needed, is referred to as secondary prevention because it is the secondary line of defense against disease. Although screening programs do not prevent the causes from initiating the disease process, they may allow diagnosis at an earlier stage of disease, when treatment is more effective.

When diseases have become symptomatic and medical assistance is sought, the goal of the clinician is to provide tertiary prevention in the form of disability limitation for patients with early symptomatic disease, or rehabilitation for patients with late symptomatic disease.

Preventive medicine seeks to enhance the lives of patients by helping them promote their health and prevent specific diseases or diagnose them early. Preventive medicine also tries to apply the concepts and techniques of health promotion and disease prevention to the organization and practice of medicine (clinical preventive services). Health is an elusive concept but means more than the absence of disease; it is a positive concept that includes the ability to adapt to stress and the ability to function in society. The three levels of prevention define the various strategies available to practitioners to promote health and prevent disease, impairment and disability at various stages of the natural history of disease. Primary prevention keeps a disease from becoming established by eliminating the causes of diseases or increasing resistance to disease.

Secondary prevention interrupts the disease process by detecting and treating it in the presymptomatic stage. Tertiary prevention limits the physical impairment and social consequences from symptomatic disease. It is not easy for prevention programs to compete for funds in a tight fiscal climate because of long delays before the benefits of such investments are noted. Specialty training in preventive medicine prepares investigators to demonstrate the cost-effectiveness and cost benefits of prevention.

二、技巧指导：目的语信息重组的几个方法（Ⅱ）

转换法（**conversion**）

转换法是在译入语中转换源语的词性、句型和语态，从而使译入语避免生硬感而变得更加顺畅的方法。转换法也是一种重组。

英译中例句：

1. These cores should be incorporated in every medical curriculum as global

requirements that would equip graduates, regardless of where they are educated, with similar universal competencies, thus securing proper quality of health care.

这一系列“核心”应作为国际化的要求结合到所有医学教育课程之中。这样可以使任何地方培养出来的毕业生都拥有相同的国际化的能力，从而保证医疗质量。

2. Many educators negatively associate standards with standardized multiple-choice tests. However, standardized tests are only one of many other means of measuring progress toward external standards such as practical examination of performance or practical demonstrations of competencies, which have been acquired during studies.

许多教育工作者不正确地将标准与标准化多选项测试混为一谈。其实标准化测试只是众多以外界标准为参照来评估进步的方式之一，例如对评估所学能力的实际操作性测试与实际演示性测试。

中译英例句：

1. 通过对颈动脉状况的筛查，既可对狭窄不甚严重的患者及早给予行为指导或药物干预，延缓其狭窄进展，又可对狭窄严重的患者实施介入治疗或手术治疗，去除其发生中风的病源，减少中风的发生及伤残。

Screening the carotid artery can give early behavioral guidance or drug intervention to patients whose cases are less severe and delay their narrowing process. It can also give interventional or surgical treatment to patients with severe stenosis, remove sources of stroke, and reduce occurrence of stroke and disability.

2. 财富的囤积必然会带来互市。于是便有了深嵌在记忆深处的牛市口、羊市街、骡马市，也才有了连接这些街道的幽僻巷陌。

Accumulations of wealth are bound to bring trade. As a result, deeply embedded in our memories are the Bull Market, the Goat Street, Mule and Horse Market, and serene alleys and quiet streets that connect these markets.

拆句法（segmentation）

拆句法用于英译汉，是把一个英语完整句分割开来，译成两个或两个以上的简单明了的汉语句子的方法。在原句的关系代词、关系副词、主语谓语连接处、并列从句连接处或转折从句连接处切断，并依照汉语表达顺序重组成汉语短句。

英译中例句：

1. Serve as a central point for sharing Canada's expertise with the rest of the world; Apply international research and development to Canada's public health programs;

and Strengthen intergovernmental collaboration on public health and facilitate national approaches to public health policy and planning.

PHAC的作用是：承当中心点，与世界其他地区分享加拿大的专业知识；申请国际研究和开发，为加拿大的公共卫生项目申请国际研究和开发项目；加强公众健康方面的政府间合作，并协助国家手段在公共卫生政策和规划方面的应用。

2. Standards in medical education are set up, by consent of experts or by decision of educational authority, as “model designs or formulations” related to different aspects of medical education, and presented in such way to make possible assessment of graduates performance in compliance with generally accepted professional requirements.

医学教育标准应征得专家同意，由教育权威决定而制订。标准应制订成为与医学教育方方面面有关的模式设计或公式设计。标准应能使对毕业生的学业评估与已经形成的专业要求相吻合。

合并法（**combination**）

合并法多用于中译英。因为英语的主、谓、宾、定、状语位置相对固定，而汉语句法结构不如英语句法结构紧密，如果将几个中文短句顺句译成英文会显得短促而僵硬。所以在翻译有些汉语短句时，需要利用介词、连词、不定式、分词结构、定语从句、独立结构等方法把汉语短句连成英文长句。

中译英例句：

根据北京安贞医院20年脑卒中病例资料分析，致死性中风仅占27%，大部分卒中病人存活且遗留偏瘫、失语等严重影响生活质量的残疾。脑卒中已对国民的生命健康造成严重威胁，并将大幅度增加疾病负担。

An analysis of cases of stroke documented by Beijing Anzhen Hospital during the past 20 years shows that fatal stroke takes up only 27% of the total cases, while the majority of stroke patients survive but are left with disabilities such as hemiplegia and aphasia that seriously affect the quality of life. Stroke seriously threatens people’s life and health and substantially increases the burden of disease.

在上面这个例句中，第一句英语用了被动语态状语合并了一个汉语分句，第二句用了并列句合并了汉语分句。

三、词汇准备

Text 1

Let's Move Active Schools 让我们动起来项目学校
take a moment 花一些时间，用一些时间
have what it takes to 具备所需的一切条件
have it easy 过得舒服，处境很好
watch one's back 注意身后，保持警惕
locker 储物柜
gangs and drugs 犯罪团伙和毒品
get each other's backs 互相保护
little-bitty 非常狭小的
get good grades 取得好成绩
pay off 有收效，获得成功
wave a wand 挥动魔法杖，施魔法
jumping jack 开合跳
push-up 俯卧撑

Text 2

WHO Representative in China 世卫组织驻华代表
2013 World No Tobacco Event 2013年世界无烟日活动
President of the Chinese Association of Tobacco Control 中国控烟协会主席
Director General of China CDC 中国疾控中心主任
distinguished guest 尊敬的各位来宾
World No Tobacco Day 世界无烟日
tobacco use 吸烟
killer 死因
tobacco-related illness 烟草相关疾病
sobering 令人警醒的；使人冷静的
smoking rates 吸烟率
ban tobacco advertising, promotion and sponsorship 禁止烟草广告、促销和赞助
WHO Framework Convention on Tobacco Control (FCTC) 《世卫组织烟草控制框架公约（FCTC）》

socially acceptable 社会可接受的

consumer product 消费品

cost-effective measures 成本效益良好的措施，成本较低的措施

State Administration of Radio, Film and TV 广播电视局，广电局

China National Tobacco Control Plan 2012-2015 《2012—2015年中国烟草控制规划》

hazard 危害；危险

addiction to tobacco use 烟草成瘾

Global Adult Tobacco Survey (GATS) 全球烟草成人调查（GATS）

high levels of exposure to indirect promotion of cigarette smoking through the entertainment media 通过娱乐媒体大量接触吸烟的间接促销

policy action 政策行动

WHO World No Tobacco Day Award 世卫组织世界无烟日奖

capacity 职位；职责

Text 3

prevention and control of noncommunicable diseases 预防和控制非传染性疾病

World Health Assembly 世界卫生大会

mortality and morbidity 疾病和死亡人数

the burden of disease 疾病负担

shared responsibility 共同责任

action plan 行动计划

stakeholder 参与方，利益相关者

annex 附件

epidemic 流行病，蔓延

obesity 肥胖，肥胖症

Obama Administration 奥巴马政府

childhood obesity 儿童肥胖

secretariat 秘书处

for the most part 在极大程度上，基本上，大多数情况下

pressing problem 紧迫问题

National Institutes of Health 美国国立卫生研究院

Obesity Research Task Force 肥胖研究专题工作组

health advocacy organizations 健康倡导组织

U.S. Federal Trade Commission 美国联邦贸易委员会
Food and Drug Administration 美国食品和药物管理局
Centers for Disease Control and Prevention 美国疾病控制和预防中心
Department of Agriculture 农业部
size up 打量，估计，判断
tackle 解决，对付
industry 工业界
non-governmental actor 非政府参与者

Text 4

opening remarks 开幕致辞
Dr. Shin Young-Soo 申英秀博士
WHO Regional Director for the Western Pacific 世界卫生组织西太平洋区域主任
Technical Advisory Group (TAG) on Immunization and Vaccine Preventable Diseases in the Western Pacific Region 西太平洋地区预防接种和疫苗可预防疾病技术咨询小组（TAG）
commend 称赞，赞扬
achieve targets 实现目标
immunization 预防接种，免疫接种
polio 脊髓灰质炎
Regional Commission for the Certification of Poliomyelitis Eradication in the Western Pacific Region 西太平洋区域根除脊髓灰质炎认证委员会
outbreak 疫情，疾病暴发
interrupted 间断的
endemic 某地特有的，地方病的
measles virus 麻疹病毒
rubella 风疹
synergize measles and rubella immunization 麻疹、风疹协同预防接种
surveillance 监测
UNICEF, United Nations Children’s Fund 联合国儿童基金会
validate 证实，验证
maternal and neonatal tetanus 孕产妇和新生儿破伤风
verify 核实，证实
hepatitis B 乙肝

infection rate 感染率

seroprevalence 血清阳性率

WHO-accredited laboratory 世卫组织认证的实验室

national regulatory authorities 国家监管部门

of assured quality 有质量保证

national schedules 全国计划免疫

mortality 死亡率，死亡人数

endorse 赞同，支持

polio endgame plan 脊髓灰质炎消灭计划

vaccine-derived poliovirus 脊灰疫苗衍生病毒

Global Vaccine Action Plan 全球疫苗行动计划

Expanded Programme on Immunization at the Regional Office （世界卫生组织西太平洋）区域办公室的预防接种扩大项目办事处

be made to order for 订制的，定做的，量身定做

equity 公平，公正，均等化

evidence-based 基于证据的，询证的

donor 捐赠者，捐献人

goals and objectives 长远目标和具体目标

vibrant 生气勃勃的，精力充沛的

Text 5

中国疾病预防控制中心 the Chinese Center for Disease Control and Prevention (China CDC)

国际防痨与肺部疾病联合会 International Union against Tuberculosis and Lung Disease (The Union)

无烟环境 smoke-free environment

启动会 launch

二手烟 secondhand smoking

暴露 exposure to

主办单位 organizer

国务院法制办 the State Council's Legislative Affairs Office

烟草危害 the harms of tobacco use

牵头 take the lead to

《国际烟草控制框架公约》 International Framework Convention on Tobacco

Control

烟草流行 tobacco epidemic

全国人大常委会 the Standing Committee of the National People's Congress

生效 take effect, go into effect, come into effect

签约和批准 sign and ratify

遏制烟草消费 curbing tobacco consumption

烟草使用对于健康危害的滞后效应 delayed manifestation of the health impact of tobacco use

烟草疾病相关死亡率 mortality of tobacco-related diseases

因病致贫 poverty caused by morbidity

正在进行的医疗体制改革 ongoing health care system reform

初衷 original intention

端口前移 start early preparation for prevention

示范行动 demonstration action

多部门的协作 multi-sectoral collaboration

Text 6

慢性病 chronic diseases, chronic illnesses

中国脑卒中大会 China Stroke Conference

处于高发势态 show a trend of high incidence

死亡原因 cause of death

脑血管病 cerebrovascular disease (CVD)

社会传染病 infectious social diseases

井喷 large eruption, outburst

刻不容缓的工作 an urgent task that admits no delay

社会经济发展核心指标 core indicators of socioeconomic development

维护民生、维护人民群众健康权益 defend/safeguard people's livelihood and right to health

把……当作头等大事来抓 give top priority to...

国家会议中心 China National Convention Center

第66届联大 the 66th UN General Assembly

国际社会 the international community

风险因素 risk factor

心脑血管疾病 cardiovascular and cerebrovascular diseases

第一位的死亡原因 the number one killer

筛查防治工程 screening, prevention and control project

司局 bureaus and departments

高危人群 high-risk populations

重大专项 major project

试点 pilot projects

颈动脉血管筛查 carotid artery screening test

健康指导 health education sessions

健康体检 physical check-ups

内科干预 internalist medical interventions

外科手术干预 surgical interventions

培训医务人员 training health workers

义诊 free consultation

健康宣教活动 health education activities

宣传册 brochure

发病 onset

高血压，糖尿病，血脂异常，心脏病 high blood pressure, diabetes, dyslipidemia, heart disease

财政、科技、社保、民政等部门 financial, technological, social security, and civil affairs departments

整合现有资源 integrate the available resources

慢病大病保障政策 health insurance policy for serious diseases and chronic diseases

脑梗死 cerebral infarction

新农合大病保障 coverage of serious diseases by the new model rural cooperative health care system

脑血管病适宜技术 the appropriate technology of cerebrovascular disease

推广，培训，科研立项 dissemination, training and research

示范基地 demonstration center

四、摘要练习

请听下面英语语篇，第一篇用源语言复述此段主要信息逻辑点及层次，第二篇用译入语复述此段主要信息逻辑点及层次。注意信息点之间的逻辑联系。

Text 1

Michelle Obama's Address to Chicago School Children at the Launch of Let's Move[1] Active Schools

28 February 2013

MRS. OBAMA: Isn't this exciting? (Applause.) Oh my goodness. Thank you, Serena[2], Allyson[3], thanks to all the athletes. And let me just tell you, I wanted to take a moment before we got into some fun, because I wanted to talk to you all—I'm in my home town. (Applause.)

So listen up, just a little serious business because all of these incredible athletes you see here—they have traveled here today to my home town because, like me, they wanted to be here with all of you amazing kids. We wanted you to know that there are millions—do you hear me, millions—of people like us all over this world who love you so much. We love you more than you can ever know. We love you so much. (Applause.)

And we care about you—I want you to hear this—we care about you. We care and believe in you. We believe that you have what it takes to accomplish anything that you want in this life. But we also want you to understand, and I want you all to listen, we want you to understand that the only difference between all of you all out there and all of us standing up here on this stage are the choices that you make in life.

It is so important for each of you to realize that every day you, and you alone, have the power to choose the life you want for yourself. Whether you spend your day watching TV or whether you use that time to pick up your books and finish your homework—see, that's your choice. Whether you fill your bodies with chips and candy or fruits and vegetables—see, that's on you. Whether you sit around all day playing video games or get up and move your bodies—these are all the choices that will determine who you will become and what you can achieve.

See, every one of these great athletes standing with me today had to make good

1 Let's Move! "让我们动起来"是一场结束美国儿童肥胖问题的运动，这场运动是由第一夫人米歇尔·奥巴马发起的。这一倡议的最初目标是："在一代人的时间内解决儿童肥胖的挑战，今天出生的孩子到达成年后将拥有健康的体重。"这场运动由第一夫人于2010年2月9日宣布开始。她指出，该运动鼓励学校提供更健康的食物、更好的食品标签，鼓励儿童参与更多的运动。

2 Serena Williams，塞雷娜·威廉姆斯，美国网坛名将，小威廉姆斯。

3 Allyson Felix，美国著名田径运动员，在2012年奥运会上代表美国参赛，赢得200米、4×100米接力和4×400米接力赛跑三枚金牌。

choices, and they had to work hard to get where they are. See, what you guys have to understand—they weren't just born faster or stronger or smarter. And maybe it's hard for you to believe, but many of us didn't have it easy growing up. I mean, some of us are from tough neighborhoods where we had to watch our backs. Or we went to schools where the books were torn and the lockers were beat up and stuff didn't always work. Yes, some of us grew up without a father—or we saw people we loved involved with gangs and drugs. And it was a struggle to get each other's backs and hang together as a family.

And let me tell you, I can tell you that growing up, my family didn't have a lot of money. We live in a little bitty apartment on the South Side of Chicago. (Applause.) South Side. (Applause.) And for most of my life growing up, I shared a tiny bedroom with my big brother. And some nights, let me tell you, it was hard to get my homework done because it was so noisy that I could barely think. And I know some of you know what that's like, right?

AUDIENCE: Yes!

MRS. OBAMA: So it was hard. So there were times when I started to doubt myself. In fact, a lot of us up on this stage grew up being told by others that we weren't good enough or smart enough to achieve our dreams. We all heard that, right? So if you guys remember just one thing from our time today, it's this: Although I am the First Lady of the United States of America—(Applause.)—listen to this, because this is the truth—I am no different from you. (Applause.)

Look, I grew up in the same neighborhoods, went to the same schools, faced the same struggles, shared the same hopes and dreams that all of you share. I am you. And the only reason that I am standing up here today is that back when I was your age, I made a set of choices with my life—do you hear me—choices.

I chose not to listen to the doubters and the haters. (Applause.) I chose to shut those voices out of my head and listen to my own voice. I chose to ignore any negative things that were happening around me, and instead focus on all the wonderful things I had going on inside of me. I chose to focus on what I could control.

So let me tell you what I did. I worked hard in school to get good grades. I listened to my teachers. I behaved in school. I learned from everyone and everything around me. I stayed active. I didn't do—I did everything that I could to keep my body healthy and fit. I did everything within my power to prepare myself for great things. And eventually all of my work paid off—I went to college, I went to law school. And because I had a good education, I could get a good job so that my family wouldn't have to worry about money and I could live in a house where my daughters could have their own rooms.

And the lesson I learned along the way is that it did not matter where I was from. It didn't matter how much my parents had. What mattered was how hard I was willing to work, and how deeply I was willing to believe in myself. (Applause.)

And one of the main reasons I wanted all of you to be here today with us is that that is true for every single one of the folks up on this stage here today. They can tell you that there is no magic to their achievements. No one waved a wand and turned these folks into champions. They turned themselves into champions by doing the hard work, getting their education, exercising every day, eating healthy, practicing their skills over and over and over again.

And we're all here today to tell you that you can do the same thing. Do you hear me—you all can do the same thing. (Applause.) You all have every reason to be hopeful about your future. Don't let anybody tell you differently. You all can make yourselves into somebody that you're proud of. You have it in you. You can be anything you want—whether it's a doctor, a teacher, a scientist, or, yes, President of the United States. You all can do that. (Applause.)

You can make your family proud of who you are and who you become. And I have the secret. Do you want to hear the secret?

AUDIENCE: Yes!

MRS. OBAMA: You have to get a good education. Do you hear me—you have to get a good education. That is the most important thing that you can do for yourselves right now. And that means that you have to go to school every day—every single day no matter what your school looks like or what's going on there, you have to be sitting at your desks, ready to learn. You've got one job at this age and that is to be the best student that you can be. (Applause.)

So listen to your teachers. Do your homework—and not just when you feel like it, but every day, no matter what's happening in your life. Remember, no one is born smart. You become smart through hard work. The more you read, the more you do math, the smarter you become. So every single one of you can become smart if you're willing to put the work in.

And finally, you guys need to take care of your bodies. You have to. That means you have to eat the right foods. It's not a joke, it's not a game—foods that will make you strong and give you energy. You've got to eat fruits. You've got to eat vegetables. You've got to use those meals, those good foods you're getting now in your schools every single day.

And you have to be active, guys. You listen to me—you've got to turn off the TV, move away from the screen. (Applause.) You've got to keep your body active, even if that means just turning on some music and dancing for an hour. Do a little dougie[1], a few jumping jacks, some push-ups. And you don't have to be an Olympic athlete to be healthy. You just have to move. That's how you'll prepare your bodies and your minds for greatness.

You know what—and now it's time for the serious stuff to end, okay? Did you all hear all the message that I had for you?

AUDIENCE: Yes!

MRS. OBAMA: You all promise me that you're going to be good students.

AUDIENCE: We promise!

MRS. OBAMA: You all promise me that you're going to eat right.

AUDIENCE: We promise!

MRS. OBAMA: You promise me you're going to get moving.

AUDIENCE: We promise!

MRS. OBAMA: And we're going to start right here and right now. (Applause.) These champions are going to lead the way by showing us how to get moving. So let's have some fun. Are you ready? (Applause.) All right, let's move! (Applause.)

复述要点提示（主要信息逻辑点及层次）

Purpose of the speech:

The First Lady of the United States calls on school kids to eat healthy and get up to do some exercises because that is how they prepare themselves for the great things they want to do in the future.

Keynotes of the speech:

The young children should know that they are loved. The First Lady repeatedly emphasized that adults love and care a lot for the school kids. They have complete faith that all these children are capable of realizing whatever plans they have made for their life.

For these young kids, the key to success is to make right choices in life. All the famous athletes standing on the stage became successful because they have made the right choices in their lives and have thus become successful. The kids must understand that they have the right to make choices and that they should always make the right choices.

The First Lady used the athletes as examples. When they were growing up, many of them experienced lots of difficulties, for example, poverty, violence, crime, poor school facility, absent parent, etc.

1 Dougie，道基舞，嘻哈舞蹈的一种，饶舌歌手道格·E. 弗雷什（Doug E. Fresh）在20世纪80年代开始表演这种舞蹈，因此以他的名字而命名。

She also used herself to demonstrate her point. She grew up in a poor neighborhood. Her family lived in a very small apartment and she and her brother had to share a bedroom.

We always start to doubt ourselves when we are faced with difficulties. It is important that we do not pay any attention to the negative things people say to us. We have to be positive and we have to have confidence in ourselves. This attitude has helped her to become the First Lady.

It is also important we always work very hard. It doesn't matter how much wealth our parents have. If we work hard in everything, for example, school, work, and exercise, we will be prepared for great things and our effort will always pay off. For example, the athletes on stage have all worked very hard to finish their education. They practiced very hard and have also done a good job controlling their diet. Eventually, they have become champions.

If the kids have the same attitude and make the right choices in life, they will be able to do anything they want to with their life. They could become doctors, teachers, scientists, or President of the United States.

The First Lady urged that all kids should get a good education. They should go to school every day. They should listen to their teachers, do their homework, and read a lot.

The First Lady urged the kids to eat healthy food, which would give their body the energy they need and keep them healthy.

The First Lady urged the kids to turn away from TV and video games, and do some exercises every day.

The First Lady asked some interactive questions to make sure that the audience got her message. Then she invited the athletes to show to the audience how to do some simple exercises.

Text 2

Remarks by Dr. Michael O'Leary, WHO Representative in China, at NHFPC[1] 2013 World No Tobacco Event

Beijing, China

30 May 2013

NHFPC Vice Minister Madame Cui Li,

Dr. Huang Jiefu, President of the Chinese Association of Tobacco Control and former Vice Minister,

Dr. Wang Yu, Director General of China CDC[2],

Distinguished guests,

Ladies and gentlemen,

Good morning.

Thank you for inviting me to be here today at this event to mark World No Tobacco Day.

As you all know, tobacco use is one of China's biggest killers. More than 1 million Chinese people die from a tobacco-related illness every year. With more than 300 million smokers in the country, it is sobering to think that the annual death toll from tobacco will increase to 3 million by 2050 if smoking rates are not reduced.

The theme for this year's World No Tobacco Day is: ban tobacco advertising, promotion and sponsorship.

The WHO Framework Convention on Tobacco Control (FCTC) requires a comprehensive ban of all forms of tobacco advertising, promotion and sponsorship.

This is because the evidence from around the world shows that comprehensive marketing bans lead to fewer people starting and continuing to smoke.

Advertising and promotion of tobacco helps to create an environment where smoking is

---

1 NHFPC全称是National Health and Family Planning Commission，中华人民共和国国家卫生和计划生育委员会，是中华人民共和国国务院的组成部门，取代原卫生部和国家计生委，具体方案在2013年3月由第十二届全国人民代表大会第一次会议审议后公布。

2 China CDC全称为the Chinese Center for Disease Control and Prevention，即中国疾病预防控制中心，简称为中国疾控中心。是由政府举办的实施国家级疾病预防控制与公共卫生技术管理和服务的公益事业单位。其使命是通过对疾病、残疾和伤害的预防控制，创造健康环境，维护社会稳定，保障国家安全，促进人民健康。

seen as socially acceptable, or "normal".

As a result, tobacco advertising, promotion and sponsorship foster an illusion that tobacco is just like any other consumer product.

But the reality is that tobacco is a lethal product: when used as intended by the manufacturers, tobacco kills up to half of its regular users.

Banning tobacco advertising, promotion and sponsorship is one of the most cost-effective measures governments can take to reduce demand for tobacco products, and in doing so, protect the health of their populations.

In China, some important steps have been taken to strengthen restrictions on tobacco marketing in recent years:

- The Advertising Law bans tobacco advertising in the mass media, including through radio, movies, TV, newspapers and magazines;
- In February 2011, the State Administration of Radio, Film and TV announced strict controls on the portrayal of smoking in movies and TV serials; and
- In December 2012, the Government of China issued the China National Tobacco Control Plan 2012-2015, which includes a strong commitment to strengthening existing bans on tobacco advertising, promotion and sponsorship.

We welcome the steps China has taken to strengthen restrictions on tobacco marketing to date.

However, further strong policy action is required to clamp down on tobacco marketing in China.

This is especially important to protect China's young people from the hazards of a lifetime of addiction to tobacco use.

Data from the Global Adult Tobacco Survey (GATS) conducted in China in 2010 shows that despite China's bans and controls, nearly 30% of young people aged 15-24 years reported noticing tobacco advertising, promotions or sponsorships in the 30 days prior to the survey.

Other studies have also shown very high levels of exposure to indirect promotion of cigarette smoking through the entertainment media in China.

This is of serious concern when we know that even brief exposure to tobacco marketing can influence adolescents.

Banning tobacco advertising, promotion and sponsorship is therefore especially important for protecting young people from the harms of tobacco.

I congratulate China CDC on the report they have produced and released today, highlighting the importance of further strong policy action in this area to protect China's public from tobacco marketing.

We look forward to continuing to work with China CDC, the National Health and Family Planning Commission, and other partners to further reform this area.

And on this note, I am delighted to announce today that WHO is this year recognizing one of our foremost partners in China's tobacco control efforts, Dr. Huang Jiefu, with a WHO World No Tobacco Day Award.

As all of you know, in both his role as President of the Chinese Association for Tobacco Control, and his former capacity as Vice-Minister of the Ministry of Health, Dr. Huang has been a leading voice for stronger tobacco control measures in China.

I congratulate Dr. Huang on his award, and hope that it serves as encouragement for other advocates for stronger tobacco control policies in China.

Thank you again for inviting me to speak today. WHO looks forward to continuing to work with all of you to achieve change on this important issue for the future of China. And may I wish you a happy—and smoke-free—World No Tobacco Day!

复述要点提示（主要信息逻辑点及层次）

主题：

中国存在大量吸烟者，需要加强工作以降低吸烟率，减少与烟草相关的死亡。中国需要制定更严格的政策，采取更有力的行动禁止烟草营销，从而减少开始和持续吸烟的人的总数。

背景：

2013年世界无烟日，国家卫生和计划生育委员会组织活动。2013年世界无烟日主题是“禁止烟草广告、促销和赞助”。

六个要点：

中国存在严重吸烟问题。每年有100多万人死于烟草相关疾病，目前有3亿多吸烟者，如不降低吸烟率，到2050年，烟草相关死亡率可能增至每年300万。

禁止烟草广告、营销和赞助活动。全球各种证据表明，发布全面烟草营销禁令可减少开始和继续吸烟的人数。烟草广告和促销让人们觉得吸烟是一种社会可接受的行为，吸烟是“正常”行为，烟草也是一种普通消费品。烟草营销禁令不但能减少烟草需求、保护人民健康，并且成本还较低。

中国已经做出的禁烟工作。中国政府历年来颁布了一系列法律法规限制烟草营销，例如《广告法》、广电局的规定等。

中国禁烟工作目前还存在的问题。2010年在中国开展的“全球烟草成人调查

（GATS）”的数据显示，近30%的15～24岁的年轻人在报告调查前一个月内看到过烟草营销活动。娱乐媒体中也存在大量的烟草间接促销内容。这些对青少年会造成更大危害，因为青少年极易受到烟草促销的影响。

世界卫生组织期待未来与中国有更多合作，期待中国在控烟这一领域取得更多成就。

世界卫生组织表彰中国控烟领域有杰出贡献的黄洁夫医生，给他颁发今年的“世界无烟日奖”。黄洁夫医生是中国控烟协会主席、卫生部前副部长。

五、英译汉练习

Text 3

Prevention and Control of Noncommunicable Diseases: Implementation of the Global Strategy

OS Surgeon General's[1] Speech at 63rd World Health Assembly

Geneva, Switzerland
20 May 2010

The United States thanks the WHO for its work on the global strategy for the prevention and control of non-communicable diseases. As the Surgeon General of the United States, I can say that we recognize that non-communicable diseases contribute significantly to mortality and morbidity worldwide, and represent an increasing proportion of the burden of disease in developing countries. Because non-communicable diseases are a significant public health issue that affect both developing and developed countries, we continue to support the WHO's Action Plan for implementing the global strategy, such as the inclusion of all stakeholders in that work, as the reduction of non-communicable diseases is a shared responsibility.

1 Surgeon General，总医官，美国公共卫生服务现役军团（United States Public Health Service Commissioned Corps, PHSCC）最高长官，授予中将军衔。PHSCC成员穿着美国海军的军官制服，但是佩戴PHSCC标志，授予美国海军一样的军官军衔，授衔资格待遇也和美军同级军衔相同，军衔由PHSCC授予。组成之初只有医生，后来加入牙医、护士、药师、工程师等专业人员，全部是军官。PHSCC的核心使命是保护、促进、改善国民的安全和健康。

We are pleased with the progress that WHO has made in implementing the action plan.

Turning to the Annex, the set of recommendations on marketing of food and non-alcoholic beverages to children should play a significant role in helping Member States promote healthier patterns of eating as part of efforts to reduce the growing epidemic of childhood obesity. This is a priority for the Obama Administration, in particular for the First Lady, who has raised awareness of childhood obesity and the importance of healthy eating.

The United States is pleased to see that the stakeholder consultation process the Secretariat implemented resulted in considerable improvement in both the structure and content of the recommendations. For the most part, the recommendations share the policy objectives that are priorities for the US Congress and the Obama Administration.

The United States is addressing the pressing problem of obesity in many ways. For example, the National Institutes of Health has established an Obesity Research Task Force, which has developed a Strategic Plan for obesity research with the input of external experts and health advocacy organizations. Our investments in obesity research and strategic planning will benefit the WHO as it implements global strategies in the prevention and control of obesity and other noncommunicable diseases.

The US Federal Trade Commission, together with the Food and Drug Administration, the Centers for Disease Control and Prevention, and the Department of Agriculture are developing standards for the marketing of foods to children in the United States.

These proposed standards were presented in December 2009, at "Sizing Up Food Marketing and Childhood Obesity", a workshop hosted by the US Federal Trade Commission, and are to be submitted to our Congress in July.

We are pleased to see the recommendations mention a range of implementation mechanisms. There is a shared responsibility for tackling the growing obesity epidemic, which means Governments, industry and non-governmental actors and individuals all have roles to play. No stakeholder should be left out.

We are pleased to support the draft resolution, as proposed and amended by Norway.

Thank you Mr. Chairman.

Text 4

Opening Remarks by Dr. Shin Young-Soo, WHO Regional Director for the Western Pacific, at the 22nd Meeting of the Technical Advisory Group (TAG) on Immunization and Vaccine Preventable Diseases in the Western Pacific Region

Manila, Philippines

25 June 2013

Distinguished participants and colleagues, ladies and gentlemen:

Welcome to the 22nd meeting of the Technical Advisory Group—or TAG—on Immunization and Vaccine-Preventable Diseases in the Western Pacific Region.

Since the previous TAG meeting in August, there has been much progress to report.

I would like to commend Member States for their hard work towards achieving targets and strengthening their immunization systems.

Let's look at some specific accomplishments:

● The Region retained its polio-free status when the Regional Commission for the Certification of Poliomyelitis Eradication in the Western Pacific in November 2012 concluded that China adequately responded to the 2011 outbreak.

● By the end of 2012, 34 countries and areas may have interrupted endemic measles virus transmission. Rubella control has also been accelerated by synergizing measles and rubella immunization and surveillance activities.

● In December 2012, WHO and UNICEF validated China's elimination of maternal and neonatal tetanus.

● Australia, China, Mongolia and New Zealand were officially verified to have achieved the regional goal of reducing hepatitis B infection rates in children to less than 1%. By 2012, the Region as a whole and at least 30 countries and areas individually achieved the less than 2% seroprevalence in five-year old children.

● WHO-accredited laboratory networks for vaccine-preventable diseases have been established with tremendous new capacities.

● The regional alliance of national regulatory authorities was established to help Member States promote the use of safe vaccines of assured quality.

● Five countries in the Region have added seven vaccines to their national schedules to reduce mortality in women and children.

These are truly impressive milestones. But still, great challenges lay ahead.

Now your expertise and wisdom are required to guide the Region on two items recently endorsed by the World Health Assembly.

First: how we should move forward so that Western Pacific countries implement the polio endgame plan by 2018.

As you know, the plan outlines activities to prevent the emergence and circulation of vaccine-derived polioviruses. Your input will be critical for successful implementation.

The second issue for the TAG is to review the proposed framework for implementation of the Global Vaccine Action Plan in the Western Pacific Region.

This global vaccine plan was endorsed by the WHA in May 2012.

Since then, the Expanded Programme on Immunization at the Regional Office has been working with Member States to identify best approaches and drafted a plan for implementing the Global Vaccine Action Plan 2011-2020.

The plan is made to order for the Region's needs with four major emphases:

1. reaching our disease reduction targets;

2. increasing equity and access to vaccination;

3. promoting evidence-based introduction of new vaccines; and

4. increasing high-level financial commitment of governments, partners and donors to ensure sustainability of immunization programmes.

Your input will be invaluable as we move forward to reach the new regional immunization goals and objectives, as well as the goals set in the Decade of Vaccines[1].

Let me close by thanking all of you for making the Expanded Programme on Immunization a vibrant and innovative force in the Western Pacific Region.

Your guidance matters greatly to make sure all of our efforts are as effective as possible—from those of governments and development agencies to those of donors and other partners.

I look forward to hearing your recommendations and wish you all a pleasant stay in Manila.

Thank you.

---

1 Decade of Vaccines，“疫苗十年”，世界卫生组织194个成员在世界卫生大会达成的共同愿景，即打造一个不受疫苗可预防疾病危害的世界，让每一个人都能享有免疫的全部好处。

六、汉译英练习

Text 5

无烟环境促进项目可有效控制二手烟暴露

中国疾病预防控制中心与国际防痨与肺部疾病联合会合作的"无烟环境促进项目"启动会致辞

中国疾病预防控制中心主任王宇
中国北京昌平中国疾病预防控制中心
2010年1月15日

尊敬的各位来宾、朋友们、同志们：

大家好！

无烟环境促进项目1月15日正式启动，我代表主办单位中国疾病预防控制中心，向积极支持本项目的卫生部、国务院法制办领导、各项目城市、政府及本项目的合作方，国际防痨和肺部疾病联合会表示衷心感谢，向参加本次启动项目的各位专家和媒体朋友们表示热烈欢迎。烟草危害是当今世界最严重的公共卫生问题之一，是人类健康所面临的巨大的，然而又是可以预防的危险因素。

为了降低烟草带来的危害以及由此而产生的巨大的经济损失，世界卫生组织牵头制定了《国际烟草控制框架公约》，这是一份为了应对烟草流行的全球化、以证据为基础的国际公约。截至2008年11月全世界已有168个国家签署并批准了这项公约。中国于2003年11月8日签署公约，是第77个签约国，并得到了全国人大常委会批准，于2006年1月8日在中国生效。各国政府的签约和批准《烟草控制框架公约》表明各国政府都认同遏制烟草消费是保护人民健康的优先重点之一，关注民众的健康是以人为本的基本目标。

虽然《国际烟草控制框架公约》的制定和实施为中国烟草控制提供了重要机遇，但同时我们也必须看到，中国的烟草控制也面临着非常严重的挑战，框架公约在中国生效的几年来，我国的烟草产量不但没有降低反而在增加。到2008年行业累计新产销卷烟已达到4 400多万箱，比2003年增长了近30%。五年的平均增长率为5.35%。

目前中国男性人群中高吸烟率和女性及儿童中的二手烟高暴露率导致每年100万人死于与烟草相关的各种疾病。到2030年，预计每年死于烟草相关疾病人数会增加至200万。由于烟草使用对于健康危害的滞后效应，目前肺癌等与烟草疾病相关死亡率也只是20世纪70年代人群烟草消费的后果。中国烟草流行的高峰是20世纪90年代以来，由于烟草使用带来危害的高峰远未到来，如果我们不控制烟草使用和二手烟的暴露，未来50年，烟草使用和带来的危害还将持续上升，这必然带来医疗费用大量增加。烟草带来的健康问题是人们因病致贫，因病返贫的一个重要因素。目前正在进行新的医疗体制改革，改革初期首先要解决卫生公平问题，保障广大群众看病就医的基本需求。随着医疗改革的推进，政府为烟草带来的慢性病治疗费用的支出也会不断增加，慢性病已成为阻碍经济发展的前三位之一。我们的初衷，不仅是解决人们看病的问题，更重要的是把端口前移，做好疾病预防工作。如果烟草使用没有得到有效控制，最终也会成为中国和世界经济发展的主要障碍。

中国疾病预防控制中心的使命是预防疾病，促进健康，中国疾控中心把烟草控制作为慢病控制重要手段，保证人们免受二手烟的危害。我们启动的无烟环境促进项目，就是要以法律为手段，通过全社会的动员，实现烟草控制。就二手烟的暴露对慢病的影响采取健康教育是一个手段，更有利的是通过政策和法律建立保障。这个项目最大的特点是项目由政府领导，项目的创新点在于通过建立起法学网和媒体网，有效地促进项目实施，建立禁止公共场所吸烟等各项法规。这种做法与单纯的健康教育还是不同的。其他国家的经验证明，只有这样才能更为有效地控制二手烟暴露，促进我国的烟草控制。我们将通过七个城市的示范行动，带动一大批城市的烟草控制立法，为出台国家层面的相关法律，推动中国的烟草控制奠定基础。

烟草控制需要长期持续努力，并全面规划实施，尤其是需要政府的牵头，多部门的协作。烟草控制工程是一项社会工程，仅靠卫生部门的力量是远远不够的，本项目也得到国务院法制办领导及项目参与政府的大力支持。我们在这里表示深深的感谢。我相信，通过多部门的共同努力，本项目的实施将为促进我国无烟环境的建设，强化我国的控烟能力，并对中国的烟草控制事业起到积极的推动作用，保障我国广大群众的健康。谢谢大家！

Text 6

团结协作，迎接慢性病的严峻挑战
陈竺部长代表卫生部在2012脑卒中[1]大会开幕式上的讲话

中国北京

2012年5月4日

尊敬的同道们、朋友们:

在这春暖花开的美好时节，我们齐聚一堂，召开“2012中国脑卒中大会”，商讨脑卒中防治工作，共商我国慢性病防控策略。我谨代表卫生部对各位同道、专家表示诚挚的问候!

当前，我国慢性疾病处于高发势态。2008年全国居民死亡原因调查显示，脑血管病已成为我国居民死亡的第一位原因。慢病是“社会传染病”，如果控制不好，未来二三十年，将会出现慢性病的“井喷”。慢病防控是一项刻不容缓的工作。降低慢病的风险，需要将其纳入社会经济发展核心指标。全国各级卫生部门要把慢病防控当作维护民生、维护人民群众健康权益的头等大事来抓，如果再不重视慢病防控工作，我们将会犯历史错误。

2012中国脑卒中大会在国家会议中心召开，共商脑卒中防治工作。过去的一年，对全世界的慢病防控工作来说，都是具有重要意义的一年。2011年9月联大召开了慢病预防和控制高级别会议。在这次大会上提出，慢性病是21世纪各国发展面临的严重挑战。国际社会将加强合作，通过各国政府和全社会的努力，减少风险因素，并创造促进健康的环境，加大国家政策保障，提高卫生系统的能力，以迎接慢性病对人类的挑战。

当前，我国慢性病处于高发阶段。其中心脑血管疾病在城乡居民主要死亡构成中已占到了40%以上。脑血管病已经成为我国第一位的死亡原因。如果不能采取及时有效措施，慢性病快速增长将成为影响人民生活水平提高和经济社会发展的巨大障碍。卫生部2009年下半年启动了脑卒中筛查防治工程，成立了有九个司局共同参与的卫生部脑卒中筛查与防治工程委员会。脑卒中高危人群筛查与防治工作列入2011年国家医改的重大专项，并先期在五省一市开始试点工作。

目前，卫生部在全国成立了90余家脑卒中筛查与防治的基地医院。据不完全统计，2010年以来，国家共开展颈动脉血管的筛查共55万例，实施健康指导和健康体

---

1 脑卒中，又称中风、脑中风，是指由于脑部供血受阻而迅速发展成的脑功能损伤。英文为stroke或cerebrovascular accident (CVA)。

检229万人次，内科干预66万人次，外科手术干预两万余例，培训医务人员近50 000人次。举行各种义诊和健康宣教活动共718场，印发脑卒中宣传册189万份，脑卒中贫困救助2 395人。

脑卒中的发病是高血压、糖尿病、血脂异常、心脏病等多种慢性病长期作用引起的，为了推进脑卒中疾病的筛查和防治工作，我想提出以下五点意见以指导脑卒中防治工作的继续向前推进：

第一，各级卫生部门要继续完善相关政策。积极协调财政、科技、社保、民政等部门，在政策和资金上给予脑卒中筛查以更多的支持。卫生系统内部要整合现有资源，充分利用基本公共卫生项目成果，推动脑卒中防控工作、医改重大项目实施，使项目资金发挥更大的效益。

第二，逐步完善包括脑卒中等慢性病大病保障政策。2012年卫生部将会同财政部、民政部在已有大病保障的基础上把包括脑梗死在内的12种大病纳入新农合大病保障范畴。切实减轻大病患者的经济负担。

第三，要充分发挥科技在卫生改革中发挥的支撑作用。要在脑血管病适宜技术推广、培训、科研立项等方面给予扶持。

第四，加强慢性病防控知识的宣传与普及。广大医务工作者要站在慢病防控第一线，传播脑卒中防控知识。

第五，建立脑卒中防控示范基地，通过脑卒中的筛查和防治体系的建设，探索适合我国国情的慢病防治工作。

资料来源：

Text 1 www.wbez.org/news/full-text-michelle-obama

Text 2 http://www.wpro.who.int/entity/china/mediacentre/speeches/2013/20130530/en/

Text 3 https://geneva.usmission.gov/2010/05/20/surgeon-general/

Text 4 www.wpro.who.int/regional_director/speeches/2011/20121113

Text 5 http://www.360doc.com/content/10/1110/09/128196_68109233.shtml

Text 6 http://zl.39.net/a/120507/2020148.html

参考答案

四、摘要练习

Text 1

米歇尔·奥巴马在"让我们动起来"项目启动仪式上对芝加哥学校儿童的致辞

2013年2月28日

奥巴马夫人：这是不是很令人兴奋？（掌声）哦，我的天啊。谢谢你们，塞雷娜、艾莉森，感谢所有的运动员。让我告诉你们，开始做好玩的事情之前，我想花点时间和大家谈谈——我回到了家乡。（掌声）

请仔细听好，我要谈一点严肃的事情，因为你们看到的所有这些了不起的运动员们，他们今天来到这里——我的家乡芝加哥，因为像我一样，他们希望能和你们这些了不起的孩子们在一起。我们想让你们知道，这个世界上有成千上万——你们听到了吗，数以百万计——像我们这样的人非常爱你们。我们爱你们的程度远超出你们的想象。我们非常爱你们。（掌声）

我们非常在乎你们——我想让你们听到这句话——我们非常关心你们。我们关心和相信你们。我们相信你们具备所需的一切条件成就任何人生目标。但是，我们也希望你们能理解，我希望大家能仔细听好，我们希望你们明白，我们所有站在这个舞台上的人和那些没有站在这个舞台上的人之间唯一的区别是在生活中做出的选择。

重要的是你们每个人都明白自己手中握有权力选择自己每天想要过的生活，这个权力完全在你自己一个人的手中。无论你们是花一天时间看电视，还是利用这段时间去拿起书本，并完成你们的功课——看，这就是你们的选择。是往自己的身体里塞满薯片、糖果，还是水果和蔬菜——看，这也是你的选择。是整天坐在那里玩游戏还是站起来活动身体——所有这些选择都将决定你们将成为什么样的人，会有怎样的成就。

看，今天和我一起站在这里的这些伟大的运动员们，他们必须做出好的选择，他们必须努力才能取得今天的成就。你们一定要明白——他们不是天生就更快、更强大或更聪明。也许你们很难相信，但我们中很多人成长的过程都非常艰难。我的意思是，我们中有些人来自治安状况不佳的社区，不得不随时警惕自己的安全。或者，当我们去上学时，用的是被撕坏的课本和被砸得破破烂烂的储物柜，很多东西都不能正常使用。是的，我们有些人成长于没有父亲的单亲家庭，又或是目睹我们所爱的人参与犯罪团伙和毒品活动，要努力拼搏才能互相保护，维持自己的家庭。

让我告诉你们，我可以告诉你们，长大过程中我的家人也没有多少钱。我们住在芝加哥南边一个非常狭小的公寓里。（掌声）芝加哥南边。（掌声）我成长过程中大部分时间都和我的哥哥共用一个小卧室。而有些夜晚，让我告诉你们，我很难完成我的功课，因为周围嘈杂得让我完全不能思考。我知道你们当中有些人知道那是什么样的情况，对吧？

观众：是的！

奥巴马夫人：所以这是很难的。所以有时候我会开始怀疑自己。事实上，站在讲台上的这些人当中，许多人都曾听到过这样的话，我们不够好或不够聪明，不能实现我们的梦想。我们都听到过这样的话，对吗？所以，如果我们今天的事情你们只记得一件，那就是：虽然我是美利坚合众国第一夫人——（掌声）——请仔细听，因为这是事实——我和你们没有什么不同。（掌声）

你们看，我和你们从小就在同一个街区长大，去上同一所学校，面临着同样的斗争，和大家有着同样的希望和梦想。我就是你们。我今天站在这里的唯一原因是，在那时，当我还是你们这个年龄时，我做出了一系列关于我的生活的选择——你们听到了吗——选择。

我选择不听怀疑或是敌视我的人的话。（掌声）我选择不听那些声音，而是听我自己的声音。我选择忽略我周围发生的所有负面的东西，专注于我自己心里计划的所有美好的事物。我选择了把重点放在我可以控制的事情上。

所以，让我告诉你们我做了什么。我在学校努力学习，取得好成绩。我在学校专心听讲，表现良好。我从大家身上和周围的一切学习。我坚持运动——所有可以保持我的身体健康的事情我都做。我做了一切在我能力范围内的事情，让自己做好准备去做伟大的事情。最终所有这些都得到了回报——我上了大学，上了法学院。因为我接受了良好的教育，我可以找到一份好工作，让我的家人不用为钱发愁，而且在我住的房子里，我的两个女儿都有自己的房间。

我一路上学到的教训是，我的出身并不重要。我的父母有多少财富并不重要。重要的是我愿意付出怎样的努力，以及我对自己有多么深厚的信心。（掌声）

我想，今天我想要你们来这里见我们的一个主要原因是，前面的话对于在这个舞台上的每一个人都是真实的。他们可以告诉你们，他们并不是靠魔法取得这些成就的。没有人挥舞着魔杖，把这些人变成冠军。是他们自己通过努力成为冠军，他们勤奋刻苦，接受教育，每天锻炼，健康饮食，一遍、一遍、又一遍练习自己的技能。

我们今天在这里要告诉你们，你们可以做到同样的事情。你们听到了吗——你们都可以做同样的事情。（掌声）你们有充分的理由对自己的未来充满希望。如果任何人告诉你们对未来不要抱有希望，不要听信他们。你们都可以使自己成为能够引以为豪的人。你们有这样的能力。你们可以实现任何人生目标——无论是成为医生、教师、科学家，或者，是的，美国总统。你们都可以做到。（掌声）

你们可以让你们的家人为你的现在和未来感到骄傲。我有个秘诀。你们想听这个秘诀吗？

观众：是的！

奥巴马夫人：一定要得到良好的教育。你们听到了吗？你们必须得到良好的教育。这是你们现在可以为自己做的最重要的事。这意味着，你们必须每天去上学——每一天，不管你们学校的外观如何，不论学校里发生什么样的事情，你们必须要坐在你们的课桌旁，准备学习。你们在这个年龄已经有了一份工作，那就是尽可能成为最优秀的学生。（掌声）

所以听老师的话，做你们的功课——不是只有想做功课时才做，而是每天都做，不管你们生活中发生了什么事。请记住，没有人天生聪明。你们通过勤奋努力变得聪明。你们读书越多，数学题做得越多，就会越聪明。因此，你们每一个人都可以变得聪明，只要你们愿意付出努力。

最后，你们要照顾自己的身体。你们必须要这么做。这意味着你们必须健康饮食。这不是一个笑话，不是一个游戏——健康饮食会让你们身体强壮，并给你们提供能量。你们一定要吃水果。你们一定要吃蔬菜。你们一定要吃学校每天提供的那些好的、健康的饭菜。

你们还要开始运动。听我说，你们一定要关掉电视，把眼睛从电视屏幕上移开。（掌声）你们一定要让你们的身体处于活动状态，即便只是打开音乐跳一个小时的舞。跳一会道基舞，做几个开合跳、几个俯卧撑。保持身体健康不需要你成为一名奥运选手。你们只需要动起来。这样可以帮助你们让身体和头脑为成就伟大的事业做好准备。

其实，现在是时候结束严肃话题了，对吗？你们听到我想传达的所有重要信息了吗？

观众：是的！

奥巴马夫人：你们都承诺要做好学生。

观众：我们承诺！

奥巴马夫人：你们都承诺要吃健康的食物。

观众：我们承诺！

奥巴马夫人：你们都承诺要开始运动。

观众：我们承诺！

奥巴马夫人：我们此时此刻就要开始了。（掌声）这些冠军将带领我们并展示如何开始运动。那么，让我们一起开心一下。你们准备好了吗？（掌声）好吧，让我们运动起来！（掌声）

Text 2

世界卫生组织驻华代表蓝睿明博士在国家卫生和计划生育委员会2013年世界无烟日活动上的致辞

中国北京

2013年5月30日

尊敬的国家卫计委副主任崔丽女士，
尊敬的中国控烟协会主席、卫生部前副部长黄洁夫医生，
尊敬的中国疾控中心王宇主任，
尊敬的各位来宾，
女士们、先生们：

早上好。

感谢各位邀请我参加今天庆祝世界无烟日的活动。

大家知道，吸烟是中国的最主要的死因之一，中国每年有100多万人死于烟草相关疾病。中国有3亿多吸烟者，如不降低吸烟率，可以预测，到2050年，烟草相关死亡率将增至每年300万，这个问题应该引起我们的警惕。

今年的世界无烟日主题是“禁止烟草广告、促销和赞助”。

《世卫组织烟草控制框架公约》（FCTC）要求全面禁止各种烟草广告、促销和赞助。

这是因为全球各种证据表明，推动这种全面营销禁令可减少开始和继续吸烟的人数。

烟草广告和促销创造了一种氛围，即，吸烟是一种社会可接受的行为，是一种“正常”行为。

烟草广告、促销和赞助活动因此让人们误认为烟草也是一种普通消费品。

然而事实却是，烟草是一种致命的产品；人们依照生产商的期望使用产品，其产品却导致半数的烟民死亡。

禁止烟草广告、促销和赞助是政府减少烟草需求、保护人民健康的最具成本效益的措施之一。

中国近年来采取了重要措施来加强对烟草销售的限制：

《广告法》禁止在大型活动中通过广播、电影、电视、报纸、杂志宣传烟草广告；2011年2月，广电局宣布严格控制电影电视剧中出现吸烟的画面；2012年12月，中国政府发布了《2012—2015年中国烟草控制规划》，对加强现有的禁止烟草广告、促销和赞助工作做出了有力承诺。

世卫组织欢迎中国目前已采取的加强限制烟草销售的措施。但中国应采取更有力的政策行动来打击烟草销售活动。更重要的是，这将保护中国的年轻人免受烟草成瘾的终身危害。

2010年在中国开展的“全球烟草成人调查”（GATS）的数据显示，尽管中国采取了禁控措施，但仍有近30%的15至24岁的年轻人反映调查前30天内见过烟草广告、促销和赞助活动。

其他研究也显示，人们通过娱乐媒体大量接触吸烟的间接促销。这令我们十分担心，因为青少年极易受到烟草促销的影响。因此，禁止烟草广告、促销和赞助对保护年轻人免受烟草危害尤其重要。

我祝贺中国疾控中心编写并于今天发布了有关报告，它强调了进一步采取更有力的政策行动来保护中国公众免受烟草促销影响的重要性。我们希望与中国疾控中心、中国卫生与计划生育委员会以及其他合作伙伴继续合作，推动这一领域的工作。

在此，我高兴地宣布，世卫组织为表彰在中国控烟领域最重要的合作者之一，特将今年的“世界无烟日奖”颁发给黄洁夫医生。众所周知，作为中国控烟协会主席、卫生部前副部长，黄医生一直领导推动中国的控烟行动。

祝贺黄部长荣获嘉奖，希望这能够推动中国制定更有力的控烟政策。

再次感谢邀请我发言。世卫组织期待着继续与大家合作，让中国未来在这一领域发生重要变化，也祝大家在无烟的世界无烟日快乐！

五、英译汉练习

Text 3

预防和控制非传染性疾病——全球战略的实施
美国公共卫生服务现役军团总医官在第63届世界卫生大会上的讲话

瑞士日内瓦
2010年5月20日

美国感谢世界卫生组织为预防和控制非传染性疾病全球战略所做的工作。身为美国公共卫生服务现役军团总医官，我可以说，我们认识到非传染性疾病导致全世界疾病和死亡人数明显增加，而且在发展中国家疾病负担中所占比例越来越大。由于非传染性疾病是一个突出的公共卫生问题，影响了发展中国家和发达国家，我们将继续支持世界卫生组织实施全球战略的行动计划，例如让所有利益相关者参与其中，因为减少非传染性疾病是大家共同的责任。

我们很高兴看到世界卫生组织在实施行动计划方面已取得进展。

行动计划的附件中有一套对儿童营销食品和非酒精饮料的建议，它们应该扮演重要的角色，帮助成员国人民形成健康的饮食习惯，以改善日益流行的儿童肥胖问题。这是奥巴马政府优先考虑的问题，尤其是第一夫人优先考虑的问题，她已经帮助人们提高了对儿童肥胖和健康饮食的重要性的认识。

美国很高兴看到，秘书处实施的利益相关者协商过程，为这些建议的结构和内容带来了相当大的改善。在大多数情况下，建议和美国国会和奥巴马政府想要实现的首要政策目标是一致的。

美国正在从许多方面解决肥胖这个紧迫问题。例如，美国国家卫生研究院已经建立了一个肥胖研究专题工作组，工作组参考外部专家和健康倡导组织的意见，开发了实施肥胖研究的战略计划。我们对肥胖研究和战略规划的投入将促进世界卫生组织实施肥胖和其他非传染性疾病的全球预防和控制战略。

美国联邦贸易委员会、美国食品和药物管理局、美国疾病控制和预防中心，以及农业部都在制定标准，管理对美国儿童进行的食品营销。

这些建议的标准于2009年12月在美国联邦贸易委员会举办的题为“评估食品营销和儿童肥胖”的研讨会上进行了介绍，并将在7月提交给美国国会。

我们很高兴看到建议中提到了一系列实施机制。对于解决日益严重的肥胖流行问题，我们都有共同的责任，这意味着各国政府、工业界和非政府性参与者和个人都要参与。所有的利益相关者应当参与。

我们很乐意支持这项由挪威提出并修订的决议草案。谢谢主席先生。

Text 4

世界卫生组织西太平洋区域主任申英秀博士在西太平洋地区预防接种和疫苗可预防疾病技术咨询小组（TAG）第22次会议上的开幕致辞

菲律宾马尼拉

2013年6月25日

尊敬的与会者和同行们，女士们、先生们：

欢迎参加简称为TAG的西太平洋地区预防接种和疫苗可预防疾病技术咨询小组第22次会议。

从上次8月的TAG会议以来，我们已经取得大量进展，在此进行报告。

我想肯定成员国为实现目标并加强他们的预防接种系统而做出的努力。

让我们来看看一些具体的成就：

- 西太平洋区域根除脊髓灰质炎认证委员会在2012年11月得出结论，中国已充分应对2011年的疫情，西太平洋地区继续维持无脊灰状态。
- 到2012年年底，34个国家和地区可能间断出现麻疹病毒的地方性流行传播。通过麻疹、风疹协同免疫接种、监测活动，风疹控制工作亦已加速。
- 在2012年12月，经世界卫生组织和联合国儿童基金会验证，中国已消除孕产妇和新生儿破伤风。
- 经正式核实，澳大利亚、中国、蒙古和新西兰已实现儿童乙肝感染率降至1%以下的区域目标。到2012年，西太平洋地区整体和至少30个国家和地区已实现了5岁儿童的血清阳性率降至2%以下的目标。
- 世卫组织认证的疫苗可预防疾病的实验室网络已经建立，大大增强了其工作能力。
- 设立国家监管部门区域联盟，协助成员国推广使用有质量保证的安全疫苗。
- 西太平洋地区的五国在全国计划免疫中增加了7种疫苗，以减少妇女和儿童的死亡率。

这些都是真正令人印象深刻的里程碑。但尽管如此，仍有巨大的挑战摆在面前。

现在需要你们的专业知识和智慧，指导最近世界卫生大会提出的本地区的两个项目。

第一，我们应该如何向前发展，使西太平洋地区国家实施2018年前脊髓灰质炎消灭计划。

正如你们所知道的，该计划包括一些活动，以防止脊灰疫苗衍生病毒的出现和流行。你们的参与会是其成功实施的关键。

TAG要关注的第二个问题是评审拟议的西太平洋地区全球疫苗行动计划实施框架。

全球疫苗行动计划由世界卫生大会于2012年5月提出。

从那时起，世界卫生组织西太平洋区域办公室的预防接种扩大项目办事处已与成员国合作，寻找最佳方法，并起草计划以实施2011—2020年全球疫苗行动计划。

该计划根据西太平洋地区的具体需求制定，强调四项内容：

1. 达到减少疾病的目标；

2. 增加疫苗接种的均等化和获取途径；

3. 提倡以科学证据为基础，引进新的疫苗；

4. 增加政府、合作伙伴和捐助者高层面的资金承诺，以确保预防接种项目的可持续性。

您的参与将是非常宝贵的，将帮助我们向前迈进，达到新的区域免疫接种长远目标和具体目标，以及疫苗十年中设定的目标。

最后请允许我感谢大家使预防接种扩大项目在西太平洋地区成为一个充满活力和创新的力量。

你们的指导意见至关重要，可以确保我们所有的努力——包括政府、发展机构、捐助者和其他合作伙伴的全部努力都实现最佳效果。

我期待着听到你们的建议，祝愿大家愉快地度过在马尼拉的日子。

谢谢。

六、汉译英练习

Text 5

Smoke-Free Environment Promotion Project Effectively Controls Exposure to Secondhand Smoking

Remarks at the Launch of Smoke-Free Environment Promotion Project, a Cooperation Project of the International Union against Tuberculosis and Lung Disease (The Union) and the Chinese Center for Disease Control and Prevention (China CDC)

Wang Yu, Director General of China CDC
China CDC, Changpin District, Beijing, China
15 January 2010

Distinguished guests, friends and colleagues,

Good morning!

The Smoke-Free Environment Promotion Project is officially launched on January 15th. On behalf of China CDC, the organizer, I'd like to express my sincere appreciation for the Ministry of Health, the officials from the State Council's Legislative Affairs Office, the project cities, the local governments, and the Union, our project partner, for their active support for the project. I'd also like to extend a warm welcome to the experts and media representatives attending the launching ceremony. The harms of tobacco use are considered one of the most serious public health problems in the world, posing great risks, which are completely preventable, to the health of humans.

In order to reduce the harm caused by tobacco use, and the consequential enormous economic losses, the World Health Organization (WHO) took the lead to develop the International Framework Convention on Tobacco Control, which is a set of evidence-based international conventions drafted in response to the globalization of the tobacco epidemic. As of November 2008, 168 countries around the world have signed and ratified the Convention. China signed the Convention on November 8, 2003 and was the 77th country to have done so. The convention was approved by the Standing Committee of the National People's Congress and took effect in China on January 8, 2006. The large number of national governments signing and ratifying the Framework Convention on Tobacco Control indicates that governments recognize that curbing tobacco consumption is a priority issue for the protection of people's health. Of course, the health of the people is an essential goal for the effort to advance the best interest of the people.

Although the development and implementation of International Framework Convention on Tobacco Control provides China with an important opportunity for tobacco control, we must also be acutely aware of the serious challenges China is facing in tobacco control. In the few years after the Framework Convention took effect in China, tobacco production in the country has not decreased, and has, instead, increased. By the end of 2008, the total annual accumulated production and sales of cigarettes in 2008 has reached 44 million cartons, increasing by nearly 30% compared with that of 2003, indicating an average growth rate of 5.35 percent over the course of five years. Currently, the high smoking rates among the Chinese male population and high exposure to secondhand smoking among children and women caused one million deaths resulting from various tobacco-related diseases each year. By 2030, the estimated annual mortality caused by tobacco-related diseases will rise to two million. Due to the delayed manifestation of the health risks of tobacco use, the incidence of lung cancer and the mortality of tobacco-related diseases we are facing now are the consequence of tobacco consumption in the 1970s. The peak of the tobacco epidemic arrived in China in the 1990s. Therefore, the peak of the harms caused by tobacco use has not yet arrived. If we do not control tobacco use and exposure to secondhand smoking, the harm caused by tobacco use will continue to grow in the next five decades, which will inevitably lead to a significant increase in medical costs. Health problems caused by tobacco have become an important factor contributing to poverty caused by morbidity. There is an ongoing health care system reform. At the beginning of the health care reform, we must first solve the health care equity problem and make sure that we meet the basic health care needs of the people. Along with the progress made in health care reform, the government will encounter growing expenditure for the treatment of chronic diseases caused by tobacco. Chronic diseases have become one of the three top obstacles to economic development. Our original intention is not only to solve the problems that people have when they seek medical help, but, more importantly, to start early preparation for prevention so as to effectively prevent illnesses. If tobacco use is not effectively controlled, it will eventually become a major obstacle to economic development in China and in the world.

It is China CDC's mission to prevent disease and promote health. China CDC uses tobacco control as an important measure to prevent chronic diseases and protect people from the harms of exposure to secondhand smoking. We started the Smoke-Free Environment Promote Project so that we will use law as the means and mobilize the whole society in order to realize the goal of tobacco control. Information and education on how exposure to secondhand smoke contributes to chronic disease will be an important measure. However, the more effective measure is policy and legal support. The most prominent feature of this project is government leadership. Innovative approaches are adopted in the project. For example, establishing the legislative network and the media network will not only effectively promote the implementation of the project, but also help develop laws and regulations banning smoking in public places. This approach differs from using health education alone. Experience from other countries shows that this is the only effective way to control exposure to secondhand smoking, and promote China's progress in tobacco control. The demonstration actions in seven cities in China will motivate many other cities to draft tobacco control legislation, thus forming the foundation for the introduction of relevant laws at the national level and the promotion of China's tobacco control campaign.

Tobacco control requires long-term sustained efforts, comprehensive planning and implementation, and, in particular, government-led multi-sectoral collaboration. Tobacco control is a social project. Therefore, the power of the health sector alone is not enough. Officials from the Legislative Affairs Office, State Council and the local governments involved in the project have all provided strong support to the project. We have the deepest appreciation for all of you! I am confident that through multi-sectoral collaboration, the project will be successfully implemented and will thus promote the smoke-free environment in China. I am also confident that the project will strengthen China's capacity in tobacco control and forcefully promote the cause of tobacco control in China. The project will help protect the health of the people in China. Thank you!

Text 6

Working in Unity and Cooperation to Meet the Challenges of Chronic Diseases

Remarks by Chen Zhu, Minister of Health,

at the Opening Ceremony of the 2012 China Stroke Conference

Beijing, China

4 May 2012

Dear colleagues and friends,

In this beautiful spring season, we are gathered here for the 2012 China Stroke Conference. We are going to have discussions on stroke prevention and chronic disease prevention and control strategies of the country. On behalf of the Ministry of Health (MOH), I'd like to extend the most sincere greetings to all the colleagues and experts!

At present, chronic diseases are demonstrating a trend of high incidence in China. According to data from the national survey of causes of death in 2008, cerebrovascular disease has become the number one killer in China. Chronic diseases are "infectious social diseases". If they are not properly managed, there will be large scale "eruptions" of chronic diseases in the next two or three decades. Chronic disease prevention and control is an urgent task that admits no delay. In order to reduce the risk of chronic diseases, they have to be incorporated in the list of core indicators of socioeconomic development. Health departments at all levels should give top priority to chronic disease prevention and control because it is essential to the protection of people's livelihood and the right to health. If we do not give chronic disease prevention and control the kind of attention it deserves, we will be making a mistake of historic proportions.

2012 China Stroke Conference is held in the China National Convention Center. We are gathered here to have discussions on the prevention and control of stroke in China. 2011 is a year of great significance for chronic disease prevention and control across the world. In September, 2011, a high-level meeting on chronic disease prevention and control was held by the 66th UN General Assembly. It was suggested at the meeting that chronic disease is a serious development challenge faced by the world in the 21st century. The international community will strengthen cooperation to reduce risk factors, create an environment that promotes health, expands protection through national policies and improves the health system's capacity to meet the challenges posed by chronic diseases through the concerted efforts of national governments and the whole society.

At present, China is in a stage of high incidence of chronic diseases. Cardiovascular and cerebrovascular diseases account for over 40% of the mortality among urban and rural residents. Cerebrovascular disease has become the number one killer in China. If effective measures are not taken promptly, the rapid growth of chronic diseases will become a huge obstacle to the improvement of living standards and socioeconomic development. MOH launched a stroke screening, prevention and control project in the second half of 2009, and established the MOH stroke screening, prevention and control project committee consisting of representatives from nine bureaus and departments. Stroke screening, prevention and control for high-risk populations was included as a major component of the health care reform in 2011 and pilot projects were started in five provinces and one city.

Currently, the MOH has set up 90 plus hospital as centers for the screening, prevention and control of stroke. According to incomplete statistical data, since 2010, a total of 550,000 carotid artery screening tests have been conducted; health education and physical check-ups have been carried out for 2.29 million person times; internalist medical interventions have been conducted for 660,000 person times; 20,000 plus surgical interventions have been performed; training of health workers was organized to cover 50,000 person times; 718 free consultation and health education activities were organized; 1,890,000 brochures on stroke were printed and distributed; 2,395 stroke patients received poverty aid.

The onset of stroke is a result of the long-term effect of chronic diseases including high blood pressure, diabetes, dyslipidemia, heart disease and others. In order to promote the screening and prevention of stroke, I'd like to make five suggestions. Hopefully, my suggestions will promote the progress of stroke prevention in China.

Firstly, health departments at all levels should continue to improve the relevant policies. We will actively coordinate the financial, technological, social security, and civil affairs departments to give more support in terms of policy and funding to stroke screening. Within the health care system, we will integrate the available resources and make full use of the outcomes of basic public health programs to promote the implementation of stroke prevention and control and major projects of health care reform so that the project funding will yield the greatest possible benefits.

Secondly, we should gradually improve government health insurance policy for serious diseases and chronic diseases such as stroke. In 2012, on the basis of existing range of coverage of serious illnesses, the Ministry of Health will work with the Ministry of Finance and Ministry of Civil Affairs to expand coverage of serious diseases in the new model rural cooperative health care system, adding 12 illness, including cerebral infarction, to the list of serious diseases covered by the system. This will help effectively reduce the financial burden of patients with serious illness.

Thirdly, we should give full play to the support provided by science and technology in health care reform. We will provide more support to the dissemination, training and research of the appropriate technology of cerebrovascular disease.

Fourthly, we should strengthen education and popularization of information on chronic disease prevention. A vast number of health workers will work on the front line of chronic disease prevention and control and help spread information on stroke prevention and control.

Fifthly, we should establish demonstration centers for stroke prevention and control. Through the construction of the stroke screening and prevention system, we will explore for chronic disease prevention and control models appropriate for China.

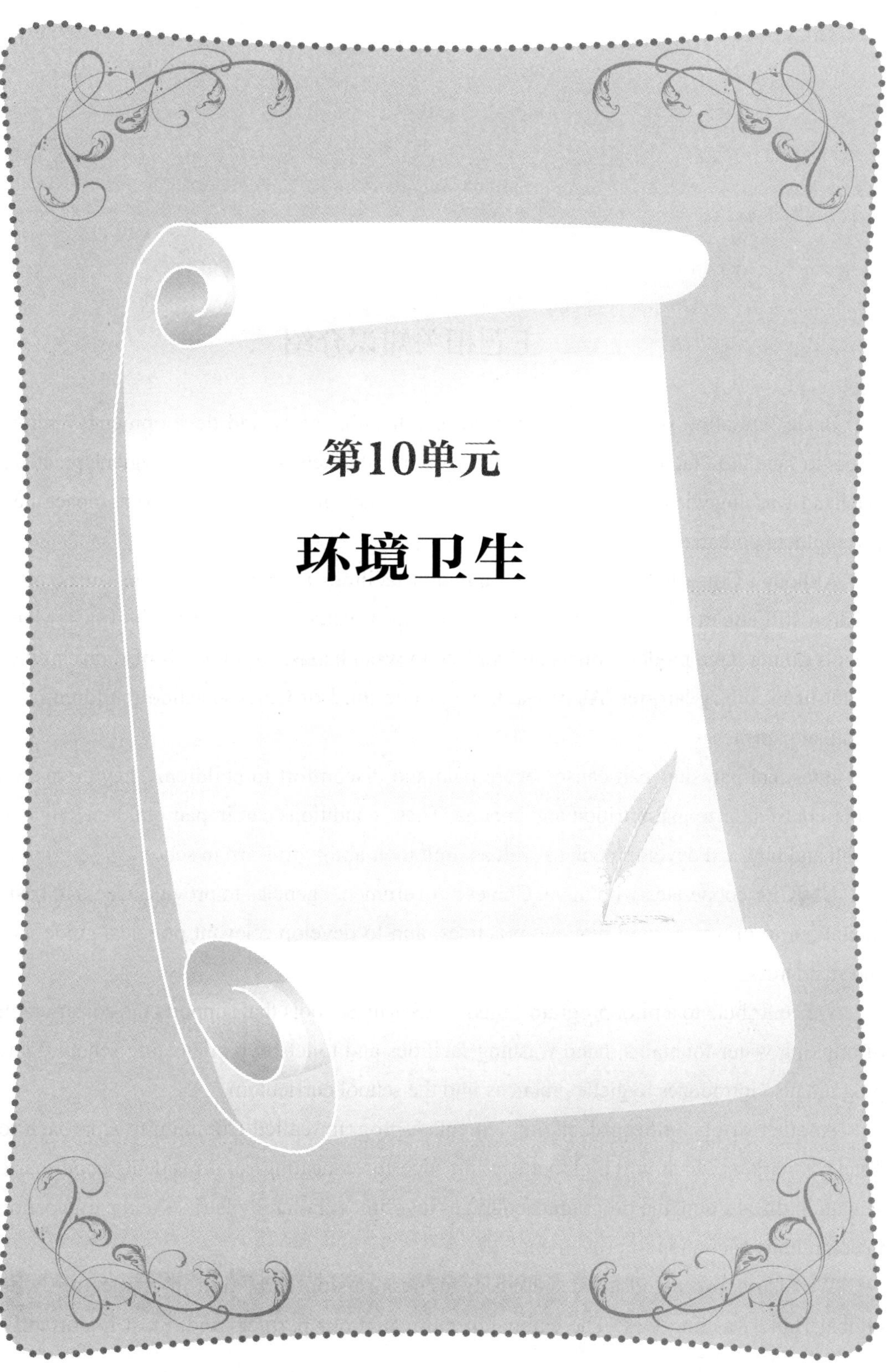

第10单元

环境卫生

一、主题相关知识介绍

Basic sanitation is necessary for children's health, safety and development. Without access to sanitation facilities, including clean water and toilets, and without hygiene practices like hand-washing with soap, children may get sick. Lack of sanitation may even impact their development potential.

Although China has improved its sanitation facilities in many geographic areas, most children still attend schools that lack adequate clean water and sanitation facilities. Many schools do not have modern toilets and a place to wash hands. Around half of rural families do not use sanitary latrines. As a result, about one-third of Chinese school children have intestinal parasites.

Intestinal parasites can cause severe pain and discomfort to children. They are also a major contributor to malnutrition and anemia. These conditions can impair children's overall health and physical development, as well as limit their ability to learn in school.

UNICEF cooperates with many Chinese government agencies to provide access to basic sanitation, to promote good hygiene practices, and to develop relevant policies, guidelines and standards.

We contribute to a pilot program called WASH-in-Schools that supports the construction of drinking water fountains, hand washing facilities and toilets at participating schools. The program also introduces hygiene practices into the school curriculum.

Another of our pilot projects implements a program called Community Approach to Total Sanitation, which is the global best practice for educating rural residents about basic sanitation. In addition, the program encourages investment in family latrines and participation in community sanitation improvement.

We also coordinated a week-long awareness-raising campaign in connection with Global Hand-washing Day. The campaign motivated our partners and, most importantly, children themselves to spread the message that people should wash their hands with soap.

UNICEF's work has also informed government policies, guidelines and standards, including: the Rural Environmental Sanitation Improvement Action, the Guidelines on Improvement of Living and Sanitation Facilities for Rural Boarding Schools, the Rural Household Sanitary Latrine Standards, and the Rural Public Sanitary Latrine Standards.

UNICEF's work to ensure access to basic sanitation and to improve hygiene practices is yielding results. With our support, more government programs and funds have been allocated to these issues.

The majority of schools participating in the WASH-in-Schools programs now offer water that meets national standards and safeguards the health of the children attending those schools. The success of the WASH-in-Schools pilot has led to its expansion into other provinces.

Inclusion in the school curriculum of hygiene practices like hand-washing with soap, and involving children in the Global Hand-washing Day campaign, has contributed to better hygiene practices among children and, ultimately, to better health.

You can help improve hygiene and sanitation for children. Take action by learning more about the importance of basic sanitation or by organizing a Global Hand-washing Day event. Or find out how you can support UNICEF's work today.

二、技巧指导：目的语信息重组的几个方法（Ⅲ）

增译法（**Amplification**）

为了符合译入语的语言表达习惯，需要在译入语中增添达意的词、词组、分句或完整句，使译入语的语言结构完整，同时又完整地表达源语的内容。

英译中例句：

Therefore, it is important to try to indicate what should be considered global and what local, where the commonality lies, and what is already global in medical education. It is clear that process of globalization of medical education will be incremental, long and arduous. It is also clear that as the different stakeholders in medical education have varying expectations, the development of international essential requirements and standards is a matter of the negotiations necessary to reach consensus. This also will require time.

因此，指明什么应被看成全球性的，什么应被看成地方性的，相同点在何处，以及医学教育中什么已经是国际化了的，这些问题非常重要。全球一体化的进程是加速的、长期的、艰辛的，这一点已显而易见。另一点也非常清楚，就是医学教育有不同的出资人，不同的出资人有不同的要求，因此制定国际基本要求和标准是一个谈判问题。谈判可以达成共识，也需要时间。（根据需要用了增译法与转换法）

中译英例句：

1. 而在绿荫深处的竹林中，一座座独具川西民居建筑风格的茅草四合院正在升起倦懒的炊烟。数声鸟鸣、几声狗吠，屋檐下闪着红光的大红灯笼，勾勒出川西平原花香人居般的农家生活。

To look further into in the depth of the green bamboos, we see blocks of rectangular courtyards in unique western Sichuan style. Cooking smoke is rising softly from the thatched roofs of the houses in the courtyards. These, together with the bird twittering, dog barking, flower blossoming, red lantern shining under the eaves of those houses, are a sketch of country life on the western Sichuan plain.（根据表达习惯增加了主语，又结合了重组法。）

2. 到武侯祠则不然，你可以观，可以群，可以乐，可以玩。

However, touring the Temple of Marquis Wu is a different experience. Here, tourists can observe history, enjoy a gathering, watch play highlights and have fun.

3. 社会主义市场经济体制初步建立，市场机制在配置资源中日益明显地发挥基础性作用，经济发展的体制环境发生了重大变化。社会保障制度、教育制度、医疗卫生制度等方面改革取得重大进展。

After the establishment of a preliminary system of socialist market economy, the market mechanism is more and more evidently performing a fundamental role in collocation resources, allowing important changes taking place in the system milieu of economic development. Meanwhile, significant progress of reform has been observed in China's social insurance, educational, medicare, and family-planning systems.

简译法（**Deletion**）

与增译法相对应，简译法是在译入语中删去不符合该语言习惯和表达方式的字与词，以避免冗言。

英译中例句：

1. While it is a formidable task for us all, I'm sure that next year at this time we'll have more awards, and more subscribers, and feel an even greater sense of accomplishment and fulfillment.

虽然我们面前的任务还很艰巨，我相信明年的此刻我们将会收获更多的奖项、更多的订单，会有更大的成就感和满足感。

2. So tonight we wish to thank you for all the wonderful ways you host us, such as providing us this fine banquet tonight. We also want to express our gratitude for the one hundred thousand Yuan upgrade of our internet services that you paid for this year.（下划线处为减掉的）

所以现在，让我们对你们的热情接待表示感谢。感谢今天的精美晚宴，同时对今年为我们的计算机升级支付费用，我们深表谢意。

中译英例句：

1. 但其时中国西医从业者寥寥无几，而且分散在中国的各个沿海城市，终因稿源和读者缺乏，上述期刊均仅出版几期即停刊。

However, these two journals ceased publication after several issues for a lack of contributors and readers, because at that time, few Chinese doctors practiced Western medicine, and these few doctors were in different coastal cities.

2. 这是一种包含多种文体、由多位作者撰写的装订成册的不定期连续出版物，所选稿件都未曾发表，阐述观点有新意，包含不同见解但言之有理。

Published in series without a set timing, this publication, with a variety of genres of writing from many contributors, has included unpublished manuscripts with new ideas that is all reasonable but different in understanding.

简化法（Simplification）

简译法指在译入语中省去不符合译入语表达习惯的字与词，与此不同，简化法是指在译入语中使用约定俗成的简称，这不仅能使译文更加地道，而且省时省力。

英译中例句：

1. In the world today, the trend towards economic globalization, a multi-polar world and IT application is gaining momentum. We live in a global village. No country can live in isolation of others like Robinson Crusoe.

当今世界，经济全球化、世界多极化、社会信息化深入发展，我们同住一个

"地球村"，没有哪一个国家能变成离群索居的"鲁滨孙"。

2. Since the beginning of time, great leaders have used their power of oratory to win and inspire followers. The speeches of George Washington, Napoleon Bonaparte, Abraham Lincoln, Mohandas Gandhi, Winston Churchill, Martin Luther King, Nelson Mandela and many others have motivated, illuminated, uplifted those who heard them.

自古以来，领袖人物们都用演讲的力量来激励追随者。乔治·华盛顿、拿破仑、林肯、甘地、丘吉尔、马丁·路德·金、曼德拉和其他很多人，都通过演讲启发、激励、鼓舞了许多听众。

3. As an ancient Chinese saying goes, "A gentleman is always ready to help others attain their goals." We believe that only by helping each other can we all attain our goals.

中国有句古话："君子成人之美。"只有美人之美，才能美美与共。

中译英例句：

1. 经济增长质量和效益显著提高，2010年国内生产总值将比2000年翻一番。

Increase will be clearly seen in the quality and benefit of economic growth: by 2010, China's GDP will double compared with the year 2000.

2. 本文以联合国环境规划署化学加工助剂专家组（PAWG）最近开展的研究工作为背景综述了消耗臭氧层物质（ODS）在化学加工过程中使用及其替代技术的现状与趋势。

Based on the research work currently carried out by the UNEP Chemical Process Agent Working Group (PAWG), the present situation and tendency of the use of Ozone Depleting Substances (ODS) in chemical process industries and their alternatives are globally summarized in this paper.

三、词汇准备

Text 1

MDG Millennium Development Goal 新千年发展目标

UNICEF United Nations International Children's Emergency Fund 联合国儿童基金会

gained access to 获得

WHO/UNICEF Joint Monitoring Programme for Water Supply and Sanitation 世界卫

生组织/联合国儿童基金会饮用水供应和卫生设施联合监测方案

diarrheal 腹泻的

sub-Saharan Africa 撒哈拉以南的非洲地区

highlight 强调、突出、突显

BRIC countries 金砖四国

piped supplies 管道自来水供应

Progress on Drinking Water and Sanitation 2012 《2012年饮用水和卫生设施进展》

diarrhoeal diseases 腹泻病

Text 2

日本国土交通省金子恭之副大臣 Mr. Kaneko Yasushi, Vice Minister of Land, Infrastructure, Transport and Tourism of Japan

韩国国土海洋部权度烨副部长 Mr. Kwon Do-Youp, Vice Minister of Land, Transport and Maritime Affairs of Korea

中日水资源交流会 Sino-Japan Workshop on Water Resources

中日河工坝工会议 Sino-Japan Symposium on River and Dam Engineering

中韩水资源交流会 Sino-Korea Workshop on Water Resources

亚洲季风区的河流修复 River Rehabilitation in the Asian Monsoon Region

水资源信息系统 Water Information System

Text 3

Asthma 哮喘

chronic obstructive pulmonary disease 慢性阻塞性肺疾病

cardiovascular disease 心血管疾病

endocrine system effects 内分泌系统的影响

neurological effects 神经系统的影响

allergies 过敏

respiratory 呼吸的

GTA resident (GTA: Great Toronto Area) 多伦多居民

hospital admissions 住院

nitrous oxide 氧化亚氮

diesel fuel 柴油燃料

kerosene 煤油

ultrafine particulates 超细微粒

sulfur dioxide 二氧化硫
carbon monoxide 一氧化碳
chronic diseases 慢性疾病
bronchitis 支气管炎
emphysema 肺气肿
asthma 哮喘
PM10 空气动力学当量直径≤10微米的颗粒物
PM2.5 可入肺颗粒物
mortality 死亡率
arrhythmias 心律失常
inflammation 炎症
wheezing 喘息
angina 心绞痛
epidemiologic study 流行病学研究
diabetes 糖尿病

Text 4

UNICEF 联合国儿童基金会
advocate 倡导
child-friendliness 易于儿童使用
open defecation 随地如厕
household latrines 家庭厕所
CLTS (community-led total sanitation) 社区主导的综合卫生
IYS International Year of Sanitation 国际环境卫生年
sustainable access 可持续地获得
sanitation and hygiene 卫生条件
programme priority 优先项目
water quality monitoring 水质检测
community-level surveillance systems 社区一级监视系统
diarrhoea 腹泻
microbial water quality 微生物的水质
ceramic filters 陶瓷过滤器
arsenic and fluoride 砷和氟
environmental degradation 环境恶化

Text 5

亚太日 The Asia-Pacific Day
人均水资源量 water resources per capita
水利建设融资难 difficulty in water project financing
水灾 water disasters
时空分布不均 uneven temporal and spatial distribution
优化配置 optimized allocation
农田灌溉用水量 irrigation water use
水库除险加固 reinforcing defective reservoirs
饮水不安全人口比例降低一半 halving the population without access to safe drinking water
农业灌溉水利用系数 agricultural irrigation water use coefficient

Text 6

爱国卫生运动 Patriotic Health Campaign
爱国卫生教育宣传活动 educational campaigns for patriotic hygiene
实施 implement, implementation
进行，做 conduct
全民健身活动 nationwide fitness activities
禁止 prohibit, prohibition
数字化 digitalize, digitalization
乱涂乱写 graffiti
废物箱或垃圾收集容器 garbage collectors， waste boxes， trash containers
绿化 green, virescence
生活垃圾、污水、粪便无害化处理 garbage, sewage, fecal detoxification treatment
环卫设施 sanitation facilities
秸秆焚烧 straw burning
医疗废弃物 medical waste
传染病 infectious diseases
监视、监察 surveillance
监测 monitor
消毒 disinfect, disinfection
动物防疫 animal epidemic prevention
结核病 tuberculosis

血吸虫病 schistosomiasis
扩大免疫规划 expanded programme on immunization, EPI immunization
精神卫生 mental health
无偿献血 voluntary blood donation
病媒生物 vector

四、摘要练习

请听下面英语语篇，第一篇用源语言复述此段主要信息逻辑点及层次，第二篇用译入语复述此段主要信息逻辑点及层次。注意信息点之间的逻辑联系。

Text 1

Millennium Development Goal Drinking Water Target Met Sanitation Target Still Lagging Far Behind

New York/Geneva
6 March 2012

The world has met the Millennium Development Goal (MDG) target of halving the proportion of people without sustainable access to safe drinking water, well in advance of the MDG 2015 deadline, according to a report issued today by UNICEF and the World Health Organization (WHO). Between 1990 and 2010, over two billion people gained access to improved drinking water sources, such as piped supplies and protected wells.

United Nations Secretary-General Ban Ki-moon said, "Today we recognize a great achievement for the people of the world. This is one of the first MDG targets to be met. The successful efforts to provide greater access to drinking water are a testament to all who see the MDGs not as a dream, but as a vital tool for improving the lives of millions of the poorest people."

The report, Progress on Drinking Water and Sanitation 2012, by the WHO/UNICEF Joint Monitoring Programme for Water Supply and Sanitation, says at the end of 2010 89 percent of the world's population, or 6.1 billion people, used improved drinking water sources. This is one percent more than the 88 percent MDG target. The report estimates that by 2015 92 percent of the global population will have access to improved drinking water.

"For children this is especially good news," said UNICEF Executive Director Anthony Lake. "Every day more than 3,000 children die from diarrheal diseases. Achieving this target will go a long way to saving children's lives."

Lake warned that victory could not yet be declared as at least 11 per cent of the world's population—783 million people—are still without access to safe drinking water, and billions without sanitation facilities.

"The numbers are still staggering," he said. "But the progress announced today is proof that MDG targets can be met with the will, the effort and the funds."

The report highlights, however, that the world is still far from meeting the part of the MDG target for sanitation, and is unlikely to do so by 2015. Only 63 percent of the world now have improved sanitation access, a figure projected to increase only to 67 percent by 2015, well below the 75 percent aim in the MDGs. Currently 2.5 billion people still lack improved sanitation.

UNICEF and WHO also cautioned that since the measurement of water quality is not possible globally, progress towards the MDG target of safe drinking water is measured through gathering data on the use of improved drinking water sources. Significant work must be done to ensure that improved sources of water are and remain safe.

"Providing sustainable access to improved drinking water sources is one of the most important things we can do to reduce disease," said WHO Director-General Dr. Margaret Chan. "But this achievement today is only the beginning. We must continue to ensure this access remains safe. Otherwise our gains will be in vain."

The report highlights the immense challenges that remain. Global figures mask massive disparities between regions and countries, and within countries.

Only 61 percent of the people in sub-Saharan Africa have access to improved water supply sources compared with 90 percent or more in Latin America and the Caribbean, Northern Africa, and large parts of Asia. Over 40 percent of all people globally who lack access to drinking water live in sub-Saharan Africa.

The report confirms that in cases where water supplies are not readily accessible, the burden of carrying water falls disproportionately on women and girls. In many countries, the wealthiest people have seen the greatest improvement in water and sanitation access, while the poorest still lag far behind.

The report provides the latest update on rural areas across the globe, highlighting the need for greater attention both to water and sanitation. In rural areas in least developed countries, 97 out of every 100 people do not have piped water and 14 percent of the population drinks surface water—for example, from rivers, ponds, or lakes.

Of 1.1 billion people who still practice open defecation, the vast majority (949 million) live in rural areas. This affects even regions with high levels of improved water access. For instance, 17 percent of rural dwellers in Latin America and the Caribbean and 9 percent in Northern Africa still resort to open defecation. Even the so-called BRIC countries, with rapidly growing economies, have large numbers of people who practice open defecation: 626 million in India, 14 million in China, and 7.2 million in Brazil.

"We have reached an important target, but we cannot stop here," the UN Secretary-General said. "Our next step must be to target the most difficult to reach, the poorest and the most disadvantaged people across the world. The United Nations General Assembly has recognized drinking water and sanitation as human rights. That means we must ensure that every person has access."

复述要点提示（主要信息逻辑点及层次）

Purpose:

Summarizing the achievements of safe drinking water, displaying the remaining problems in this regard, and planning for future.

Achievements:

WHO/UNICEF Joint Monitoring Programme for Water Supply and Sanitation has a report entitled "Progress on Drinking Water and Sanitation 2012". It says by the end of 2010, 89 percent of the world's population used improved drinking water sources. Since MDG target is 88 percent, so the target has been met by 1 extra percent. This proves that MDG goals can be met.

Remaining problems:

● At least 11 percent of the world's population, that is 783 million people, still have no access to safe drinking water, and billions without sanitation facilities.

● Only 63 percent of the world now have improved sanitation access. By 2015 the figure can increase only to 67 percent, yet the MDGs is 75 percent. Currently 2.5 billion people still lack improved sanitation.

● Sanitation target is still lagging far behind MDG target of safe drinking water, and is not yet possible, so improved drinking water sources is seen as a progress, for this can reduce diseases. This is a beginning and need to cautiously continue.

● The biggest challenge is the global massive disparities between regions and countries, and within countries. In sub-Saharan Africa only 61 percent of people have improved water supply sources while the figure in Latin America and the Caribbean, Northern Africa, and large parts of Asia is 90%.

● Rich people have more access to improved water sources while the poor have less or least.

● In rural areas of the least developed countries, 97 out of every 100 people do not have piped water and 14 per cent of the population drinks surface water.

So the goal is to help the poorest and the most disadvantaged people across the world, because drinking water and sanitation are human rights.

Text 2

Chinese Minister of Water Resources, Chen Lei's Speech at the Signing Ceremony of the China, Japan and Korea Joint Statement during the 5th World Water Forum

20 March 2009

Excellencies,
Distinguished guests,
Ladies and gentlemen,

I am delighted to attend the signing ceremony of the China, Japan and Korea Joint Statement during the 5th World Water Forum, together with Mr. Kaneko Yasushi, Vice Minister of Land, Infrastructure, Transport and Tourism of Japan, and Mr. Kwon Do-Youp, Vice Minister of Land, Transport and Maritime Affairs of Korea.

First of all, on behalf of the PRC Ministry of Water Resources, I would like to convey my sincere gratitude to all the guests, including officials from the Ministry of Land, Infrastructure, Transport and Tourism of Japan and the Ministry of Land, Transport and Maritime Affairs of Korea, as well as experts, entrepreneurs and media friends from Japan and Korea that are present at this ceremony.

Water is a fundamental natural resource and a strategic economic resource. It is also a control factor of the ecological environment. With intermingled impacts of global climate change and rapid economic and social development, constantly emerging water problems such as drought and water shortage, flood and waterlogging, water pollution and soil erosion, have proposed great challenges to the entire Asian-Pacific Region and even the whole world. Therefore, water crisis of all kinds can only be properly dealt with and addressed through effective coordination and close cooperation of all countries of the world.

All situated in North-East Asia, China, Japan and Korea are close neighbors only separated by a strip of water and have kept extensive exchanges and effective cooperation in water field for a long time. The regular exchange mechanisms between the Ministry of Water Resources of China with the Ministry of Land, Infrastructure, Transport and Tourism of Japan include "Sino-Japan Workshop on Water Resources" and "Sino-Japan Symposium on River and Dam Engineering". The "Sino-Korea Workshop on Water Resources" is the exchange mechanism between the Ministry of Water Resources of China and the Ministry of Land, Transport and Maritime Affairs of Korea. These exchange mechanisms play an important role in enhancing mutual understanding, exchanging experiences and boosting cooperation of the three countries.

During the 4th World Water Forum held in Mexico in 2006, China, Japan and Korea successfully hosted the joint sessions of "Flood Management", "River Rehabilitation in the Asian Monsoon Region" and "Water Information System", and also announced the proposal of joint sessions to the international community that won positive feedback from international water field.

In order to cope with water problems in North-East Asia together and further cooperation on water related issues, China, Japan and Korea are willing to further our efforts on sharing of technologies and experiences, widen our cooperation areas and deepen our partnership. We are also considering to establish an annual meeting mechanism for water ministers of our three countries on a regular basis, whereby we shall carry out joint studies on specified key areas, strengthen exchange and cooperation in water field, tackle water problems faced by us with concerted efforts, and advance towards common development. I am confident that, through common efforts and sincere cooperation of the three countries, we will surely accomplish new breakthroughs and progresses in finding solutions for major water problems and key water areas, and make further contributions to solve global water problems and sustainable utilization of water resources.

复述要点提示（主要信息逻辑点及层次）

讲话背景：

水资源是生态环境的基础性资源，在发展中占有重要地位。然而在气候变化和经济社会发展的影响下，水资源相关问题已变成全世界的挑战。世界各国需共同努力解决此问题。

问题现状：

中日韩三国一衣带水，在水利领域一向有着良好的交流和合作。交流的机制已经形成，即中日水资源工作坊、中日河流与水坝工程大会和中韩水资源工作坊。三国之间的交流机制对加深了解、推动合作起到了重要作用，并在国际社会得到良好反馈。各方充分认识到水资源对经济发展、生态环境、全球气候变化的重要影响。

前景：

为了共同应对东北亚的水资源问题，三国愿进一步加强合作，深化交流，进一步完善定期会晤机制。三方应加强联合研究，更好地解决共同面临的水问题。

五、英译汉练习

Text 3

Air Pollution and Health

Air pollution affects our health in many ways, particularly our lungs, heart and blood vessels. Research has linked air pollution to a number of health concerns like:

- Asthma;
- Chronic obstructive pulmonary disease;
- Cardiovascular disease;
- Lung cancer;
- Endocrine system effects;
- Neurological effects; and
- Allergies.

In addition, air pollutants typically increase the severity or frequency of common respiratory and cardiovascular medical conditions or illnesses.

According to the most recent scientific research, there is no “safe level” for air pollution. In other words, there is no level below which air pollution poses no adverse health effects. Air pollution poses a health risk all year long, not just in the hot summer months. These health impacts severely impact our quality of life and place unnecessary strain on the health care system.

Poor air quality reduces quality of life for all GTA residents, especially for children and the elderly, and for those with respiratory and cardiovascular problems. Negative health effects increase as air pollution worsens. Studies show that even modest increases in air pollution can cause small, but measurable increases in emergency room visits, hospital admissions and death.

The harmful effects of air pollution are primarily the result of exposure to five common air pollutants:

- Nitrous oxide;
- Ozone (ground-level ozone is not directly emitted but is produced when sunlight combines with hydrocarbons and nitrogen oxide, two compounds produced by cars, trucks, industrial processes, and power-generating plants, and found wherever gasoline, diesel fuel, kerosene, oil, or natural gas are combusted);
- Fine and ultrafine particulates;
- Sulfur dioxide; and
- Carbon monoxide.

These pollutants contribute to the air pollution mix commonly known as smog. They arise from the combustion of fossil fuels in vehicles, from heating of buildings, and from the production of electricity. Depending on exposure time, health status, genetic background, and the concentration of pollutants, air pollution can:

- Make it harder to breathe;
- Irritate your eyes, nose and throat;
- Worsen chronic diseases such as bronchitis, emphysema and asthma;
- Cause heart attacks, heart failure and other forms of heart disease due to constricted blood vessels, altered heart rates and rhythms, and blood clotting; and
- Lead to premature death.

WHAT IS THE CONNECTION BETWEEN AIR POLLUTION AND CARDIOVASCULAR HEALTH?

While many people are aware of the connection between air pollution and respiratory illness, over the last decade a growing body of evidence has led to increased concern of the effects of air pollution on heart disease and stroke.

Of special interest are several environmental air pollutants that include carbon monoxide, oxides of nitrogen, sulfur dioxide, ozone, lead, and particulate matter (PM10 and PM2.5). These pollutants are associated with increased hospitalization and mortality due to cardiovascular disease, especially in persons with congestive heart failure, frequent arrhythmias, or both.

Air pollution is thought to increase the inflammation of blood vessels which is of particular concern for people who suffer from poor cardiovascular health as their ability to handle the inflammation is already compromised.

WHAT ARE THE SHORT TERM EFFECTS OF AIR POLLUTION ON MY HEALTH?

People already suffering from respiratory or cardiac problems are the most likely to feel the short term effects of air pollution. These effects can arise after exposure to high levels of pollutants over a period ranging from several minutes to several weeks.

Exposure to pollution can exacerbate preexisting health problems in those who are vulnerable and in serious cases lead to hospitalization or death. Symptoms are those of the preexisting illness, including:

● Irritation and inflammation of the respiratory tract;

● Wheezing;

● Tightness in the chest;

● Pain while deep breathing;

● Difficulty breathing;

● Increased shortness of breath on exertion.

You will not necessarily experience all these symptoms, and you may have symptoms that are not on the list. For this reason you should be alert to the symptoms you have already learned to recognize due to your health condition.

The onset of these symptoms may also be caused by a host of other factors that you should also watch for, including heat, humidity, viruses, seasonal pollen (e.g., ragweed), and misuse of medication.

People with existing illnesses may have the following specific symptoms:

● People with asthma or COPD may notice an increase in cough, wheezing, shortness of breath or phlegm;

● People who have suffered from heart failure may experience increased shortness of breath or welling in the ankles and feet;

● People with heart rhythm problems may notice increased fluttering in the chest and feeling lightheaded;

● People with angina or coronary artery disease may have an increase in chest or arm pain.

WHAT ARE THE LONG TERM EFFECTS OF AIR POLLUTION ON HEALTH?

Most epidemiological investigations have looked at the effects of short term rather than long term exposure. Studies have shown an increased risk of lung cancer or cardiovascular and cardiopulmonary disease in populations living in highly polluted cities. What's more, long term exposure could interfere with pregnancy (low birth weight and premature birth) and lung development in children.

In addition to respiratory and cardiovascular vulnerabilities, a 2010 national epidemiologic study found a correlation PM2.5 exposure and increased rates of adult diabetes (even after adjustment for other risk factors like obesity and ethnicity on diabetes rates).

A Government of Canada study assessed the annual number of excess deaths due to current air pollution levels in Canada associated with both short- and long-term exposure to air pollution.

Estimated Number of Excess Deaths in Canada Due To Air Pollution (10 pages, Air Health Effects Division, Health Canada, and Meteorological Service of Canada, Environment Canada, Gatineau, Quebec, April 2005).

Results found that based on non-accidental mortality counts and National Air Pollution Surveillance data and pollutant-mortality concentration response functions from epidemiological studies the annual excess number of deaths associated with short-term exposure was estimated to be 1,800, with long-term exposure was estimated to be 4,200, resulting in a total excess deaths estimate of 5,900 people.

To mitigate these effects, we must work together to decrease current air pollution levels, for example by ensuring reductions of industrial air pollutants, reducing energy use from buildings and ensuring increased use of public transit. Our efforts would also protect the health of those who are most vulnerable to the effects of air pollution.

Text 4

On Environmental Hygiene and Individual Hygiene

UNICEF

While gains were made in sanitation coverage over the last 15 years, some regions and countries are not on track to meet the MDG sanitation target by 2015. It is now clear that new approaches are necessary to sustainably increase coverage levels.

UNICEF is increasingly emphasizing sanitation, expanding its own programmes of support in countries around the world and advocating for an increased focus on sanitation by governments and funding partners. The focus of UNICEF support is to help develop improved programming models and to provide support to government partners for taking successful models to scale. This approach involves significant work at the field level while engaging governments and other stakeholders at national level. UNICEF is also active in the development of improved sanitation technology: developing and promoting latrines and toilets that are affordable but also satisfy criteria for safety, effectiveness, sustainability, environmental impact and child-friendliness.

New community-based approaches for sanitation promotion are showing considerable promise in some countries. Instead of focusing on latrine construction, these approaches stress the elimination of open defecation in communities. Communities are encouraged to carry out an analysis of existing defecation patterns and threats, and to use local resources to build low-cost household latrines and ultimately eliminate the practice of open defecation.

These approaches have been especially successful in Cambodia, Zambia and other countries (where the approach is called community-led total sanitation, or CLTS). In India, where the approach—called total sanitation—is being applied on a large-scale, the MDG target for sanitation will likely be met and exceeded. The model is also being introduced with successful results in Bolivia, Ethiopia, Indonesia, Nigeria and other countries.

Recognizing the impact of sanitation on health, the environment, poverty reduction and economic and social development, the United Nations declared 2008 as the International Year of Sanitation (IYS). The IYS initiative placed a spotlight on the seriousness of the global sanitation crisis and kick-started efforts to accelerate progress for meeting the Millennium Development Goal (MDG) target of halving, by 2015, the proportion of the world's population without sustainable access to basic sanitation.

IYS focuses on five key messages that underline both the benefits of improved sanitation and the need for action:

1. Sanitation is vital for human health. Poor sanitation and hygiene causes death and disease.

2. Sanitation generates economic benefits. Improved sanitation has positive impacts on economic growth and poverty reduction.

3. Sanitation contributes to dignity and social development. Sanitation enhances dignity, privacy and safety, especially for women and girls.

4. Sanitation helps the environment. Improved disposal of human waste protects the quality of drinking-water sources and improves community environments.

5. Improving sanitation is achievable. Working together, households, communities, governments, support agencies, civil society and the private sector have the resources,

technologies and know-how to achieve the sanitation target.

Improving access to safe water and sanitation facilities leads to healthier families and communities. However, when people are also motivated to practice good hygiene—especially hand-washing with soap—health benefits are significantly increased. Because the evidence on the importance of hand-washing with soap is clear, UNICEF has made it a programme priority.

Education and communication are important components of a hygiene promotion programme. All people have a right to know about the relationship between water, sanitation, hygiene and the health of themselves and their families. However, education alone does not necessarily result in improved practices. Knowing about the causes of disease may help, but new hygiene practices may be too unfamiliar, too difficult, or take too much time, especially for poor people. Promoting behavioural change is a gradual process that involves working closely with communities, studying existing beliefs, defining motivation strategies, designing appropriate communication tools and finally encouraging practical steps towards positive practices. Communities should be fully engaged in the process at all stages using participatory processes, and special attention should be given to building on local knowledge and promoting existing positive traditional practices.

Behavioural change is necessary not only at the community level, but among decision makers as well. All stakeholders—from politicians and government officials to field workers and people themselves—must be encouraged to recognize the importance of hygiene.

Sanitation and Hand-washing

The best way to address faecal contamination of drinking water is by preventing it from happening in the first place. Well-constructed latrines that are used regularly prevent the contamination of water supplies. Regular hand-washing after defecation and before handling water (or food) minimizes the risk that water used and stored in the home is contaminated with dirty hands. For these reasons, UNICEF stresses sanitation and hygiene promotions as the first line of defence for protecting drinking water from faecal contamination.

Water Quality Monitoring

As water quality problems become more serious and widespread, water quality monitoring becomes a more important component of national efforts in this sector. These efforts can be complemented by community-level surveillance systems, where people are empowered with the knowledge and tools necessary to monitor the quality of their own water sources. UNICEF and its partners are playing an increasingly active role in supporting governments and communities in this important area.

Household Water Treatment and Safe Storage

There is an increasing body of evidence demonstrating that household water treatment along with improved water storage and handling significantly improves microbial water quality and has a greater impact on diarrhoea than previously thought. In recognition of this, UNICEF country WASH programmes are increasingly providing support in this area. Activities include the promotion of safe water storage and handling practices and household water treatment. UNICEF is also involved in the development of appropriate technologies for household water treatment. Example of household water treatment supported by UNICEF is ceramic filters.

Arsenic and Fluoride

For over a decade, UNICEF has worked closely with governments and other partners in countries where fluoride and arsenic are serious problems, including Bangladesh, India, China, Vietnam and elsewhere. UNICEF programmes support testing and mapping initiatives, developing improved water quality monitoring systems, raising awareness in communities about the issue, helping people find alternative safe water sources, and promoting filters and other technologies that help people treat water themselves.

Freshwater Management

In the case of arsenic and fluoride, most of the health problems are caused by naturally occurring forms of the contaminants. An increasing number of water quality problems, however, originate from human-made pollution and general environmental degradation.

六、汉译英练习

Text 5

中华人民共和国水利部部长陈雷在第五届世界水论坛"亚太日"上的致辞

2008年3月20日

各位阁下，

女士们、先生们，朋友们：

今天，我很高兴参加"亚太日"活动，与亚洲各国的同行们一道，围绕解决水问题、推动亚太地区可持续发展，交流经验，分享成果，探讨对策。

水，是人类生存与发展的生命线，是实现经济社会可持续发展的重要物质基础。亚太地区是一个充满活力、具有巨大发展潜力的地区，但在水资源领域却面临着一系列挑战：亚太地区人口占世界的61%，而水资源总量仅为世界的1/3，人口快速增长导致人均水资源量下降、水资源短缺问题突出、水与卫生普及率不高、水资源管理能力薄弱、水利建设融资难等问题，每年有大约5.6亿农村人口得不到安全饮用水，1980年至2006年，因水灾死亡的人口达60万，占世界水灾死亡总数的80%。因此，有效减轻水旱灾害损失、促进水资源可持续利用，是我们共同关注的重大问题，也是亚太地区共同面临的紧迫任务。

中国是世界上人口最多的发展中国家，也是水资源相对短缺的国家。人多水少，水资源时空分布不均，与生产力布局不相匹配，已成为影响中国经济社会可持续发展的突出问题。

中国政府高度重视解决水问题，把节约资源、保护环境作为基本国策，坚持以人为本，坚持人与自然和谐，对水资源进行合理开发、高效利用、综合治理、优化配置、全面节约、有效保护和科学管理，以水资源的可持续利用保障经济社会的可持续发展。中国30年来以年均1%的用水低增长率，保障了年均近10%的经济高速增长；在连续30年保持农田灌溉用水量零增长的情况下，粮食产量提高近50%，养活了占世界21%的人口。这是十分了不起的成就，也是对世界发展与繁荣做出的重大贡献。

当前和今后一个时期，中国致力于全面建设小康社会，加快推进现代化进程。中国政府高度重视水问题，把水利摆在更加突出的位置，将在2010年底前完成大中型和重点小型水库除险加固任务，解除病险水库对人民群众生命财产的威胁；提前

6年实现联合国千年宣言确定的饮水不安全人口比例降低一半的目标，并在2013年底全面解决农村饮水安全问题；2020年基本完成大型灌区续建配套和节水改造任务，新增和恢复有效灌溉面积554万公顷，使农田有效灌溉面积达到6 333万公顷，农业灌溉水利用系数由现在的0.46提高到0.55。到2020年，中国全面建设小康社会目标实现之时，防洪安全将得到可靠保障，城乡居民普遍享有安全清洁的饮用水，水环境和水生态状况显著改善，水利信息化和现代化水平明显提高。

女士们、先生们!

多年来，亚太各国和地区致力于解决水问题，积极探索和构建适合本国国情的经济发展模式。中国政府真诚希望加强亚太地区在水领域的对话、交流与合作，共同推动本地区水领域的发展，促进世界的和谐与亚太地区经济社会的可持续发展。

最后，衷心感谢“亚太日”活动的主办方！祝本次活动取得圆满成功！

Text 6

国家卫生城市标准（节选）

一、爱国卫生组织管理

（一）认真贯彻落实《国务院关于加强爱国卫生工作的决定》，将爱国卫生工作纳入辖区各级政府议事日程，列入社会经济发展规划，具有立法权的城市应当制订本市的爱国卫生法规，其他城市应当制订市政府规范性文件。城市主要领导高度重视，各部门、各单位和广大群众积极参与爱国卫生工作。

（二）辖区内各级爱卫会组织健全，成员单位分工明确、职责落实。爱卫会办公室独立或相对独立设置，人员编制能适应实际工作需要，爱国卫生工作经费纳入财政预算。街道办事处及乡镇政府配备专兼职爱国卫生工作人员，社区居委会及村委会协调做好爱国卫生工作。

（三）制订爱国卫生工作规划和年度计划，有部署、有总结。积极开展卫生街道、卫生社区、卫生单位等创建活动。辖区范围内建成不少于1个省级以上的卫生乡镇（县城）。在城乡广泛开展爱国卫生教育宣传活动。

（四）畅通爱国卫生建议与投诉平台，认真核实和解决群众反映的问题。群众对卫生状况满意率≥90%。

二、健康教育和健康促进

（五）以《中国公民健康素养——基本知识与技能》为主要内容，广泛开展健康教育和健康促进活动。居民健康素养水平达到卫生事业发展规划要求。

（六）健康教育网络健全，各主要媒体设有健康教育栏目。车站、机场、港口、广场和公园等公共场所设立的电子屏幕和公益广告等应当具有健康教育内容。社区、医院、学校等积极开展健康教育活动。

（七）广泛开展全民健身活动，机关、企事业单位落实工作场所工间操制度。80%以上的社区建有体育健身设施。经常参加体育锻炼的人数比率达到30%以上。每千人口至少有2名社会体育指导员。

（八）深入开展禁烟、控烟宣传活动，禁止烟草广告。开展无烟学校、无烟机关、无烟医疗卫生机构等无烟场所建设。室内公共场所、工作场所和公共交通工具设置禁止吸烟警语和标识。

三、市容环境卫生

（九）市容环境卫生达到《城市容貌标准》要求。建成数字化城管系统，并正常运行。城市主次干道和街巷路面平整，主要街道无乱张贴、乱涂写、乱设摊点情况，无乱扔、乱吐现象，废物箱等垃圾收集容器配置齐全，城区无卫生死角。城市河道、湖泊等水面清洁，岸坡整洁，无垃圾杂物。建成区绿化覆盖率≥36%，人均公园绿地面积≥8.5平方米。城市功能照明完善，城市道路装灯率达到100%。

（十）生活垃圾收集运输体系完善，垃圾、粪便收集运输容器、车辆等设备设施全面实现密闭化，垃圾、粪便日产日清。主要街道保洁时间不低于16小时，一般街道保洁时间不低于12小时。建筑工地管理符合《建筑施工现场环境与卫生标准》要求。待建工地管理到位，规范围挡，无乱倒垃圾和乱搭乱建现象。

（十一）生活垃圾、污水、粪便无害化处理设施建设、管理和污染防治符合国家有关法律、法规及标准要求。推行生活垃圾分类收集处理，餐厨垃圾初步实现分类处理和管理，建筑垃圾得到有效处置。省会城市和计划单列市实现生活垃圾全部无害化处理，生活污水全部收集和集中处理；其他城市和直辖市所辖行政区生活垃圾无害化处理率≥90%，生活污水集中处理率≥85%。

（十二）生活垃圾转运站、公共厕所等环卫设施符合《城镇环境卫生设施设置标准》《城市公共厕所卫生标准》等要求，数量充足，布局合理，管理规范。城市主次干道、车站、机场、港口、旅游景点等公共场所的公厕不低于二类标准。

（十三）集贸市场管理规范，配备卫生管理和保洁人员，环卫设施齐全。临时便民市场采取有效管理措施，保证周边市容环境卫生、交通秩序和群众正常生活秩序。达到《标准化菜市场设置与管理规范》要求的农副产品市场比例≥70%。

（十四）活禽销售市场的卫生管理规范，设立相对独立的经营区域，按照动物防疫有关要求，实行隔离宰杀，落实定期休市和清洗消毒制度，对废弃物实施规范处理。

（十五）社区和单位建有卫生管理组织和相关制度，卫生状况良好，环卫设施完善，垃圾日产日清，公共厕所符合卫生要求。道路平坦，绿化美化，无违章建筑，无占道经营现象。市场、饮食摊点等商业服务设施设置合理，管理规范。

（十六）城中村及城乡接合部配备专人负责卫生保洁，环卫设施布局合理，垃圾密闭收集运输，日产日清，清运率100%。有污水排放设施。公厕数量达标，符合卫生要求。路面硬化平整，无非法小广告，无乱搭乱建、乱堆乱摆、乱停乱放、乱贴乱画、乱扔乱倒现象。无违规饲养畜禽。

四、环境保护

（十七）近三年辖区内未发生重大环境污染和生态破坏事故。

（十八）贯彻落实《中华人民共和国大气污染防治法》，环境空气质量指数（AQI）或空气污染指数（API）不超过100的天数≥300天，环境空气主要污染物年均值达到国家《环境空气质量标准》二级标准。贯彻落实《秸秆禁烧和综合利用管理办法》，秸秆综合利用率达到100%，杜绝秸秆焚烧现象。区域环境噪声平均值≤60分贝。

（十九）贯彻落实《中华人民共和国水法》《中华人民共和国水污染防治法》等法律法规，集中式饮用水水源地一级保护区水质达标率100%，安全保障达标率100%，城区内水环境功能区达到要求，未划定功能区的无劣五类水体。

（二十）医疗废弃物统一由有资质的医疗废弃物处置单位处置，无医疗机构自行处置医疗废物情况。医源性污水的处理排放符合国家有关要求。

五、重点场所卫生

（二十一）贯彻落实《公共场所卫生管理条例》，开展公共场所卫生监督量化分级工作。公共场所卫生许可手续齐全有效，从业人员取得有效健康合格证明。

（二十二）小餐饮店、小食品店、小浴室、小美容美发、小歌舞厅、小旅店等经营资格合法，室内外环境整洁，硬件设施符合相应国家标准要求，从业人员取得有效健康合格证明。

（二十三）贯彻落实《学校卫生工作条例》，学校和托幼机构教室、食堂（含饮用水设施）、宿舍、厕所等教学和生活环境符合国家卫生标准或相关规定。加强传染病、学生常见病的预防控制工作，设立校医院或卫生室，配备专职卫生技术人员或兼职保健教师。开展健康学校建设活动，中小学健康教育开课率达100%。

（二十四）贯彻落实《中华人民共和国职业病防治法》，用人单位作业场所职业病危害因素符合国家职业卫生标准。按照《职业健康监护技术规范》要求，对从事接触职业病危害作业的劳动者开展职业健康检查，开展职业健康教育活动。近三年未发生重大职业病危害事故。

六、食品和生活饮用水安全

（二十五）贯彻落实《中华人民共和国食品安全法》，建立健全食品安全全程监管工作机制，近三年未发生重大食品安全事故。

（二十六）食品生产经营单位内外环境卫生整洁，无交叉污染，食品储存、加工、销售符合卫生要求。对无固定经营场所的食品摊贩实行统一管理，规定区域、限定品种经营。

（二十七）餐饮业、集体食堂餐饮服务食品安全监督量化分级管理率≥90%。食品从业人员取得有效的健康合格证明。落实清洗消毒制度，防蝇、防鼠等设施健全。

（二十八）牲畜屠宰符合卫生及动物防疫要求，严格落实检疫程序。

（二十九）按照《生活饮用水卫生监督管理办法》要求，市政供水、自备供水、居民小区直饮水管理规范，供水单位有卫生许可证。二次供水符合国家《二次供水设施卫生规范》的标准要求。开展水质监测工作，出厂水、管网末梢水、小区直饮水的水质检测指标达到标准要求。

七、公共卫生与医疗服务

（三十）贯彻落实《中华人民共和国传染病防治法》，近三年未发生重大实验室生物安全事故和因防控措施不力导致的甲、乙类传染病暴发流行。按期完成艾滋病、结核病、血吸虫病等重点疾病预防控制规划要求。

（三十一）以街道（乡、镇）为单位适龄儿童免疫规划疫苗接种率达到90%以上。疫苗储存和运输管理、接种单位条件符合国家规定要求。制订流动人口免疫规划管理办法，居住满3个月以上的适龄儿童建卡、建证率达到95%以上。

（三十二）开展慢性病综合防控示范区建设。实施全民健康生活方式行动，建设健康步道、健康食堂（餐厅）、健康主题公园，推广减盐、控油等慢性病防控措施。

（三十三）贯彻落实《中华人民共和国精神卫生法》，健全工作机构，完善严重精神障碍救治管理工作网络，严重精神障碍患者管理率达到75%以上。

（三十四）辖区内疾病预防控制机构设置合理，人员、经费能够满足工作需要，疾病预防控制中心基础设施建设达到《疾病预防控制中心建设标准》要求，实验室检验设备装备达标率达到90%以上。

（三十五）无偿献血能够满足临床用血需要，临床用血100%来自自愿无偿献血。建成区无非法行医、非法采供血和非法医疗广告。

（三十六）每个街道办事处范围或3万～10万服务人口设置一所社区卫生服务中心，每个乡镇设置一所政府举办的乡镇卫生院。基层医疗卫生机构标准化建设达标率达到95%以上。

（三十七）辖区婴儿死亡率≤12‰，5岁以下儿童死亡率≤14‰，孕产妇死亡率≤22/10万。

八、病媒生物预防控制

（三十八）贯彻落实《病媒生物预防控制管理规定》，建立政府组织与全社会参与相结合的病媒生物防控机制，机关、企事业单位和社区定期开展病媒生物预防控制活动，针对区域内危害严重的病媒生物种类和公共外环境，适时组织集中统一控制行动。建成区鼠、蚊、蝇、蟑螂的密度达到国家病媒生物密度控制水平标准C级要求。

（三十九）掌握病媒生物滋生地基本情况，制定分类处理措施，湖泊、河流、小型积水、垃圾、厕所等各类滋生环境得到有效治理。

（四十）开展重要病媒生物监测调查，收集病媒生物侵害信息并及时进行处置。重点行业和单位防蚊蝇和防鼠设施合格率≥95%。

资料来源：

Text 1 http://www.who.int/mediacentre/news/releases/2012/drinking_water_20120306/en/

Text 2 http://www.mwr.gov.cn/english/speechesandarticles/chenlei/200907/t20090714_59299.html

Text 3 http://www.cleanairpartnership.org/air_pollution_and_your_health

Text 4 http://www.who.int/iris/handle/10665/23567

Text 5 http://www.kouyi.org/field/environment/889.html

Text 6 http://www.nhfpc.gov.cn/jkj/s5898/201405/a8ce63259ee640729671917865467a88.shtml

参考答案

四、摘要练习

Text 1

千年发展目标的饮用水具体目标得以实现　但卫生设施目标仍相距甚远

纽约/日内瓦

2012年3月6日

联合国儿童基金会与世卫组织今日发布的一份报告显示，全世界已实现将无法持续获得安全饮用水的人口比例减半的千年发展目标，这远早于2015年千年发展目标的最后期限。1990至2010年之间，20亿以上的人口获得了经过改良的饮用水源，如自来水供应和受保护的水井。

联合国秘书长潘基文说，“今天，我们赞赏为世界人民取得的一项伟大成就。

这是千年发展目标中率先实现的其中一项。为改善获得饮用水做出了成功努力，这是向所有认可千年发展目标的人们提供的一个证据，他们未将该目标看作空想，而是将其作为改善数百万最贫困人民生活的一个重要工具”。

世卫组织/联合国儿童基金会饮用水供应和卫生设施联合监测方案《2012年饮用水和卫生设施进展》报告提到，到2010年年底，全世界89%的人口，或者说61亿人使用了经过改善的饮用水源。这比千年发展目标确立的88%的目标高出一个百分点。这份报告估计，到2015年，全球将有92%的人口获得经改善的饮用水。

“这对于儿童而言尤其是个好消息”，联合国儿童基金会执行主任安东尼·雷克说，“每天有3 000名以上的儿童死于腹泻病。实现这一目标对挽救儿童生命大有裨益。”

雷克提醒人们，至少有11%的世界人口（7.83亿人）仍无法获得安全的饮用水，还有数十亿人没有卫生设施，因此现在还不能宣布取得了胜利。

“这些数字依旧高得骇人”，他说，“但今天宣布的进展证明，只要有毅力、努力和资金，千年发展目标就能够实现。”

然而，该报告强调，在实现千年发展目标的卫生设施具体目标方面，全世界依旧相差甚远，并不太可能在2015年前成功实现。目前，全世界仅有63%的人口可以获得良好的卫生设施，预测数据显示，到2015年时仅可能提高到67%，大大低于千年发展目标中确定的75%的目标。目前，仍有25亿人缺乏良好的卫生设施。

联合国儿童基金会和世卫组织还提醒到，由于无法在全球衡量水质，在安全饮用水的千年发展目标方面取得的进展是通过收集经改善的饮用水源使用数据来衡量的。必须做大量的工作，确保改良水源既做到安全又保持安全。

“提供可持续获得的改良饮用水源是我们为减少疾病而能做的最重要的事情之一”，世卫组织总干事陈冯富珍博士说，“但现在取得的这项成就仅仅是个开始。我们必须继续保持所获水源的安全性。否则，我们的收获也将付诸东流。”

报告强调了依旧存在的巨大挑战。全球数据掩盖了区域和国家之间以及一国之内存在的巨大差异。

与拉丁美洲和加勒比海、北非及亚洲大部分地区90%或更高的比例相比，在撒哈拉以南的非洲，仅有61%的人能够获得经改善的饮用水供应水源。全球40%以上不能获得安全饮用水的人口生活在撒哈拉以南的非洲。

该报告证实，在无法易于获得水供应的地区，提运水的重担会过多地落在妇女和女孩的肩上。在许多国家，最富裕的人们在获得饮用水和卫生设施方面获得的改善最大，而最贫穷者依旧远远落后。

本报告提供了全球农村地区方面的最新情况，突出说明在饮用水和卫生设施方面需要给予更多关注。在最不发达国家的农村地区，每100人中就有97人不能得到自来水，并且14%的人口饮用源自河流、池塘或湖泊等的地表水。

在依旧进行露天排便的11亿人中，绝大部分（9.49亿）生活在农村地区。这甚至会影响到饮用水获得情况已有大幅改善的地区。例如，拉丁美洲和加勒比海有17%的农村居民以及北非有9%的农村居民仍旧在露天排便。即便是在所谓的经济出现迅速增长的金砖国家，仍有大量人口在露天排便：印度6.26亿人、中国1 400万人以及巴西720万人。

“我们已经实现了一项重要目标，但我们不能在此停滞不前”，联合国秘书长说，“下一步我们必须锁定全世界最难覆盖、最贫穷和最弱势的人。联合国大会已将饮用水和卫生设施当作人权。这就意味着，我们必须确保每一个人都能够得到。”

Text 2

中华人民共和国水利部部长陈雷
在第五届世界水论坛中日韩三国联合声明签字仪式上的讲话

2009年3月20日

各位阁下，
尊敬的各位来宾，
女士们、先生们：

今天，我很高兴能与日本国土交通省金子恭之副大臣和韩国国土海洋部权度烨副部长共同出席第五届世界水论坛中日韩三国联合声明签字仪式。

首先，请允许我代表中华人民共和国水利部，向前来出席签字仪式的日本国土交通省和韩国国土海洋部的官员，以及日韩两国的专家、学者、企业界代表和新闻界朋友表示衷心的感谢！

水是基础性的自然资源和战略性的经济资源，是生态环境的控制性要素。在全球气候变化和经济社会快速发展双重因素的交织作用下，干旱缺水、洪涝灾害、水体污染、水土流失等水问题日益凸显，已成为亚太地区，乃至全世界共同面临的挑战，只有通过世界各国的协调配合和紧密合作，才能有效应对和解决各种水危机。

中日韩三国同属东北亚地区，是一衣带水的友好邻邦，长期以来在水利领域有着广泛的交流与良好的合作。中国水利部与日本国土交通省在水资源领域的定期交流机制包括“中日水资源交流会”和“中日河工坝工会议”。中国水利部与韩国国土海洋部在水资源领域的交流机制为“中韩水资源交流会”。这些交流机制对加深相互了解、交流经验、推动合作发挥了重要作用。在2006年墨西哥举行的第四届世界水论坛期间，中日韩三国还成功举行了“洪水管理”、“亚洲季风区的河流修复”和“水资源信息系统”联合分会，并向国际社会宣读了联合分会的倡议，在国际水利界产生了很好的反响。

为了共同应对本地区面临的水问题，加强涉水事务合作，中日韩三国愿意进一步分享技术经验、拓宽交流领域、深化合作关系，着手建立一年一次的中日韩三国水利部长定期会晤机制。通过该机制，三国将选取重点领域开展联合研究，加强水利领域的交流协作，协力解决共同面临的水问题，促进共同发展。我相信，通过三国的共同努力和通力合作，一定能够在重大水问题和关键水领域取得新的突破和进展，为解决全球水问题，实现水资源可持续利用做出新的贡献!

五、英译汉练习

Text 3

空气污染与健康

空气污染在许多方面影响着我们的健康，尤其影响我们的肺、心脏和血管。研究表明，空气污染导致许多健康问题，如：

- 哮喘；
- 慢性阻塞性肺疾病；
- 心血管疾病；
- 肺癌；
- 内分泌系统的问题；
- 神经系统问题；
- 过敏。

此外，空气污染物通常会加重常见呼吸系统和心血管系统疾病，或增加患病的频率。

最新的科学研究表明，空气污染没有“安全级”的说法。换言之，空气污染危害健康，不存在不威胁健康的等级。空气污染一年到头都会让健康面临危险，这个危险不仅仅只在炎热的夏季。这些影响健康的因素，严重影响我们的生活质量，给卫生保健系统不必要的压力。

空气质量差，降低了所有GTA居民的生活质量，尤其是儿童和老人的生活质量，也降低了那些有呼吸系统和心血管问题的人的生活质量。对健康有害的负面效果随空气污染恶化而加重。研究表明，即使空气污染有一点点细微的恶化，也能显著增加急诊室的就诊人数、住院人数和死亡人数。

空气污染的有害影响主要是人暴露于五种常见空气污染物中的结果：

●氧化亚氮；

●臭氧（地面臭氧不是直接排放产生的，而是因为碳氢化合物和氮氧化物在阳光的照射下产生的，这两种化合物产生于汽车、卡车、工业生产过程，以及发电厂发电过程，同时这些化合物在任何燃烧汽油、柴油、煤油、石油或天然气的地方都能找到）；

●细微和超细颗粒物；

●二氧化硫；

●一氧化碳。

这些污染物汇合形成空气污染的混合物，俗称雾霾。他们出自车辆燃烧的化石燃料、建筑物供暖，以及电力生产。依照暴露在污染物中的不同时间、自身健康状况、遗传背景和污染物的浓度，空气污染可以：

●让人难以呼吸；

●刺激人的眼、鼻、喉；

●加剧慢性疾病如支气管炎、肺气肿和哮喘；

●由于导致血管收缩、心率和心律改变以及凝血而引发心脏病、心脏衰竭以及其他形式的心血管病；

●导致过早死亡。

空气污染和心血管健康之间的联系是什么？

虽然很多人都知道空气污染与呼吸系统疾病之间的关系，在过去的十年中，已经有越来越多的证据让人们对空气污染对心脏病和中风的影响更加关注。

特别令人关注的是几种空气污染物，包括一氧化碳、氮氧化物、二氧化硫、臭氧、铅和颗粒物（PM10和PM2.5）。这些污染物与住院率增加、心血管疾病死亡相关，特别与充血性心脏衰竭、频发心律失常患者，或者这两种病都有的患者相关。

空气污染被认为会增加血管炎症，为那些心血管状况不佳的人所特别关注，因为他们的身体对炎症的抵抗力已经下降。

空气污染对健康的短期影响是什么？

已经患有呼吸系统疾病或心脏病的人最有可能感受到空气污染的短期影响。暴露在高浓度的污染物后几分钟至几周时间，影响就会发生。

暴露于污染之中会诱发那些易感人群身上已经存在的健康问题，在严重的情况下甚至会导致急症住院或死亡。预先已存在的疾病症状包括：

●呼吸道红肿和炎症；

- 气喘；
- 胸闷；
- 深呼吸疼痛；
- 呼吸困难；
- 劳累时气喘加重。

不是每一个人都一定会经历所有这些症状，你的症状这里可能没有提及。因此，你应该警惕自己已经意识到的身体不适。

上述症状也可能是其他种种因素造成的，例如温度、湿度、病毒、季节性花粉（例如豚草）和错用药物，这些你都应该注意。

已经患病的人可能有以下具体症状：

- 患有哮喘或慢性阻塞性肺病的人可能会咳嗽加剧、喘息加重、呼吸急促或有痰；
- 患有心衰的人可能感到呼吸急促加剧，脚和脚踝肿胀；
- 心律有问题的人会感到心跳加快，头昏眼花；
- 有心绞痛或冠状动脉疾病的人胸痛或手臂痛会加剧。

空气污染对健康的长期影响是什么?

大多数流行病学调查观察暴露于污染物中的短期影响，未观察长期影响。研究表明，生活在高度污染的城市的人群患肺癌、心血管疾病与肺心病的风险增加。更重要的是，长期暴露于污染之中可能会干扰妊娠（导致出生体重低、早产）并影响孩子的肺部发育。

除了呼吸系统和心血管系统易受感染，加拿大2010全国流行病研究发现，暴露于PM2.5之中与成人糖尿病患病率增加相关（即使调整了肥胖和种族等导致糖尿病发病率的其他危险因素之后也是如此）。

加拿大政府的一个研究评估了当前加拿大空气污染水平导致死亡人数超常与短期和长期暴露于空气污染之中的相关关系。

加拿大由于空气污染造成的超长死亡数评估长10页，参与单位包括空气对健康影响部、健康加拿大、加拿大气象局、加拿大环境局，2005年4月在魁北克加蒂诺发表。

结果发现，根据非意外死亡数记录、国家空气污染监测数据，以及来自流行病学研究的污染物——死亡率浓度响应函数，每年与短期暴露相关的超常死亡人数估算为1 800人，与长期暴露相关的死亡人数估算达到了4 200人，总共死亡人数估算为5 900人。

为了减轻这些影响，我们必须共同努力，降低目前的空气污染水平，例如确保工业空气污染减少，减少建筑的能源消耗，鼓励多用公共交通方式。我们所做的努力也会保护那些最易受空气污染影响的人的健康。

Text 4

关于环境卫生与个人卫生

联合国儿童基金会

过去的15年中，我们在提高卫生设施覆盖率方面取得了很大成绩，但是一些国家和地区还没有走上在2015年之前实现千年发展目标的轨道。现在很清楚，要可持续地增加覆盖率，需要新的方法。

联合国儿童基金会正日益加强对环境卫生的关注，在全世界范围内扩大自己支持的项目，并倡导政府及资金合作伙伴提高对环境卫生的重视。联合国儿童基金会支持的重点是帮助开发改善项目的模式，并为推广成功的模式向政府合作伙伴提供支持。在鼓励国家级政府及其他利益相关各方的同时，这种模式在项目所在地还需要做大量的工作。联合国儿童基金会也积极发展改善卫生条件的技术：开发并推广成本低且安全、有效、可持续、环保和易于儿童使用的标准的公厕和户厕。

在一些国家，以社区为基础的新的卫生设施推广方法卓有成效。这些方法不再专注于厕所的建设，而是强调禁止在社区随地大小便。鼓励社区对现有的如厕方式及其危险性进行分析，利用当地资源建造低成本的家庭厕所，并最终消除随地如厕的习惯。

这些方法已经在柬埔寨、赞比亚和其他一些国家获得了显著成效（这种方式被称为社区主导的综合卫生，或CLTS）。这种综合卫生模式在印度被广泛使用，千年发展目标中的环境卫生目标将可能在那里被实现甚至超越。这种模式也被成功地推广到玻利维亚、埃塞俄比亚、印度尼西亚、尼日利亚和其他一些国家。

考虑到环境卫生对健康、环境、减贫及经济和社会发展的影响，联合国宣布2008年为国际环境卫生年（IYS）。国际环境卫生年的目标是强调全球环境卫生危机的严重性，并再接再厉，加速实现在2015年之前将无法可持续地获得基本卫生设施的人口比例减少一半的千年发展目标。

国际环境卫生年注重五个关键讯息，强调改善环境卫生的效益和行动的必要性：

1. 环境卫生对人类健康至关重要。卫生条件差和不良的卫生习惯引起疾病和死亡。

2. 环境卫生创造经济效益。改善环境卫生对经济增长和减少贫困具有积极的影响。

3. 环境卫生提高尊严和促进生活发展。环境卫生增强尊严、保护隐私和安全感，特别是对妇女和女童。

4. 环境卫生有助于环境保护。加强对人类排泄物的处理，以保护饮用水源并改善社区环境。

5. 改善环境卫生是可以实现的。家庭、社区、政府、资助机构、民间团体和私营公司共同努力，拥有实现环境卫生目标的资源、技术和方法。

提高安全用水和卫生设施的覆盖率可以促进家庭和社区的健康。而如果人们培养出讲卫生的好习惯，尤其是用肥皂洗手的习惯，保健效益就将显著提高。因为已经有证据清楚地显示出用肥皂洗手的重要性，联合国儿童基金会将其列为优先项目。

教育和沟通是卫生宣传项目的重要组成部分。所有人都有权利知道水、环境卫生和个人卫生与自己和家庭之间的关系。但是，仅教育本身并不一定能改善行为习惯。了解疾病的成因可能会有所帮助，但是新的卫生习惯对很多人来讲可能太陌生、太困难或太花时间，尤其是对穷人来说。促进行为改变是个渐进的过程，需要与社区密切合作；研究现有的信仰；制定激励策略；设计适当的交流工具并鼓励采取实际的步骤建立正确的行为习惯。应该鼓励社区充分参与整个过程的各个阶段，并应特别注意学习当地的地方知识，推广现存的好的传统习惯。

行为的改变不仅在基层社区是必要的，对决策者也是必要的。所有相关各方——从政治家和政府官员到实施项目的当地工作者和人民大众，都必须认识到个人卫生的重要性。

环境卫生与洗手

解决粪便污染饮用水这一问题的最好办法就是首先预防它的发生。建筑适当的厕所通常可以防止供水污染。每次如厕之后和处理水或食物之前洗手可以将不干净的手污染家里使用和储存的水的风险降至最低。由于这些原因，联合国儿童基金会强调，宣传环境卫生和个人卫生是预防饮用水被粪便污染的第一道防线。

水质检测

随着水质问题日益严重和普遍，水质检测成为这个领域的国家重点工作。这些工作可以得到社区一级监视系统的辅助。社区工作者掌握了检测他们自己水源的知识和必要的工具。联合国儿童基金会及其合作伙伴发挥着越来越积极的作用，在这一重要领域中支持政府和社区的工作。

家庭用水处理与安全储存

越来越多的证据显示，采用家庭用水净化与改善水储存和操作方式一起，可以明显改善含微生物的水的水质，并且对腹泻的影响超过以前的认知。意识到这点，联合国儿童基金会“中国—联合国儿童基金会爱生学校全方位环境改善”项目不断增加向这一领域提供支持。项目活动包括促进安全的储水和操作，以及家庭用水净化处理。联合国儿童基金会还参与开发适当的家庭用水净化处理技术。例如由联合国儿童基金会支持的家庭用水处理案例：陶瓷过滤器。

砷和氟

十多年来，联合国儿童基金会与各国政府及其他合作伙伴在氟和砷问题严重的国家紧密合作，这些国家包括孟加拉、印度、中国、越南及其他地方。联合国儿童基金会项目支持检查并规划行动、开发改良的水质检测系统、提高社区对该问题的认知、帮助人们寻找替代性安全水源，并推广过滤器和其他帮助人们自己净化水质的技术。

淡水的管理

与砷和氟相关的多数的健康问题是由自然形成的污染物造成的。然而，日益增加的水质问题则是因为人类制造的污染和总体的环境恶化造成的。

六、汉译英练习

Text 5

Chinese Minister of Water Resources, Chen Lei’s Speech on “The Asia-Pacific Day” of the 5th World Water Forum

20 March 2008

Excellencies,
Ladies, gentlemen and dear friends,

Today, I am delighted to attend the Asian-Pacific Day where we can exchange experiences, share outcomes and conduct discussions with colleagues from other Asian-Pacific countries in conquering water problems and promoting sustainable development in the Asian-Pacific region.

Water is the lifeline for the livelihood and development of human being and a critical material foundation for sustainable social and economic development. The Asian-Pacific region is an area full of energy and has huge development potentials. Nevertheless, the water sector in the Asian-Pacific region is confronted with a great deal of challenges. Population of the Asian-Pacific region occupies 61% of the world total, whereas its water resources only account for 1/3 of the world total. As a result of rapid population increase, problems are emerged such as reduction of water resources per capita, severe water shortage, limited access to water and sanitation and low capacity in water management and difficulty in water project financing. Approximately 560 million rural population are unable to access to safe drinking water. From 1980 to 2006, water disasters in Asia Pacific resulted in 600,000 deaths, accounting for 80% of the world total. Thus, reducing losses of flood and drought disasters and sustainable utilization of water resources are not only issues of our common concern but also pressing tasks for all Asian-Pacific countries.

China is a developing country with largest population in the world and relatively scarce water resources. With large population but limited water resources plus uneven temporal and spatial distribution of water resources and the consequent mismatch between such distribution and the layout of productivity, it has become the predominant problem that has great impact on sustainable development of economy and society of China.

The Chinese Government attaches great attention to finding solutions for water issues and regards resource conservation and environmental protection as the basic national policies. In line with the philosophies of human orientation and harmony between man and nature, the Chinese water sector endeavors to ensure sustainable economic and social development with sustainable utilization of water resources, i.e., rational development, efficient utilization, integrated management, optimized allocation, all-round conservation, effective protection and scientific management of water resources. Over the past 30 years, China has sustained a nearly 10% annual economic growth rate at an annual growth rate of 1% in water use. For 30 consecutive years, China has increased grain output by nearly 50% with zero increase of irrigation water use, and fed 21% of the world population. These are marvelous achievements and significant contributions that China has made for world development and prosperity.

Currently and hereafter, China is devoted to constructing a well-off society in an all-round way and accelerating to drive the process of modernization. The Chinese Government attaches high importance to water issues and puts the water sector in the more outstanding place. We shall complete the task of reinforcing large, medium and key small defective reservoirs by the end of 2010, and thereby eliminate their threats to people's lives and properties. China will realize the UN Millennium Development Goal of halving the population without access to safe drinking water 6 years ahead of time, and completely solve rural difficulty in accessing safe drinking water by the end of 2013. Continuous and supplementary construction and water-saving renovation of large irrigation areas will be completed by 2020 when effectively irrigated farmland in China will extend by 5.54 million hectare and the total effectively irrigated farmland will reach 63.33 million hectare, and agricultural irrigation water use coefficient will-go up from 0.46 to 0.55. By 2020 when the goal of building a well-off society in an all-round way becomes a reality in China, the Chinese people will be safely protected from floods, have access to safe and clean drinking water in both urban and rural areas, enjoy remarkably improved water environment, water ecology and enhanced informationization and modernization of the water sector.

Ladies and gentlemen,

For many years, Asian-Pacific countries have been committed to addressing water problems, and actively exploring and developing economic development patterns tailored to their respective national situations. The Chinese Government sincerely hopes to enhance dialogues, exchanges and cooperation in water field among Asian-Pacific countries, with joint efforts for promoting development of the water sector in this region, as well as harmony of the world and sustainable development of economy and society in the Asian-Pacific region.

Finally, I would like to express my heartfelt gratitude to the host of the Asian-Pacific Day, and wish this event a great success!

Text 6

National Standards of City Sanitation (Excerpts)

Ⅰ. Organizational Management of the Patriotic Health Promotion

1. Administrations shall seriously implement the "Decision of the State Council on Strengthening the Patriotic Health Promotion", bring the patriotic health promotion work into the working schedule of the government at all levels, and into social and economic development plans. Cities that have legislative power shall formulate its own patriotic sanitation regulations, while other cities will formulate its City Hall normative rules. The main city government leaders shall attach great importance to patriotic health promotion, and all governmental departments and citizens are encouraged to actively participate in hygiene and health promotion.

2. Patriotic Health Campaign Committee at all levels shall improve their organizational functions; clarify their division of responsibilities and work. Offices of Patriotic Health Campaign Committee shall be set up independently or relatively independently, and their staffs shall meet the needs of actual work. The funds for health promotion shall be included into the committee's budget. Community offices and township governments shall have their own full-time or part-time hygiene and health promoters. Community neighborhood committees and village committees shall coordinate with the promotion.

3. Governments involved shall formulate work program and annual plan with implementation procedures and ending-program report requirements for hygiene and health promotion. They shall actively organize campaigns on establishing clean streets, clean communities, and clean units. In the area under their jurisdiction, they shall established no less than one model clean town or township awarded by the provincial government or above. Their educational campaigns for hygiene and health shall reach as many citizens as possible in the urban and rural areas.

4. Administrations shall create an easy access to a platform for suggestions and complaints concerning hygiene and health, carefully verify and solve the problem complained by citizens, and ensure that the citizen's satisfaction rate be≥90%.

Ⅱ. Health Education and Health Promotion

5. Based on "China Citizen Health Literacy—Basic Knowledge and Skills", we conduct extensive campaigns on health education and health promotion, with a goal that the residences' health literacy level meet the requirements of the plans of health development.

6. Administrations shall improve health education network and require that all major media establish columns on health education. The already established electronic screens and public service announcements at railway station, airports, harbors, squares and parks shall include contents of health education. Communities, hospitals, and schools shall actively conduct health education activities.

7. Administrations shall conduct nationwide fitness activities. Government departments, enterprises, and institutions shall implement workplace break-time exercise program. More than 80% of communities shall build sports and fitness facilities. People who often participate in physical exercise will reach 30% of the population. Every thousand people shall have at least 2 social sports instructors.

8. Administrations shall have in-depth advocacy activities for prohibition of smoking, tobacco control, and prohibition of tobacco advertisement, as well as establishing smoke-free schools, government departments, and medical institutions. Indoor public places, workplaces

and public transportation areas shall have signs of warnings for prohibition of smoking.

Ⅲ. City Hygiene and Sanitation

9. The appearance and environment of the city shall achieve "Urban Appearance Standards". Digital city management system shall be established and operate normally. The urban primary and secondary roads, streets and lane paths shall be even and neat; the main streets have no chaotic posting, graffiti, and arbitrary stalls, as well as have no arbitrary litters and spits; Cities shall be fully equipped with garbage collectors such as waste boxes and trash containers; the city will have all corners cleaned. Urban rivers and lakes shall have clean surface, the river banks be clean and tidy with no garbage. The city's already constructed areas shall have ≥36% of green coverage, and the per capita green area of the park will be ≥8.5 square meters. The urban road lighting coverage will reach 100%.

10. Administrations shall improve garbage collection and transportation system, so that garbage and feces collection as well as transportation containers, vehicles, equipment and facilities can be fully sealed up, and garbage and feces can be cleaned up every day. The main streets must be kept clean in no less than 16 hours, while ordinary streets must be kept clean in no less than 12 hours. Construction site management shall satisfy "Environment and Health Standards for Construction Sites". The to-be-built construction sites must have standardized enclosures, and have no arbitrary dumping and arbitrary temporary constructions.

11. The construction and management of garbage, sewage, fecal detoxification treatment facilities as well as pollution prevention shall meet the requirements of relevant laws, regulations and standards. Administrations shall implement classified garbage collection and disposal, initially realize kitchen garbage classification and management, and effectively dispose construction wastes. Provincial capitals and chosen cities shall achieve detoxification of domestic garbage; their sewage shall be completely collected and treated together. Other cities and administrative districts under the jurisdiction of municipalities will achieve detoxification treatment of ≥90% of their domestic garbage, and their collective sewage treatment rate shall reach≥85%.

12. Waste transportation stations, public toilets and other sanitation facilities shall meet the "Standards for Urban Public Sanitation Facility Installation" and "Standards for Urban Public Toilet Sanitation". Abundant in quantity, they shall be reasonably laid out in the city and well managed in accordance with the standards. Toilets in cities' primary and secondary roads, railway stations, airports, harbors, tourist attractions and other public places shall meet at least Types 2 standard.

13. Bazaars shall have complete set of sanitation facilities, standardized management, administrative staff and cleaning staff. Temporary convenient markets shall have effective management measures to ensure the surrounding neighborhood clean, their traffic in order, and their normal life undisturbed. Agricultural markets that have met the requirement of "Structure and Management Standards of the Standardized Agricultural Markets" shall reach the rate of ≥70% of all markets.

14. In accordance with the hygiene standards, live poultry markets shall establish relatively independent business area, have a segregated slaughtering area in accordance with relevant requirements of animal epidemic prevention, implement the system of periodical closing for cleaning and disinfection, and practice standardized waste treatment.

15. Communities and units are required to establish their sanitation and hygiene management systems, to ensure their sanitation and hygiene conditions to be good, their sanitation facilities in good shape, their garbage well disposed every day, and their public toilets met the sanitation requirements. Their streets shall be even, their areas covered with greens, with no illegal construction and no vendors selling in public areas. Markets, food stalls and other commercial services are arranged at reasonable places and management of them standardized.

16. Villages inside the city and the junction areas between the city and the rural areas shall have cleaning staff for sanitation and hygiene. Their sanitation facilities shall be reasonably laid out, and garbage bags sealed up in transportation and 100% removed and disposed every day. They shall have sewage disposal facilities. The number of their public toilets shall meet the standards of quantity and sanitation requirements. Their streets shall be even, with no illegal small advertisement on their walls, no arbitrary temporary constructions, no arbitrary chaotic heaping, parking, sticking, scribbling, dumping, and littering. No violation on rearing livestock.

Ⅳ. Environmental Protection

17. Within 3 year, the jurisdictional regions shall have no major accidents of environmental pollution and ecological damage.

18. Administrations shall implement "Air Pollution Prevention and Control Law of the People's Republic of China" to ensure their Ambient Air Quality Index (AQI) or Air Pollution Index (API) lower than 100 and last for≥300 days, and their annual average ambient air pollutants satisfy Level 2 standard of China's "Ambient Air Quality Standards". They shall implement the "Prohibition of Straw Burning and Methods of Its Comprehensive Utilization and Management" to ensure the rate of their comprehensive utilization of straws

to reach 100%, so as to eliminate straw burning. The average of their environmental noise shall be≤60 dB.

19. Administrations shall implement "Water Law of the People's Republic of China" and "Water Pollution Prevention Law of the People's Republic of China". At Level 1 protection area of the centralized drinking water source, the water quality shall 100% satisfy the standard and 100% satisfy the safety insurance standards. The functional areas of water environment within the city shall meet the requirements, while the areas whose function has not been designated shall not have sub-level v water bodies.

20. Medical waste shall be treated and disposed only by qualified medical waste disposal departments. No medical institutions can dispose their medical wastes by themselves. Iatrogenic sewage discharge and treatment shall comply with the relevant national requirements.

Ⅴ. Sanitation and Hygiene of Five Places of Special Attention

21. Administrations shall implement "Regulations on the Administration of Sanitation at Public Places" and conduct quantification and grading work in surveillance of sanitation and hygiene in public places. Public places shall have complete and valid sanitation licenses, and their employees shall have valid health certificates.

22. Small restaurants, small grocery stores, small public bathrooms, small beauty salons, small dance halls, and small hotels shall have legal business qualifications. Their indoor and outdoor environment shall be clean, hardware facilities shall meet relevant national standards, and their employees shall have health certificates.

23. Administrations shall implement "School Sanitation and Hygiene Regulations". The classrooms, dining-rooms (including drinking water facilities), dormitories, and washrooms of schools, nurseries and kindergartens shall meet the national sanitation and hygiene standards or regulations. Educational institutions shall have their own campus hospitals or clinics, equip them with full-time doctors or part-time health-care personnel, and strengthen prevention against infectious diseases and common diseases. Schools shall organize activities on healthy school building, and provide health education to 100% of all students.

24. Administrations shall implement "Occupational Disease Prevention Law of People's Republic of China". At workplaces, elements of occupational hazards shall satisfy the national occupational health standards. According to "Occupational Health Surveillance Technique Specifications", workers exposed to occupational hazards shall have occupational health examination and vocational health education. Workplaces shall not have major accidents of occupational hazards in three years.

Ⅵ. Safety of Food and Drinking Water

25. Administrations shall implement "Food Safety Law of the People's Republic of China", establish and improve their food safety supervision mechanism, and ensure that no major food safety accidents would happen in 3 years.

26. Food production mills and business shall ensure their outdoor and indoor surroundings clean, avoid cross contamination, and guarantee that their food storage, processing, and sales meet the hygiene requirements. The food vendors who have no fixed place for business shall be managed by unified administration. They can only sell in designated areas and the items they sell shall be restricted.

27. The supervision and quantified classification management rate of food safety in the catering industry and collective canteens shall be greater than 90%. The employees in the catering service shall have valid health certificates. All catering business shall follow systematic procedures of cleaning and disinfection, and guarantee that their protective facilities against flies and rodents in good condition.

28. Livestock slaughters shall meet the requirements of sanitation and of animal epidemic prevention. The quarantine procedures shall be strictly implemented.

29. In accordance with the "Administrative Regulations for Supervision of Drinking Water", municipal water supply, self-prepared water supply, and residential drinking water supply shall have standardized management; these units shall have administrative permits. Secondary water supply shall meet the requirements of the national "Sanitation Standards of the Secondary Water Supply Facilities". All parties involve shall conduct water quality monitoring and insure that the water from the water plants, from network pipes, drinking water from the residential area satisfy the standards of water quality testing indicators.

Ⅶ. Public Health and Medical Services

30. Administrations shall implement the "Law of the People's Republic of China on the Prevention and Treatment of Infectious Diseases," and ensure that in 3 years no major laboratory bio-accidents or outbreaks of Type A and B infectious diseases would occur. They shall complete on time the prevention and control plan for serious diseases such as AIDS, tuberculosis, and Schistosomiasis.

31. The rate of EPI vaccination to school-age children designated to community or township shall reach 90%. Vaccine storage, vaccine transportation, and units that are designated to give vaccine shall satisfy the national requirements. The administration shall establish administrative methods for migrant immunization program management, create immunization cards for children at the age of more than 3 months, and ensure 95% of the

children have the cards.

32. The administration shall establish demonstration zones of comprehensive prevention and control of chronic diseases; start actions for national healthy lifestyle; construct health trails, healthy canteens (restaurants), health theme parks; and promote alt reduction, oil control and other chronic diseases prevention and control measures.

33. The administrations shall implement "Mental Health Law of People's Republic of China", improve working mechanism, and improve the management of severe mental disorder treatment networks, so as to ensure the management rate of patients with severe mental disorders to reach 75%.

34. The institutions of disease prevention and control shall have good institutional mechanism; their personnel and funding shall meet operational needs; the infrastructure of disease prevention and control centers shall achieve "Standards for the Construction of Disease Control and Prevention Center"; the equipment rate of examination equipments in their laboratory shall reach at least 90%.

35. Voluntary blood donation shall meet the needs of clinical use; clinical blood use shall be 100% from voluntary blood donation. The established areas shall not have illegal clinical practice, illegal blood collection and illegal medical advertisement.

36. One community health care service center shall be established in every community or district that has a population of 30-100 thousand people. Each township shall have a township clinic funded by the government. The construction of standardized primary health care institutions shall 95% meet with the required standards.

37. The infant mortality rate in each district must be≤12‰; the mortality rate of children under five years of age must be≤14‰, and the maternal mortality rate must be ≤22 / 10 million.

Ⅷ. Prevention and Control of Vectors

38. The administration shall implement the "Regulations on Administration of Vector Prevention and Control," establish prevention and control mechanisms that involve participation of all society. Government departments, enterprises, institutions and communities shall have vector prevention and control activities on a regular basis, and organize timely collective actions against vector species that seriously threaten public outdoor environment. In the established areas, the density of rats, mosquitoes, flies, and cockroaches shall satisfy Standard Grade C prescribed by the requirement of the national vector density control.

39. The administration shall know well the local situation of vector reproduction sites

and develop classified measures of control, to ensure the possible sites of vector reproduction such as lakes, rivers, ponds, garbage stations, and toilets be effectively treated.

40. The administration shall have monitoring investigation on vectors, collect information on vectors infraction and timely solve the problem. The anti-mosquito and rodent facilities in the key industries and units shall reach a qualification rate of ≥95%.

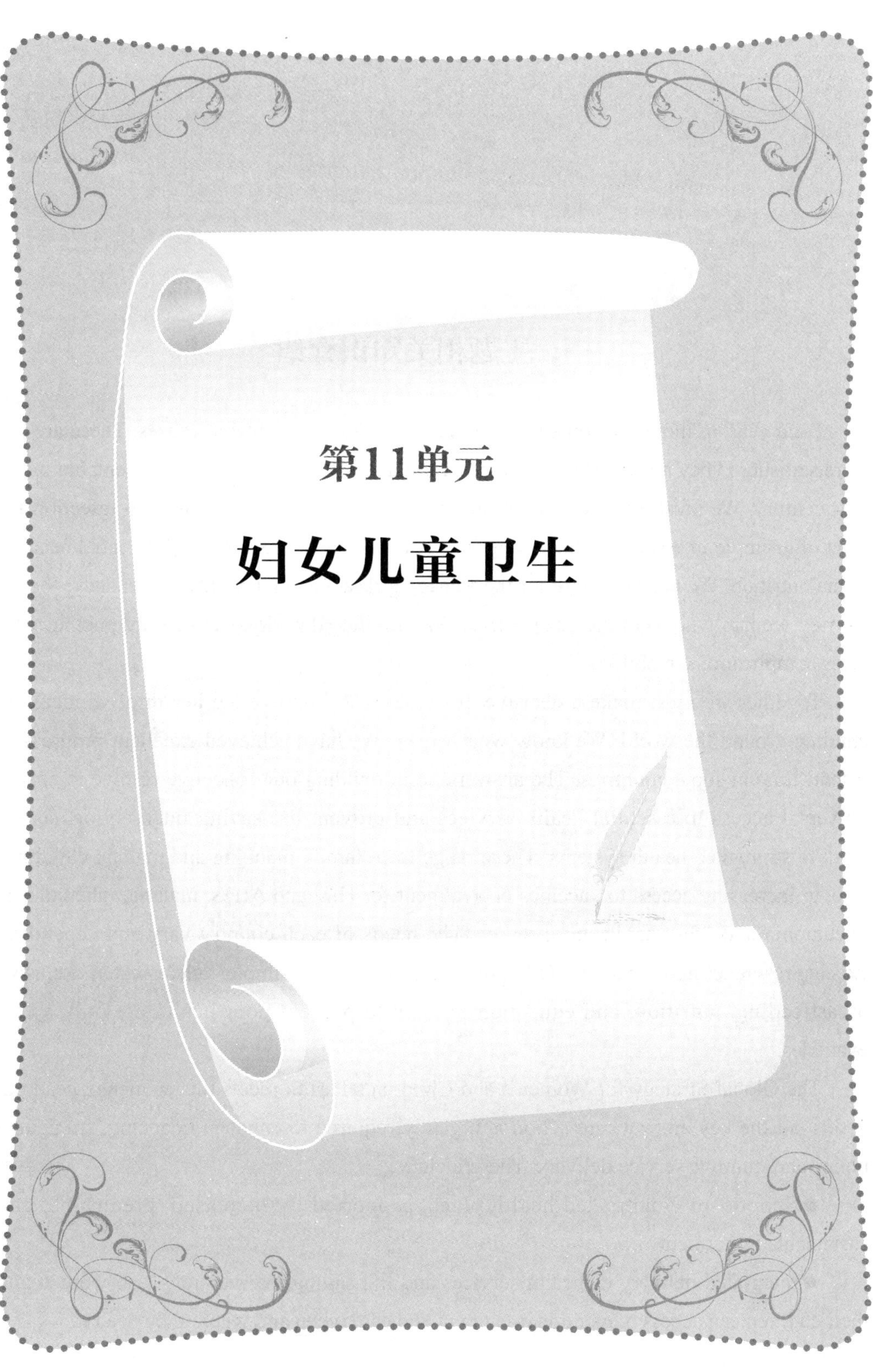

第11单元

妇女儿童卫生

一、主题相关知识介绍

Each year, millions of women and children die from preventable causes. These are not mere statistics. They are people with names and faces. Their suffering is unacceptable in the 21st century. We must, therefore, do more for the newborn who succumbs to infection for want of a simple injection; for the young boy who will never reach his full potential because of malnutrition. We must do more for the teenage girl facing an unwanted pregnancy; for the married woman who has found she is infected with the HIV virus; and for the mother who faces complications in childbirth.

Together we must make a decisive move, now, to improve the health of women and children around the world. We know what works. We have achieved excellent progress in a short time in some countries. The answers lie in building our collective resolve to ensure universal access to essential health services and proven, life-saving interventions as we work to strengthen health systems. These range from family planning and making childbirth safe, to increasing access to vaccines or treatment for HIV and AIDS, malaria, tuberculosis, pneumonia and other neglected diseases. The needs of each country vary and depend on existing resources and capacities. Often the solutions are very simple—clean water, exclusive breastfeeding, nutrition, and education on how to prevent poor health are only a few examples.

The Global Strategy for Women's and Children's Health meets this challenge head on. It sets out the key areas where action is urgently required to enhance financing, strengthen policy and improve service delivery. These include:

● Support to country-led health plans, supported by increased, predictable and sustainable investment.

● Integrated delivery of health services and life-saving interventions—so women and their children can access prevention, treatment and care when and where they need it.

- Stronger health systems, with sufficient skilled health workers at their core.
- Innovative approaches to financing, product development and the efficient delivery of health services.
- Improved monitoring and evaluation to ensure the accountability of all actors for results.

We thank the many governments, international and non-governmental organizations, companies, foundations, constituency groups and advocates who have contributed to the development of this Global Strategy. This is a first step. It is in all our hands to make a concrete difference as a result of this plan. I call on everyone to play their part. Success will come when we focus our attention and resources on people, not their illnesses; on health, not disease. With the right policies, adequate and fairly distributed funding, and a relentless resolve to deliver to those who need it most—we can and will make a life-changing difference for current and future generations.

二、技巧指导：目的语信息重组的几个方法（Ⅳ）及译前准备

（一）目的语信息重组的几个方法（**IV**）

包孕法（**Reversion**）

包孕法多用于英译汉，指在把英语长句译成汉语时，将英语后置修饰成分按照汉语的正常语序放在中心词之前，使修饰成分在汉语句中形成前置包孕。但汉语中修饰成分不宜过长，因为在汉语中，过长的前置修饰语会造成汉语句子成分混乱不清。

英译中例句：

1. There are also standards for human rights, bringing the pressure of world opinion on states that violate generally accepted standards of behavior.

人权方面也有标准。这些标准给违背公认行为标准的国家带来世界舆论的压力。

2. With the efforts of national and international experts, as well as all level project staff, the draft schemes for medical financial assistance in the four project districts have been completed. In the annual review of the project, the DFID team provided some comments and

suggestions regarding the revision of the proposals.

在国内和国际专家以及各级项目工作人员的努力下，四个项目区的医疗救助草案已经完成。在该项目的年度审查中，英国国际发展部就有关方案的修订提供了一些意见和建议。

插入法（Embedment）

插入法本是笔译中常用到的一种方法，指在译入语中使用破折号、括号、前后逗号，也就是用同位语、插入语、定语从句等，把难以处理的句子成分用插入语的方式来处理。口译中借用了其运用同位语、插入语、定语从句这些方式处理复杂的情况。

中译英例句：

1. 过去的三年，是新中国成立以来卫生事业发展史上极为不平凡的三年。三年来，深化医改这一事关13亿人民健康福祉的重大民生工程取得了明显成效。

The past three years are three extraordinary years in the history of public health development since the founding of People's Republic of China. In these three years, the in-depth medicare reform, a major livelihood project that is critical to the health and wellbeing of the 1.3 billion people, has obtained remarkable achievements.（将原文中带长定语的同位语用同位插入语方式译出）

2. 在定性资料的获取方面，课题组在2002年11月至12月期间，选取北京（代表大城市）、深圳（代表沿海经济发达的开放地区）、绍兴（代表南方小城市）、咸阳（代表西北地区中等城市）作为代表城市。

In finding the qualitative data, the research group selected, during the time of November and December of 2002, Beijing, (representing big cities), Shenzhen (representing the open, developed coastal regions), Shaoxing (representing small cities in southern China), and Xianyang (representing the medium-ranged cities in the northwestern China) as representative cities.

解释法（Explanation）

在翻译与文化现象有关的句子时常用解释法。在翻译成语、典故、俚语、俗语等特殊文化词语，或在民族文化积淀中形成的专有名词、专用词组、缩略语和固定搭配的时候，经常会有对等、对应译法都无法解决的情况，在这种时候，就要用到解释法。

英译中例句：

1. A chain is no stronger than its weakest link.

链条的坚固程度取决于它最薄弱的环节。

2. All work and no play makes Jack a dull boy; all play and no work makes Jack a mere boy.

只工作，不玩耍，聪明孩子要变傻；尽玩耍，不学习，聪明孩子没出息。

3. Better wear out shoes than sheets.

宁可运动磨破鞋子，不愿生病磨破床单。

4. The Christmas season fills our hearts with gratitude for the many blessings in our lives. And with those blessings comes a responsibility to reach out to others.

圣诞节期间，回顾生活中得到的诸多福佑，我们的心中充满了感激。而上帝给我们福佑的同时，也给了我们责任：我们要向他人伸出援手。

（这句话用顺译法译出效果会非常笨拙且不清楚："圣诞节向我们心中注满我们对生活中诸多福佑的感激。与那些福佑一同到来的是一种接触到他人的责任。"）

中译英例句：

她有沉鱼落雁之容，闭月羞花之貌。

She is so beautiful that the fish is amazed to fail swimming, the swallow falls from shocking, the moon hides behind the cloud for comparison and the flower is shy for competition.

（二）译前准备

译前准备有两个组成部分：1. 长期译前准备；2. 临时译前准备。长期译前准备即平时的日常训练、自我训练，以及专业知识与文化知识储备、词汇量储备等。临时译前准备指接到具体翻译任务之后所做的案头工作。

翻译的质量与翻译之前的准备工作是成正比的，这是因为已有储备的专业知识和特定场合下的背景知识可以影响译员对信息的注意、理解、记忆和转换速度。熟悉的信息容易抓住译员的注意力，而不熟悉的信息即使听见了，译员也会因不熟悉而想记也记不住。大家可以试一试：找一份与自己专业无关的、完全陌生的、晦涩难懂的中文材料，一人念出，其他人用中文复述，你会发现复述的结果不理想。因为其中很多信息你不懂，所以没听明白而记不住。不准备就上翻译场，无疑是打无准备之仗，胜算的概率很小。所以必须要提早准备。

职场上技能再好的译员碰到不熟悉的内容之时，也会要求至少半个月的准备时间。因此在接到口译任务后，首要任务就是了解此次会议或谈话的上下文。泛泛来讲，就是以前曾讨论过的内容、关键词、人物关系、时间与地点等。以城市贫困人口社区卫生服务项目培训为例，这是一个30人左右的小会议，时间4天整。以前曾有过概念会议，这次是操作培训。因此译员首先要上网查询这个领域概念是什么，发展的来龙去脉是怎样的，以前此项目在何时何地都做了哪些工作、开过哪些会议，在会议上讨论过什么议题、结果如何。其次要找主办方尽可能地了解情况。通常这些项目都会有一些以往的资料，会有本次会议的日程安排，主办方或承办方介绍，参会人员名单、头衔、背景介绍或科研成果介绍，演讲人名单和发言标题等；有时还会有演讲人的发言稿、发言提纲、讲义或PPT文档。如果译者拿得到这些东西，首先应该尽可能地了解，尽可能地记下并熟悉上下文、中英文关键词与术语；拿不到太多材料的时候，就只能依靠前期在网上用关键词的方式搜索来的相关知识和术语。

再以一个研二的口译工作坊为例。这次的任务是音乐学院萨克斯管系的大师班大型现场授课外加小型音乐会。因为是外籍教师授课，又涉及现场展示、指导演奏方式，所以能索要到的书面材料只是三位授课者的背景材料和几个曲目信息。受训学生完全没有背景知识。因此任务提前一个月告知学生，他们在互联网上阅读了有关萨克斯管乐器的知识、乐曲的信息，团队尽可能全面地收集了一般乐理知识、五线谱知识、萨克斯管乐器构造的术语，吹奏方法的术语、曲目信息、乐曲表达的内容等，并以互助抽背的方式背熟了上述材料。索要到的中文、英文材料都翻译过了并熟记，一些学生还找了相关资料进行视译练习。能够准备的都尽可能充分地准备了。在材料准备阶段了解了讲者之后，还见过了讲者本人，有过短暂的交谈，多少熟悉了一下讲者的口音。最后在实战中的确用到了很多背记过的术语和概念，因而工作起来非常顺利。

综上所述，译前准备包括：

1. 用关键词搜索任务话题的各种信息并熟记；
2. 准备双语专业术语；
3. 索要各种会议资料并熟悉其内容，此时除了专业术语以外还要注意缩写词、人员名字以及与之相关的职务名称；
4. 做与该话题相关的双语视译练习；
5. 了解发言者的口音和说话风格，了解听众的构成。

三、词汇准备

Text 1

preventable deaths 可阻止死亡

MDG Millennium Development Goals 千年发展目标

maternal health 孕产妇保健

Global Strategy 全球性战略

take coordinated action 采取协调一致的行动

high priority 高度优先，优先考虑

affordable and accessible 可负担与无障碍

indigenous populations 原住民

commitment 承诺，许诺，承担义务

the ECOSOC Ministerial Review on Global Health 联合国经济及社会理事会对全球卫生的部长级审查

UNGA Special Session 联大特别会议

the Maputo Plan of Action 马普托行动计划

CARMMA the Campaign on Accelerated Reduction of Maternal Mortality in Africa 非洲孕产妇死亡率加速降低运动

the African Union Summit Declaration 2010 for Actions on Maternal, Newborn and Child Health 2010非洲联盟首脑会议孕产妇、新生儿和儿童健康行动宣言

Text 2

stable, peaceful and productive societies 稳定、和平、有生产力的社会

parasitic diseases 寄生虫病

mortality and fertility rates 死亡率和生育率

cost-effective 有成本效益的

functioning health systems 运转良好的卫生系统

immunizations 免疫接种

integrated management of childhood illness 儿童疾病综合管理

The Paris Declaration 《巴黎宣言》

The Accra Agenda for Action 《阿克拉行动议程》

The Monterrey Consensus 《蒙特利尔共识》

newborn and postnatal care 分娩和产后护理

emergency obstetric 产科急诊
oral rehydration therapy 口服补液疗法
zinc supplements 锌补充剂
ready-to-eat food 即食食品
malaria 疟疾
disease-specific program 特定疾病规划
The Expanded Programme on Immunization 扩大免疫规划
women's empowerment 妇女赋能

Text 3

UNAIDS 联合国艾滋病规划署
prevalence 感染率
antiretroviral drug 抗反转录病毒药
case detection 病例发现率
the Secretary-General's Special Envoy to Stop TB 联合国秘书长控制结核特使
global immunization strategy 全球疫苗接种战略
the Integrated Management of Childhood Illness 儿童期疾病综合管理战略
formula of oral rehydration salts 口服补液盐配方

Text 4

create synergies 创造凝聚力
economic returns 经济效益
disease eradication and elimination 消灭和根除疾病
measles 麻疹
rubella 风疹
neonatal tetanus 新生儿破伤风
high and equitable coverage 高覆盖和公平覆盖
available vaccines 可用疫苗
immunization services 免疫接种服务
allocating adequate human and financial resources 分配足够的人力和财政资源
foster alignment 加强协调
mobilize more financial resources 动员更多财务资源
substantive agenda item 实质性议程项目
accountability framework 问责框架

Text 5

妇幼健康优质服务示范工程 Demonstration Project of Excellent Maternal and Child Health Services

孕产妇死亡率 pregnant mortality

缺陷防治 defect prevention

突出 highlight

资源优化整合 optimal integration

规范 standardize

专科 specialties

管理制度 administrative system, management system

产科学 obstetrics

产房 delivery ward

新生儿科学 neonatology

新生儿 newborn infants

漏洞 loopholes

急救转诊网络 emergency referral network

剖宫产 caesarean

母乳喂养 breastfeeding

乙肝母婴传播 mother to child transmission of Hepatitis B

宫颈癌 cervical cancer

叶酸预防神经管缺陷 supplement of folic acid to prevent neural tube defects

孕前优生健康检查 pre-pregnancy eugenic health checks

投诉举报 complaint and report

Text 6

缠足 foot-binding

卫生部 The Ministry of Health

人力资源和社会保障部 The Ministry of Labor and Social Security

妇幼保健司 The Department of Community Health and Maternal & Child Health Care

就业促进司 The Department of Labor and Wages

全国总工会女职工委员会 The Women Worker's Committee of the All-China Federation of Trade Unions

中国女企业家协会 The China Women Entrepreneurs Association

全国女律师协会 China Women Judges Association

女医师协会 Society of Chinese Women Doctors
妇女能顶半边天 women can hold up half the sky

四、摘要练习

请听下面英语语篇，第一篇用源语言复述此段主要信息逻辑点及层次，第二篇用译入语复述此段主要信息逻辑点及层次。注意信息点之间的逻辑联系。

Text 1

Global Strategy for Women's and Children's Health (Excerpt 1)

Foreword by the United Nations Secretary-General Ban Ki-moon

With just five years left to achieve the Millennium Development Goals (MDGs), global leaders must intensify their efforts to improve women's and children's health. The world has failed to invest enough in the health of women, adolescent girls, newborns, infants, and children. As a result, millions of preventable deaths occur each year.

We have made less progress on MDG 5, improving maternal health, than any other. Yet we now have an opportunity to achieve real, lasting progress—because global leaders increasingly recognize that the health of women and children is the key to progress on all development goals.

This Global Strategy requires that all partners unite and take coordinated action. Everyone has an important role to play: governments, civil society, community organizations, global and regional institutions, donors, philanthropic foundations, the United Nations and other multilateral organizations, development banks, the private sector, the health workforce, professional associations, academics and researchers.

Real progress is entirely possible. In fact, it has already been made in some of the world's poorest countries, where a high priority has been accorded to women and children within national health agendas.

Meanwhile, innovations in technology, treatment and service delivery are making it easier to provide better and more effective care, and both new and existing financing mechanisms are making care more affordable and accessible. By investing even more in these efforts, we will see major improvements. Already, 10,000 fewer children are dying each day than in 1990.

Now is the time for all partners to join forces in a concerted effort. This means scaling up and prioritizing a package of high-impact interventions, strengthening health systems, and integrating efforts across diseases and sectors such as health, education, water, sanitation and nutrition. It also means promoting human rights, gender equality and poverty reduction.

All actors should work to optimize current investments. All are accountable for their commitments and need to raise the additional, predictable funding required to deliver basic health services and meet the health-related MDGs.

This strategy focuses on the time when women and children are most vulnerable. For pregnant women and newborns alike, the greatest risk of death comes during childbirth and in the first few hours and days afterwards. Adolescents are also vulnerable, and we must make sure they're given control over their life choices, including their fertility. This requires a focus on the most vulnerable and hardest-to-reach women and children: the poorest, those living with HIV/AIDS, orphans, indigenous populations, and those living furthest from health services.

It needs building on our health and human rights commitments. The Global Strategy builds on commitments made by countries and partners at several events: the Programme of Action agreed to at the International Conference on Population and Development; the Beijing Declaration and Platform for Action agreed at the Fourth World Conference on Women, the ECOSOC Ministerial Review on Global Health; the UNGA Special Session, "Healthy Women, Healthy Children: Investing in Our Common Future"; and the 54th session of the Commission on the Status of Women. It also builds on regional commitments and efforts, such as the Maputo Plan of Action, the Campaign on Accelerated Reduction of Maternal Mortality in Africa (CARMMA), and the African Union Summit Declaration 2010 for Actions on Maternal, Newborn and Child Health.

复述要点提示（主要信息逻辑点及层次）

With just five years left to achieve the MDGs, global leaders must renew their commitment and invest enough in the health of women, adolescent girls, newborns, infants, and children, because millions of preventable deaths still occur each year.

This means that progress on MDG 5, that is improving maternal health, is not enough. Since the global leaders have now recognized more that the health of women and children is the key to progress on all development goals, there will be solution.

This Global Strategy requires that all partners take coordinated action. The governments, civil society, community organizations, global and regional institutions, donors, philanthropic foundations, the United Nations and other multilateral organizations, development banks, the private sector, the health workforce, professional associations, academics and researchers will work together.

Approaches for progress:

● Give a high priority to women and children within national health agendas.

● Make innovations in technology, treatment and service delivery for more effective care, as well, combine both new and existing financing mechanisms to make care more affordable and accessible.

● Prioritize a package of high-impact interventions, strengthen health systems, and integrate efforts across diseases and sectors such as health, education, water, sanitation and nutrition.

● Promote human rights, gender equality and poverty reduction.

● Raise the additional, predictable funding required to deliver basic health services and meet the health-related MDGs.

● Focuses on the time when women and children are most vulnerable. Focus on the most vulnerable and hardest-to-reach women and children: the poorest, those living with HIV/AIDS, orphans, indigenous populations, and those living furthest from health services.

● Build our health and human rights commitments. The Global Strategy builds on commitments in events: such as the Programme of Action, the Beijing Declaration and Platform for Action, the ECOSOC Ministerial Review on Global Health, and so on.

Text 2

Global Strategy for Women's and Children's Health (Excerpt 2)

Foreword by the United Nations Secretary-General Ban Ki-moon

Investing in the health of women and children makes good sense

Women and children play a crucial role in development. Investing more in women's and children's health is not only the right thing to do, it also builds stable, peaceful and productive societies. Increasing investment has many benefits.

It reduces poverty. Charging women and children less, or nothing, for health services improves access to care and enables poorer families to spend more money on food, housing, education and activities that generate income. Healthy women work more productively, and stand to earn more throughout their lives. Addressing under nutrition in pregnant women and children leads to an increase of up to 10% in an individual's lifetime earnings. In contrast, poor sanitation leads to diarrhea and parasitic diseases, which reduce productivity and prevent children from going to school.

It stimulates economic productivity and growth. Maternal and newborn deaths slow growth and leads to global productivity losses of US$15 billion each year. By failing to address under-nutrition, a country may have a 2% lower GDP than it otherwise would. In contrast, investing in children's health leads to high economic returns and offers the best guarantee of a productive workforce in the future. For example, between 30% and 50% of Asia's economic growth from 1965 to 1990 has been attributed to improvements in reproductive health and reductions in infant and child mortality and fertility rates.

It is cost-effective. Essential health care prevents illness and disability, saving billions of dollars in treatment. In many countries, every dollar spent on family planning saves at least four dollars that would otherwise be spent treating complications arising from unplanned pregnancies. For less than US$5 (and sometimes as little as US$1) childhood immunization can give a child a year of life free from disability and suffering.

It helps women and children realize their fundamental human rights. People are entitled to the highest attainable standard of health.This fundamental principle of development and human rights is affirmed by many countries in a range of international and regional human-rights treaties.

Working together to accelerate progress is key elements of the Global Strategy

We know what works. Women and children need an integrated package of essential interventions and services delivered by functioning health systems. Already, many countries are making progress. In Tanzania, for instance, deaths of children under five have fallen by 15%-20% because of widespread use of interventions such as immunizations, vitamin A supplements and integrated management of childhood illness. Sri Lanka has reduced maternal mortality by 87% in the past 40 years by ensuring that 99% of pregnant women receive four antenatal visits and give birth in a health facility.

We know what we need to do. In line with the principles of the Paris Declaration, the Accra Agenda for Action and the Monterrey Consensus, all partners must work closely together in the following areas:

Country-led health plans. Partners must support existing, costed national health plans to improve access to services. Such plans cover human resources, financing, and delivery and monitoring of an integrated package of interventions.

A comprehensive, integrated package of essential interventions and services. Partners must ensure that women and children have access to a universal package of guaranteed benefits, including family-planning information and services, antenatal, newborn and postnatal care, emergency obstetric and newborn care, skilled care during childbirth at appropriate facilities, safe abortion services (when abortion is not prohibited by law), and the prevention of HIV and other sexually transmitted infections. Interventions should also include: exclusive breastfeeding for infants up to six months; vaccines and immunization; oral rehydration therapy and zinc supplements to manage diarrhea; treatment for the major childhood illnesses; nutritional supplements (such as vitamin A); and access to appropriate ready-to-eat foods to prevent and treat malnutrition.

Integrated care improves health promotion and helps prevent and treat diseases such as pneumonia, diarrhea, HIV/AIDS, malaria, tuberculosis, and non-communicable diseases.

Stronger links must be built between diseases-specific programs (such for HIV/AIDS, malaria and tuberculosis) and services targeting women and children (such as the Expanded Programme on Immunization, sexual and reproductive health and the integrated management of childhood illness). Partners should coordinate efforts with those working in other sectors to address issues that impact on health, such as sanitation, safe drinking water, malnutrition, gender equality and women's empowerment.

Health systems strengthening. Partners must support efforts to strengthen health systems to deliver integrated, high-quality services. They should extend the reach of existing services,especially at the community level and to the underserved, and manage scarce resources more effectively. They also need to build more health facilities to give vulnerable people access to medical expertise and drugs.

Health workforce capacity building. Partners must work together to address critical shortages of health workers at all levels. They must provide coordinated and coherent support to help countries develop and implement national health plans that include strategies to train, retain and deploy health workers.

Coordinated research and innovation. Partners must find innovative ways to provide high quality care and to expand research programs that develop new interventions, such as vaccines, medicines and diagnostic devices. They must develop, fund and implement a prioritized and coordinated global research agenda for women's and children's health, and strengthen research institutions and systems in low- and middle-income countries.

复述要点提示（主要信息逻辑点及层次）

因为妇女儿童在发展中的关键作用，加大对妇女儿童健康的投资力度，有助于创造稳定、和谐和富有生产力的社会环境。

●促进减贫。减少或完全取消对妇女和儿童的卫生保健收费，增加贫困家庭获得医疗救助的机会，使他们能够把更多的钱用在食品、住房、教育和创收活动上。

●促进生产力和经济增长。孕产妇和新生儿死亡减慢经济发展速度，每年导致全球生产力损失高达150亿美元。处理不好营养不良问题导致国家国内生产总值下降，比预期减少2%。

●具有成本效益。基本卫生保健对于疾病和残疾的预防起到积极的作用，从而可节省数十亿美元的治疗费用。

●帮助妇女和儿童认识到应享有的基本人权。人人有权享有达到最高标准的健康状态。这一发展和人权的基本原则在一系列国际和区域人权条约中得到许多国家的认可。

齐心协力地加快进展是全球战略的关键。运转良好的卫生系统提供综合性一揽子基本干预措施和服务是能够奏效的措施。《巴黎宣言》、《阿克拉行动议程》和《蒙特利尔共识》原则要求所有合作伙伴在以下领域紧密合作：

国家主导的卫生计划。计划涵盖人力资源、融资以及提供和监督实施综合性一揽子干预措施。

全面、综合的一揽子基本干预措施和服务，包括计划生育宣传和服务，产前、分娩和产后护理，产科急诊和新生儿护理，分娩期间提供熟练照护，安全堕胎服务，以及艾滋病毒和其他性传播感染的预防。干预措施包括：六个月以下婴儿纯母乳喂养、疫苗和免疫接种、采用口服补液疗法和锌补充剂管理腹泻疾病、主要儿童疾病的治疗、营养补充等。

综合保健。有助于肺炎、腹泻、艾滋病、疟疾、结核和非传染病等疾病的预防和治疗。加强特定疾病规划。

加强与其他部门协调，解决如环境卫生、安全饮用水、营养不良、两性平等和赋予妇女权力等对健康有影响的问题。

加强卫生系统。扩大现有服务的可及范围，尤其是社区一级和服务不到位的地区，更有效地管理稀缺匮乏资源。让弱势群体获得好的卫生设施，专业医学服务和药物。

卫生人员的能力建设。协助协调各国制定和实施国家卫生计划，找到培养、留住和使用卫生工作者的方针策略。

协调研究和创新。

五、英译汉练习

Text 3

Address by Dr. Margaret Chan, Director-General to the 61st World Health Assembly

Mr. President, honourable ministers, excellencies, distinguished delegates, ladies and gentlemen,

You have before you a report on the monitoring of achievements. As you all know, I have made the health of the African people and of women my two overriding priorities when measuring the effectiveness of our work. And rightly so. Progress is least in Africa. Progress for women is hardest.

Let me comment on overall progress. At the end of last year, better data and statistical methods allowed WHO and UNAIDS to chart the evolution of the HIV/AIDS epidemic with greater precision.HIV incidence peaked in the late 1990s. Prevalence has been level since 2001. In a significant trend, deaths from AIDS have declined during the past two years.

Evidence now allows us to conclude, with confidence, that this decline in mortality is linked to dramatic recent increases in access to antiretroviral drugs. The access of women to treatment is at least as good as that for men. Globally, close to three quarters of people receiving antiretroviral drugs are in Africa, where the epidemic is disproportionately severe.

This demonstrates that something as complex as antiretroviral therapy can indeed be introduced in resource-constrained settings. But we are still running behind this devastating, unforgiving epidemic. The numbers remain staggering: an estimated 33.2 million people living with HIV and 2.5 million newly infected in 2007 alone. Clearly, we must seize every opportunity for prevention. This is the only way to catch up and eventually get ahead.

Tuberculosis has a good diagnostic and treatment strategy, and we have solid evidence that the approach works. Progress remains steady, though the rate of case detection has slowed compared with recent years.

Poor medical practices, which contribute to the development of drug resistance, are a major concern. Earlier this year, WHO issued a report showing that multi-drug resistant TB has reached the highest levels ever recorded.

Even more worrisome is the continuing occurrence of extensively drug-resistant TB, which is virtually impossible to treat. To allow this form of TB to become widespread would be a setback of epic proportions. For these patients, our treatment options effectively go back to the era that predates the advent of antibiotics.

Next month, I will be joining the UN Secretary-General at the first-ever global leadership forum on scaling up the response to the co-epidemics of HIV and TB. This is yet another example of the growing engagement of world leaders in health issues.

The forum takes place at a time when several high-burden countries are showing very promising increases in the numbers of people accessing integrated HIV/TB services. Leadership, also from the Secretary-General's Special Envoy to Stop TB, former president Mr. Jorge Sampaio of Portugal, can take this momentum a step further.

For malaria, we are finally seeing solid progress. Rapid declines in mortality in parts of Africa show the power of recommended strategies to deliver dramatic results. This year we commemorated the first-ever world malaria day, a sign of global commitment to tackle this disease.

On that occasion, the Secretary-General and his Special Envoy, Mr. Ray Chambers, challenged the international community to embark on an ambitious plan to reduce malaria deaths by the end of 2010. If we can do this, we will boost the prospects for better health in Africa in a tremendous way.

Last year, global mortality of young children dipped below 10 million for the first time in recent years. You will be considering a report on the global immunization strategy, one of the best success stories in public health. I want to thank all partners concerned, also in the Measles Initiative, and extend my very special appreciation to UNICEF and the GAVI Alliance.

Also, we are clearly seeing the broad-based impact of the Integrated Management of Childhood Illness, which has now been adopted as the principal child survival strategy in 100 countries. Of these, 49 have extended coverage to more than half of the country's districts. In just two years, the number of countries reaching this level of coverage has doubled. I congratulate these countries on their great efforts.

Research has given us an additional boost towards achievement of the goal for reducing childhood mortality. The use of zinc to treat diarrhoea, along with a new formula of oral rehydration salts, will help save the lives of millions of children. Earlier this year, research coordinated by WHO demonstrated that home-based treatment of pneumonia—the number one killer of young children—is just as effective as hospital care, and possibly even safer. Given my commitment to primary health care, evidence that supports community and home-based care pleases me most especially.

Yet, as is so often the case in public health, when one thick layer of morbidity and mortality begins to thin, it reveals more starkly another critical problem. This is the case with newborn mortality, another big problem we need to address. Once again, research has demonstrated that something as simple as skin-to-skin contact with mothers—so-called "kangaroo" mother care—can save the lives of pre-term babies.

We also need to save the lives of mothers. As the report before you notes, progress in improving women's health is disappointingly slow. This is especially true for maternal health, where mortality has remained stubbornly high despite more than 20 years of efforts.

I personally find this lack of progress outrageous. Does the value society places on women so small that their lives are simply dismissed as expendable? If the answer is no, then we absolutely must double our efforts to make sure that the health of women is protected.

I know that social and cultural changes take time. But I have also seen some studies of microfinancing schemes for women that have produced rapid improvements in their social status, in their control over household decisions, and in their spending on family health. In some studies, an unexpected bonus has been a decline in domestic violence.

I firmly believe we need to explore every option that can potentially raise the status of women, protect their health, and free them to realize their human potential and their great capacity as agents of change.

Text 4

65th World Health Assembly WHA65.17

Agenda item 13.12

26 May 2012

Global Vaccine Action Plan

The Sixty-fifth World Health Assembly,

Having considered the report on the draft global vaccine action plan;

Recognizing the importance of immunization as one of the most cost-effective interventions in public health, which should be recognized as a core component of the human right to health;

Acknowledging the remarkable progress made in immunization in several countries to ensure that every eligible individual is immunized with all appropriate vaccines, irrespective of geographical location, age, gender, disability, educational level, socioeconomic level, ethnic group or work condition;

Applauding the contribution of successful immunization programmes in achieving global health goals, in particular in reducing childhood mortality and morbidity, and their potential for reducing mortality and morbidity across the life-course;

Noting that the introduction of new vaccines targeted against several important causes of major killer diseases such as pneumonia, diarrhoea and cervical cancer can be used as a catalyst to scale up complementary interventions and create synergies between primary health care programmes; and that beyond the mortality gains, these new vaccines will prevent morbidity with resulting economic returns even in countries that have already succeeded in reducing mortality;

Concerned that, despite the progress already made, disease eradication and elimination goals such as the eradication of poliomyelitis, the elimination of measles, rubella, and maternal and neonatal tetanus cannot be met without achieving and sustaining high and equitable coverage;

Concerned that low-income and middle-income countries where the adoption of available vaccines has been slower may not have the opportunity to access newer and improved vaccines expected to become available during this decade;

Alarmed that globally routine immunization services are not reaching one child in five, and that substantial gaps persist in routine immunization coverage within countries;

Recalling resolutions WHA58.15 and WHA61.15 on the global immunization strategy,

1. ENDORSES the Global Vaccine Action Plan;

2. URGES Members States:

(1) to apply the vision and the strategies of the Global Vaccine Action Plan in order to develop the vaccines and immunization components of their national health strategy and plans, paying particular attention to improving performance of the Expanded Programme on Immunization, and according to the epidemiological situation in their respective countries;

(2) to commit themselves to allocating adequate human and financial resources to achieve the immunization goals and other relevant key milestones;

(3) to report every year to the regional committees during a dedicated Decade of Vaccines session, on lessons learnt, progress made, remaining challenges and updated actions to reach the national immunization targets;

3. REQUESTS the Director-General:

(1) to foster alignment and coordination of global immunization efforts by all

stakeholders in support of the implementation of the Global Vaccine Action Plan;

(2) to ensure that the support provided to the Global Vaccine Action Plan's implementation at regional and country level includes a strong focus on strengthening routine immunization;

(3) to identify human and financial resources for the provision of technical support in order to implement the national plans of the Global Vaccine Action Plan and monitor their impact;

(4) to mobilize more financial resources in order to support implementation of the Global Vaccine Action Plan in low-income and middle-income countries;

(5) to monitor progress and report annually, through the Executive Board, to the Health Assembly, until the Seventy-first World Health Assembly, on progress towards achievement of global immunization targets, as a substantive agenda item, using the proposed accountability framework to guide discussions and future actions.

Tenth plenary meeting, 26 May 2012

A65/VR/10

六、汉译英练习

Text 5

国家卫生计生委关于实施妇幼健康优质服务示范工程的通知（节选）

为提高妇幼健康服务水平，保证人民群众获得优质的妇幼健康服务，切实维护人民群众健康权益，国家卫生计生委决定，从2014年起，在全国实施妇幼健康优质服务示范工程，通过引导、示范和推广，全面提升妇幼健康服务水平。

一、指导思想和工作目标

妇幼健康优质服务示范工程要全面贯彻《中华人民共和国母婴保健法》《中华人民共和国人口与计划生育法》和《2011—2020年中国妇女儿童发展纲要》，坚持为人民健康服务方向，坚持"儿童优先、母亲安全"宗旨，坚持妇幼卫生工作方针，提高妇幼健康服务与管理水平，满足广大妇女儿童的健康需求。

妇幼健康优质服务示范工程的总体目标是：推动各级政府更加重视妇幼健康工作，全面提升妇幼健康服务质量和管理水平，切实改善妇幼健康服务的公平性与可及性，不断提高妇女儿童健康水平，保障避孕节育的有效性、安全性和及时性，打造优质服务新品牌，使人民群众更加满意，促进妇幼健康事业又好又快发展。具体包括5个方面：

——领导重视好。各级政府把妇幼健康工作纳入经济社会发展总体规划和政府目标责任考核，建立有效的协调工作机制和稳定的投入保障机制。

——规范管理好。妇幼健康服务体系健全，机构建设标准规范。管理制度、工作制度、技术规范、操作流程完善，监督管理有力，制度执行到位。

——服务质量好。妇幼健康服务机构环境温馨，医疗保健服务水平不断提高，妇幼健康服务质量明显提升。

——指标落实好。妇女儿童核心健康指标持续改善，妇幼健康服务工作指标显著提高，圆满完成各项工作任务。

——人民满意好。群众口碑好，树立妇幼健康优质服务品牌，服务对象满意度逐步提高。

二、主要内容

（一）强化落实政府职责。各级政府高度重视妇幼健康工作，将其纳入当地经济和社会发展规划，将孕产妇死亡率、婴儿死亡率、5岁以下儿童死亡率、避孕节育服务有效率、出生缺陷防治措施落实率等妇幼健康核心指标纳入政府目标责任考核，制定妇幼健康事业发展规划并组织实施，明确各相关部门职责，建立协调工作机制，实施妇幼健康目标管理。落实妇幼健康服务各项工作经费，保障各项任务顺利完成。

（二）坚持正确发展方向。坚持“以保健为中心，以保障生殖健康为目的，保健与临床相结合，面向群体、面向基层和预防为主”的妇幼卫生工作方针。为妇女儿童提供从出生到老年、内容涵盖生理和心理的主动、连续的医疗保健服务与健康管理，强化公共卫生责任，突出群体保健功能，有效落实区域妇幼健康服务指标。

（三）加强服务体系建设。地方政府举办独立的妇幼健康服务机构，推进妇幼保健与计划生育技术服务资源优化整合。全面实施机构标准化建设，保障基本业务用房，配置基本医疗设备，落实人员编制与经费，配备专业技术人员，重视人才队伍建设，特别是助产士等紧缺人才培养。机构内部科室设置规范，逐步加强妇幼健康重点专科建设。

（四）健全完善规章制度。完善妇幼健康服务相关管理制度、工作规范、技术标准、操作流程等，健全监督、评价制度。各相关医疗机构建立健全产科、产房、新生儿科和计划生育技术服务管理制度，规范工作流程。妇幼健康服务机构严格执行医疗服务的相关法律法规和管理规定，其他提供妇幼健康服务的医疗机构认真落实妇幼保健工作的相关要求，各级业务主管部门对制度落实情况进行督导检查。

（五）强化日常监督管理。认真贯彻执行《母婴保健法》和《人口与计划生育法》，把母婴保健和计划生育技术服务监督执法纳入综合监督执法，加强监督检查，严格机构、人员和技术准入，规范服务行为。建立妇幼健康服务定期巡查和不定期抽查制度，查找管理漏洞，通报突出问题，加强内部管理。推进信息化建设，提高信息化管理水平。

（六）不断提升服务水平。加强对基层妇幼健康工作的业务指导、培训与评价。加强妇幼健康人才培养，采取多种方式进行岗位培训和继续医学教育。制定辖区妇幼健康人员业务培训规划并组织实施，加强适宜技术和新技术培训及推广。开展群众满意度调查，以群众需要为目标，改善服务设施，改进服务流程，广泛开展便民惠民服务，方便群众接受妇幼健康服务，不断适应群众对妇幼健康服务的需求。

（七）切实保证服务质量。建设辖区危急重症孕产妇和新生儿救治中心，健全急救转诊网络，确保绿色通道通畅。妇幼健康服务机构建立服务质量、医疗安全评价体系，加强机构内部管理和基础质量管理，加强重点环节、重点区域、重点人员管理，改进服务质量，确保医疗安全。严格落实首诊负责、三级医师查房、疑难病例讨论、会诊、术前讨论、死亡病例讨论、交接班等核心制度，规范病历书写，促进合理检查、合理用药、合理治疗。合理控制剖宫产率，积极倡导母乳喂养。

（八）全面实现任务目标。降低孕产妇死亡率、婴儿死亡率、5岁以下儿童死亡率，提高免费计划生育技术服务率工作指标。规范实施农村孕产妇住院分娩补助，农村妇女宫颈癌乳腺癌检查，增补叶酸预防神经管缺陷，预防艾滋病、梅毒、乙肝母婴传播，“降低孕产妇死亡和消除新生儿破伤风”、贫困地区儿童营养改善和新生儿疾病筛查等妇幼重大公共卫生服务项目。推进免费孕前优生健康检查项目，落实孕产妇、儿童健康管理基本公共卫生服务项目，因地制宜开展妇幼健康民生项目，保质保量完成各项目目标。

（九）主动接受社会监督。以《医疗机构从业人员行为规范》为重点，深入开展医务人员职业道德和法制纪律教育，加强行风建设，提升医德医风水平。加强对群众的健康教育，传播健康知识，提高群众健康素养。全面推行妇幼健康服务机构院务公开制度，通过设置意见箱、开通热线电话和网上信箱等多种形式，畅通投诉举报渠道，主动接受社会各界监督，不断改进工作。

（十）树立行业良好形象。弘扬良好职业道德、服务意识和奉献精神，为妇女儿童提供人性化服务和人文关怀。树立先进典型，加大对爱岗敬业、勤奋工作、无私奉献先进典型的宣传报道力度，特别是宣传长期扎根基层、少数民族和边远地区服务群众的先进事迹，展现广大妇幼健康工作者精神面貌，塑造好形象，传递正能量。

Text 6

中国驻卡尔加里总领事刘永凤
在国际妇女论坛卡城分会主题年会上的演讲

2011年2月8日

各位尊敬的来宾：

大家晚上好。能出席今天晚上的活动，尤其是能和在座这么多优秀的女性相聚，我感到很荣幸。

特别令我高兴的是，这次年会以庆祝中国农历新年为主题。我想，友谊的最好体现莫过于相互分享彼此的重要节日。借此机会，我愿向你们介绍一下现代中国妇女事业的发展状况。

同西方社会一样，直到20世纪初，男性在中国社会中仍占据主导地位，女性几乎没有话语权，也不享受任何权益。中国妇女受压迫最明显的标志——缠足，在20世纪初仍屡见不鲜。我的奶奶便是缠足的受害者之一，忍受了常人无法想象的痛苦和屈辱。

可喜的是，100年前，辛亥革命推翻了中国的封建帝制，1949年，新中国成立后，中国政府采取了一系列措施提倡和保障男女平等，中国妇女地位得到了显著提升。

一是从法律上提供保障。中国宪法规定女性享有一切与男性同等的权利。中国政府还出台了各项法律法规，保护妇女在财产、继承、婚姻、受教育等社会生活方方面面的平等权益。

二是从组织上提供保障。中国政府设立了各种机构、组织来保障妇女权益。如卫生部、人力资源和社会保障部分别设立了妇幼保健司和就业促进司，以促进妇女健康和男女收入平等。为确保各行各业、各民族妇女的平等权益，各类非政府组织也纷纷成立。1949年成立的全国妇联将促进各少数民族妇女同胞的社会地位平等作为其工作的重要内容之一。近年来，在中国还先后组建了全国总工会女职工委员会、中国女企业家协会、全国女律师协会、女医师协会等妇女组织。目前，中国共有约27 000个妇女儿童权益保护机构，致力于保障和提高妇女的权利和地位。

实际上，几乎每一个企、事业单位和各级政府机关内部，都有妇女组织。驻卡尔加里总领馆也有一个妇女工作小组，严萍女士就是这个小组的组长，她也参加了今天的活动。

在中国政府和全国人民的共同努力下，60年来，中国妇女事业的发展取得了显著成就：

首先是妇女在中国的社会地位大幅提升。根据去年的统计，适龄女童小学入学率达99.54%；普通高校本专科在校女生比例占学生总数的49.86%，略高于女性在总人口中所占48.47%的比例；妇女人才在就业人口中所占比例达45.4%；在公务员中的比例达到40%以上。孕产妇死亡率从1950年的15‰下降至2003年的0.5‰。

其次是社会对女性的看法发生了巨大改变。以前，中国家庭更注重对男孩子的培养，而现在，中国家庭在培养子女时，不会因性别不同而存在差异。之前提到的女性在高等院校所占比例便很好地说明了这一转变。如果你看看周围，也会发现在卡尔加里留学的女生与男生几乎一样多。家庭、学校鼓励女生参加各类学术、体育、艺术活动，很多女生都能在公平竞争中取得优异成绩。

中国城市的妇女大都受过良好教育，她们自信，有职业理想，收入不菲。她们中有医生、律师、法官、企业家，甚至宇航员。过去10年，福布斯中国10大首富榜单中每年至少有一名女性，这对我们大家都是一个巨大的鼓舞！

在当今中国社会，男性已不被认为比女性更优越。妻子或女友收入更高的情况比比皆是。中国妇女结婚后不改用丈夫的姓，有时孩子甚至继承母亲的姓。“结婚”对于中国现代女性来说，已成为一个选项，而非必须完成的任务。

当然，和其他国家一样，尽管中国的妇女事业取得了长足的发展，但在某些地区，尤其是某些农村地区，性别歧视仍然存在。很多农村妇女的收入远低于男性，她们仍从属于丈夫，担任了照料家庭的传统角色。

但是，我相信男女平等是完全可以实现的。虽然还有很长的路要走，但我们不会放弃。我们已经取得了重大成绩，我们会继续坚持我们的努力。

国际妇女论坛等国际组织为我们提供了沟通、联系的舞台，相信通过这张网络，我们能发挥更大潜能，为改善全世界妇女地位做出更大贡献。

中国有句话，“妇女能顶半边天”，相信我们的男同胞们能够胜任顶起另外半边天的重任！

最后，感谢主办方给我这个机会与大家分享我的一些想法。恰逢中国农历新年，祝各位身体健康、家庭幸福、事业进步！

资料来源：

Text 1 http://www.who.int/pmnch/activities/jointactionplan/201009gswch_chinese.pdf

Text 2 http://www.who.int/pmnch/activities/jointactionplan/201009gswch_chinese.pdf

Text 3 http://apps.who.int/gb/e/e_wha61.html

Text 4 http://apps.who.int/iris/bitstream/10665/87770/1/A65_R17-ch.pdf

Text 5 http://www.moh.gov.cn/fys/s3581/201408/918e1c39782e415a9a7eaf0b96eaace2.shtml

Text 6 http://www.fmprc.gov.cn/mfa_chn/dszlsjt_602260/t800672.shtml

参考答案

四、摘要练习

Text 1

促进妇女儿童健康全球战略（节选1）

导言

联合国秘书长潘基文

距实现千年发展目标的最后期限只有五年的时间，全球领导人必须加紧努力，改善妇女和儿童的健康。在促进妇女、少女、新生儿和婴幼儿的健康方面，世界没能给予足够的投资，致使每年有数百万人因可预防的疾病而死亡。

我们在实现千年发展目标五（改善孕产妇保健）方面的进展，落后于其他任何千年发展目标。然而，我们现在有机会实现真正、持久的进展，因为全球领导人日益认识到，妇女和儿童的健康是实现所有发展目标的关键所在。

本全球战略要求所有合作伙伴团结起来，采取协调一致的行动。每个人都可以发挥重要的作用：政府、民间社会、社区组织、全球和区域机构、捐助者、慈善基金会、联合国和其他多边组织、开发银行、私营部门、卫生部门、专业协会、学术界和研究人员。

真正取得进展是完全有可能的。事实上，世界上一些最贫穷的国家已经取得了进展。这些国家对妇女和儿童问题给予了高度重视，将其列入国家卫生议程。

同时，通过在技术、治疗和服务提供方面采用创新办法，使提供优质高效的医疗服务更加便捷易行，新的和现有的融资机制则可增强医疗可负担性和可获得性。我们在这些方面再加大力度，情况就会大有改观。与1990年相比，现在每天的儿童死亡人数已减少1万。

所有合作伙伴齐心协力、共同行动的时刻已经到来。这意味着要强化一揽子具有重大影响的干预措施并确定优先顺序，强化卫生系统，并对不同疾病和不同部门的努力进行整合，如卫生、教育、水务、环境卫生和营养。它还意味着促进人权、两性平等和减贫。

所有行动者应努力优化现有投资。所有方面应对自己的承诺负责，并且需要筹措更多可预测的资金，用于提供基本卫生服务，实现与卫生相关的千年发展目标。

本战略着眼于妇女和儿童最为脆弱的时期。在分娩过程和婴儿出生头几个小时及最初几天中，孕妇和新生儿都会面临最大的死亡风险。青少年也很脆弱，我们必须确保他们拥有人生选择的自主权，包括生育自主权。这需要重点关注最脆弱、最难触及的妇女和儿童：最贫穷的妇女儿童、携带艾滋病毒和患有艾滋病的妇女儿童、孤儿、原住民妇女儿童和最难以获得卫生服务的妇女儿童。

它需要建立在我们对卫生与人权的承诺的基础上。全球战略建立在各国和合作伙伴在若干活动中所做出的承诺的基础上。这些活动包括在国际人口与发展会议上商定的《行动纲领》、在第四次世界妇女大会上商定的《北京宣言和行动纲领》、经社理事会全球卫生问题部长级审查会议、联合国大会特别会议“妇女健康、儿童健康：为我们共同的未来投资”，以及联合国第54届妇女地位委员会会议。全球战略还以区域承诺和努力为基础，如《马普托行动计划》、加速降低非洲孕产妇死亡率运动，以及2010年关于孕产妇、新生儿和儿童健康的非盟首脑会议宣言。

Text 2

促进妇女儿童健康全球战略（节选2）

导言

联合国秘书长潘基文

投资妇女儿童健康是明智之举

妇女和儿童在发展中起着至关重要的作用。加大对妇女儿童健康的投资力度，不仅仅是我们分内的职责，还有助于创造稳定、和谐和富有生产力的社会环境。

促进减贫。减少或完全取消对妇女和儿童的卫生保健收费，可增进贫困家庭获得医疗的机会，使他们能够把更多的钱用在食品、住房、教育和创收活动上。健康妇女的工作更有成效，在整个生命历程中有可能赚取更多的收入。解决孕妇和儿童营养不良问题，可导致个人的终生收入增加幅度高达10%。与此相反，卫生条件恶劣则会导致腹泻和寄生虫病缠身，致使生产力降低，儿童无法上学读书。

促进生产力和经济增长。孕产妇和新生儿死亡使经济发展的速度减慢，每年导致全球生产力损失金额高达150亿美元。处理不好营养不良问题，可导致国家国内生产总值比预期减少2%。相反，投资儿童健康可带来巨大的经济回报，为未来的生产力大军提供最佳保障。例如，在1965至1990年期间，亚洲经济增长率在30%～50%之间不等，可归因于生殖卫生得到改善，婴幼儿死亡率和生育率有所下降。

具有成本效益。基本卫生保健对于疾病和残疾的预防起到积极的作用，从而可节省数十亿美元的治疗费用。在许多国家，在计划生育上每花费1美元至少可节省

4美元本来要用于计划外怀孕造成的并发症治疗的资金。儿童免疫接种的费用不到5美元（有时还不到1美元），却可为儿童争取1年的健康生命，免受残疾和病痛的折磨。

帮助妇女和儿童认识到应享有的基本人权。人人有权享有可达到的最高标准的健康。这一发展和人权的基本原则在一系列国际和区域人权条约中得到许多国家的认可。

齐心协力，加快进展是全球战略的关键要素

我们知道什么措施能够奏效。对于妇女和儿童，需要有运转良好的卫生系统为其提供综合性一揽子基本干预措施和服务。许多国家现已开始取得进展。例如，在坦桑尼亚，由于免疫接种、维生素A补充、儿童疾病综合管理等干预措施得到普遍采用，5岁以下儿童死亡率降低15%～20%。在过去40年里，通过确保99%的孕妇接受4次产前检查，并且在卫生设施中分娩，斯里兰卡孕产妇死亡率下降了87%。

我们知道需要做什么。根据《巴黎宣言》、《阿克拉行动议程》和《蒙特利尔共识》所载原则，所有合作伙伴必须在以下领域紧密合作：

国家主导的卫生计划。合作伙伴必须支持现有的并已列入经费预算的国家卫生计划，以增加获得服务的机会。此类计划涵盖人力资源、融资以及提供和监督实施综合性一揽子干预措施。

全面、综合的一揽子基本干预措施和服务。合作伙伴必须确保妇女和儿童能获得整个一揽子保障的利益，包括计划生育宣传和服务，产前、分娩和产后护理，产科急诊和新生儿护理，在有关设施分娩期间提供熟练照护，安全的堕胎服务（如果法律不禁止堕胎），以及艾滋病毒和其他性传播感染的预防。干预措施也应包括：对不足6个月大婴儿进行纯母乳喂养、疫苗和免疫接种、采用口服补液疗法和锌补充剂管理腹泻疾病、主要儿童疾病的治疗、营养补充（如维生素A），以及获得适当的即食食品以预防和治疗营养不良。

综合保健改善健康促进，有助于肺炎、腹泻、艾滋病、疟疾、结核和非传染病等疾病的预防和治疗。必须加强特定疾病规划（如艾滋病、疟疾和结核规划）与着眼于妇女和儿童的保健服务（如扩大免疫规划、性和生殖卫生、儿童期疾病综合管理）之间的联系。

合作伙伴应加强与其他部门的协调，以解决对健康有影响的一些问题，如环境卫生、安全饮用水、营养不良、两性平等和赋予妇女权力。

加强卫生系统。合作伙伴必须支持努力加强卫生系统，以提供高质量的综合性服务。应扩大现有服务的可及范围，特别是在社区一级和服务不到位的地区，并且应对稀缺匮乏的资源予以更加有效的管理。还需要建立更多的卫生设施，使弱势群

体获得医学专业知识和药物。

卫生部门能力建设。合作伙伴必须齐心协力，解决各级卫生工作者严重短缺问题。必须提供协调一致的支持，协助各国制定和实施国家卫生计划，包括如何培养、留住和使用卫生工作者的方针策略。

五、英译汉练习

Text 3

世界卫生组织总干事陈冯富珍博士在第六十一届世界卫生大会上的讲话

主席先生，尊敬的各位部长，阁下，尊敬的各位代表，女士们、先生们：

各位面前有一个关于监测成就的报告。众所周知，在衡量我们的工作时，我会优先考虑非洲人民的健康和妇女健康。我的想法是对的。非洲的进展最小。妇女的问题最难。

我讲讲总体的进展。去年底，更好的数据和统计方法使世卫组织和联合国艾滋病规划署可以更准确地描绘出艾滋病毒和艾滋病流行的演变情况。20世纪90年代晚期，艾滋病毒感染达到高峰。2001年以后感染率一直保持平稳。一个重要趋势是，在过去两年里，艾滋病导致的死亡人数在下降。

现有证据允许我们充满信心地做出结论，死亡率的下降与最近大幅度提高抗反转录病毒药物的获得有关。至少妇女在获得治疗的情况上与男性是相同的。全球范围内，在使用抗反转录病毒药物的人中，有近四分之三在非洲，艾滋病在那里极为严重。

这表明，我们确实可以将抗反转录病毒药物治疗这样复杂的疗法引入资源短缺的地区。当然，我们的脚步还是落后于这个毁灭性的无情流行病。数据仍然是惊人的：估计有3 320万人携带艾滋病病毒生存，仅2007年新感染人数就达到250万。很明显，我们必须抓住每个机会进行预防。这是我们赶上并最终超过这个流行病的唯一途径。

对结核病，已有良好的诊断和治疗战略，而且我们有足够证据显示，这个方法是有效的。我们在稳步取得进步，尽管与最近几年相比，发现病患的速度开始降低。

造成抗药性的不良医疗行为，是一个需要关注的问题。今年早些时候，世卫组织发布的一个报告表明，耐多药结核病发病率已达到近年最高纪录。

更令人担忧的是广泛抗药结核病持续发生，该病几乎无法治疗。如果这种形式的结核病广泛传播，就将是一个极大规模的挫折。对于这类患者，我们的治疗选择实际上回到了抗生素出现以前的时期。

下个月，我将与联合国秘书长一起参加首次全球领导人论坛，讨论加强应对艾滋病毒和结核病这两个共存流行病的问题。这也是世界领导人现在越来越多参与卫生事务的另一例证。

此次论坛召开之时，也是很多负担沉重的国家正在努力使更多人口获得艾滋病和结核病综合医护服务之时。领导人可以把这个趋势再往前推动一下。与会的还有联合国秘书长控制结核特使、葡萄牙前总统乔治·桑帕约先生。

在疟疾方面，我们终于取得了实质性的进展。非洲部分地区死亡率快速下降，这表明所建议的战略产生了明显的效果。今年，我们庆祝了第一个世界疟疾日，它标志着全球战胜这一疾病的决心。

当时，秘书长及其特使雷·钱伯斯先生要求国际社会实施一个雄心勃勃的计划，即到2010年年底降低疟疾死亡率。如果我们能这样做，就会极大地促进非洲健康，获得更好的未来。

去年，全球幼儿死亡率是近年来首次下降到低于1 000万。你们将讨论一个关于全球疫苗接种战略的报告，它是公共卫生领域最成功的经验之一。我要对所有合作伙伴表示感谢；对于麻疹行动，我特别要感谢联合国儿童基金会以及疫苗和免疫全球联盟。

同时，我们清楚地看到儿童期疾病综合管理战略的广泛影响，它现在已经被100个国家采纳，成为主要的儿童生存战略，其中有49个国家将其涵盖范围扩展到国内半数以上地区。短短两年间，达到这一涵盖水平的国家的数目翻了一番。我祝贺这些国家做出的巨大努力。

研究工作向我们展示了在实现降低儿童死亡率目标方面的新进展。配合口服补液盐配方，使用锌来治疗腹泻，将有助于拯救千百万儿童的生命。今年早些时候，由世卫组织协调的研究工作表明，在家治疗婴幼儿的头号致死疾病肺炎，与在医院治疗同样有效，甚至可能更安全。我一直致力于初级卫生保健，因此，支持以社区和家庭为基础的治疗的证据尤其让我高兴。

然而，正如公共卫生中常见的情况，当一个方面的发病率和死亡率开始下降，就会暴露出更加令人震惊的另一个方面的重大问题。新生儿死亡率即是如此，这是我们需要处理的又一个重大问题。研究工作也再度表明，一些简单的方式，例如与母亲的肌肤之亲，即所谓的“袋鼠式”母亲护理法，可以拯救早产儿生命。

我们还需要拯救母亲的生命。如大家面前的报告所指出的，改善妇女健康进展缓慢，令人感到失望。在孕产妇健康方面，情况尤其如此，经过20多年的努力，死亡率仍然居高不下。

我个人认为，这一缺乏进展的局面令人难以容忍。社会难道如此看轻妇女的价值，以至她们的生命被视为可有可无？如果答案是否定的，那么我们绝对有必要加倍努力，确保妇女的健康受到保护。

我知道社会和文化改革需要时间。但我还看到了一些研究报告，表明妇女小额信贷计划极大地提高了她们的社会地位，增加了她们对家庭决定的控制权，增加了她们的家庭健康费用。在一些研究中，一个意想不到的好处是家庭暴力减少了。

我坚信，我们需要探讨每一种选择，只要它有可能提高妇女的地位，保护她们的健康，释放她们作为人的潜能，开发她们作为变革动力的巨大能力。

Text 4

第六十五届世界卫生大会　WHA65.17

议程项目13.12

2012年5月26日

全球疫苗行动计划

第六十五届世界卫生大会，

审议了有关全球疫苗行动计划草案的报告；

认识到免疫接种作为最具成本效益的公共卫生干预措施之一十分重要，应承认其为享有健康的人权的核心组成部分；

确认一些国家已经在确保每个符合条件的个人均能接种所有适合疫苗而不论其地理位置、年龄、性别、是否残疾、教育水平、社会经济地位、民族或工作条件方面取得突出进展；

赞赏成功免疫规划在实现全球卫生目标特别是减少儿童死亡率和发病率以及有可能在整个生命历程降低死亡率和发病率方面所做出的贡献；

注意到针对几种主要死因疾病如肺炎、腹泻和宫颈癌的重要病因推出了新疫苗，这有可能促进补充干预措施的扩大并在初级卫生保健规划之间创造协同效应；而且除降低死亡率外，这些新疫苗还将预防发病，从而产生经济效益，即使在已经成功降低死亡率的国家也是如此；

担忧虽然已经取得了进展，但如果不实现并保持高覆盖和公平覆盖，消灭和消除疾病的目标如消灭脊灰和消除麻疹、风疹以及产妇和新生儿破伤风的目标将无法实现；

担忧采用可获得疫苗速度较慢的低收入和中等收入国家或许没有机会获得今后

十年预计会出现的新疫苗和改进疫苗；

对每五位儿童就有一位未获得全球常规免疫服务而且各国内部常规免疫接种覆盖仍存在巨大空白感到震惊；

忆及有关全球免疫战略的WHA58.15和WHA61.15号决议，

1. 批准全球疫苗行动计划；

2. 敦促会员国：

（1）使用全球疫苗行动计划确定的前景和战略，以制定其国家卫生战略和计划的疫苗和免疫接种相关内容，尤其要注意增进扩大免疫规划的绩效，并使其符合各自国家的流行病学形势；

（2）致力于为实现免疫接种目标和其他相关关键里程碑分配足够的人力资源和资金；

（3）每年向区域委员会有关疫苗十年的专门会议报告其获得的经验教训、取得的进展、仍然存在的挑战及为实现国家免疫目标而采取的最新行动；

3. 要求总干事：

（1）加强协调所有利益攸关方的全球免疫工作以支持全球疫苗行动计划的实施；

（2）确保为落实全球疫苗行动计划向区域和国家层面提供的支持将特别重视将常规免疫问题纳入在内；

（3）确定提供技术支持的人力资源和资金以实施全球疫苗行动计划的国家计划并监督其影响；

（4）动员更多财务资源，以支持低收入和中等收入国家落实全球疫苗行动计划；

（5）监督进展情况并每年通过执委会以实质性议程项目向卫生大会报告实现全球免疫目标的进展情况，利用建议的问责框架指导讨论和未来的行动，直至第七十一届世界卫生大会。

第十次全体会议，2012年5月26日
A65/VR/10

六、汉译英练习

Text 5

National Health Planning Commission's Advice on Implementation of the Demonstration Project of Excellent Maternal and Child Health Services (Excerpt)

To improve maternal and child health services, ensure civilian access to quality maternal and child health services, and safeguard people's right of health, the National Health and Family Planning Commission (NHFPC) have decided to implement demonstration project of excellent maternal and child health services from 2014. Maternal and child health services will be thoroughly improved through guidance, demonstration and promotion.

I. Guiding Principles and Objectives

Excellent service demonstration project of maternal and child health will fully implement "Law of the People's Republic of China on Maternal and Infant Health Care", "Law of the People's Republic of China on Population and Family Planning", and "2011-2020 China Women and Children Development Program". It will follow the idea of serving to promote people's health, adhere to the principle of "child's priority and maternal safety", adhere to the policy of maternal and child health, so as to improve the administration of maternal and child health service and satisfy the needs of health of women and children.

The target of the Demonstration Project of Excellent Maternal and Child Health Services is to promote governments at all levels to pay more attention to maternal and child health; fully upgrade service quality of and administrative ability for maternal and child health; reach equity of and accessibility to maternal and child health service, constantly improve health of women and children; guarantee effectiveness, security and timeliness of contraception; build new service brand for the satisfaction of residents, so as to promote a fast development of maternal and child health service. This includes the following 5 aspects:

● Leaders' close attention. Governments at all levels will include maternal and child health program into their overall economic and social development plan and evaluation of governmental implementation of objectives. They will establish effective mechanism of coordination and stable mechanism for guaranteeing investment.

● Standardized management. This means a sound system for maternal and child health service and standardized institution-building. The management system, working mechanism, technical specifications, and operational process will be all good; their supervision is effective and the implementation of rules will be well done.

● Good service quality. Maternal and child health services will have friendly surroundings and environment and constantly improve their professional capability, so that their service quality will be improved significantly.

● Good implementation of targets. The main health indicators for women and children will continue to improve, the required indicators for maternal and child health care will be significantly improved, and all tasks will be successful completed.

● People's satisfaction. The services will create good public reputation so that customer satisfaction will gradually grow.

II. The Main Content

1. Strengthening the fulfillment of Government's responsibility. Government at all levels will pay serious attention to maternal and child health program and include it into the local economic and social development plan. They will take pregnant mortality, infant mortality, mortality of children under the age of five, contraceptive service efficiency, and implementation rate of birth defect prevention into the evaluation of governmental goals and responsibilities. They will make plans for the development of maternal and child health care and organize their implementation by clarifying the responsibility of individual departments, establishing a coordinating work mechanism, and implementing target management of maternal and child health. Meanwhile, identification of fund for maternal and child health services is a guarantee for the successful completion of all tasks.

2. Adhering to the correct direction of development. Governments will adhere to the guidelines of "focusing on health care, safeguarding reproductive health as purpose, combining health care and clinical care, targeting at the grass-roots population for their maternal and child health. For women and children, governments will provide them, from birth to old age, active and continuous medical care services and health management covering physical and psychological aspects. They will strengthen their responsibility for public health, highlight the function of population health, and effectively accomplish the regional indicators for maternal and child health services.

3. Strengthening the construction of service system. Local governments will establish independent maternal and child health service institutions, so as to promote optimal integration of resources for maternal and child health care and family planning medical facilities. Local governments will comprehensively accomplish construction of institutional standardization, guarantee premises for their basic program, allocate basic medical

equipments, determine their staffing and funding, equip themselves with professionals and technicians, and pay high attention for their talent team construction, in particular training of personnel that is in urgent shortage, such as midwives. Maternal and child health care institutions will have standardized departments and standardized facilities. The governments will gradually strengthen construction of key maternal and child health specialties.

4. Improving rules and regulations. Governments will improve their administrative regulations, program rules, technical standards, working procedures, supervision system and evaluation system. All relevant medical institutions will establish and improve their administrative system of obstetrics departments, delivery wards, neonatology departments, and family planning technical services, as well as standardize their workflows. Maternal and child health care institutions must strictly enforce laws and regulations related to medical service while other institutions that also provides maternal and child health services must execute all requirements related to the maternal and child health. Departments at all levels must conduct supervision and inspection on the implementation of their rules.

5. Strengthening daily supervision and administration. Related institutions will seriously abide by the "Law of PRC on Maternal and Infant Health Care" and "Law on Population and Family Planning", by including supervision on maternal and child health service and family planning technical service into their integrated surveillance and law enforcement, strengthening supervision and inspection, strictly examine admittance of organization, personnel and techniques, and standardizing service behaviors. They will establish a routine of regular inspection and random checks, look for loopholes in management, report problems to related parties, strengthen internal administration, promote informationization, and improve information management.

6. Raising service standards. This means to give better professional guidance, training and assessment to institutions that provide basic maternal and child health service. Governments will enhance personnel training on maternal and child health, job training and continuing medical education in various ways. They will make plans on personnel professional training and implement it, and strengthen training of appropriate technology and promotion of new technologies. Targeting at the needs of people, they will conduct satisfaction survey, improve services facilities and process of service, provide a wide range of services for people's convenience, for them to have easy access to maternal and child health services, so as to constantly adapt to people's demand for maternal and child health services.

7. Ensuring the quality of service. Governments will construct treatment center for critically severe pregnant women and newborn infants in their administration areas, as well

as improve emergency referral networks to ensure green channels unobstructed. Maternal and child health care institutions will establish an evaluation system for service quality and medical safety. They will enhance agency's internal management and infrastructure management, strengthen management of key links, key areas, and the needy, improve service quality, and ensure medical safety. They will strictly implement the core system of initial diagnosis responsibility, three-level ward rounds, difficult case discussion, consultation of doctors, and preoperative discussions, death case discussions, and shift changes. They will standardize medical record writing and promote rational examination, rational drug use, and proper treatment. They will reasonably manipulate the rate of caesarean, and actively promote breastfeeding.

8. Fully achieving all mission objectives. The objectives are that related institutions will reduce maternal mortality, infant mortality, and mortality rate of children under five years of age; improve service rate of free family planning technical service. They will standardize and implement the fundamental programs such as subsidies for rural pregnant women's hospitalized childbirth, screening of rural women's cervical cancer and breast cancer, supplement of folic acid to prevent neural tube defects, prevention of the spread of AIDS, syphilis and hepatitis b disease, reduction of maternal mortality, elimination of neonatal tetanus, improvement of the nutrition of children in the poverty-stricken areas, and neonatal diseases screening. They will promote free pre-pregnancy eugenic health checks, implement basic public health services for management of maternal and child health, livelihood projects for maternal and child health undertaken in accordance with the local conditions, and guarantee to complete the goal with good quality and quantity.

9. Actively accepting supervision by citizens. Related institutions will abide by the "Specification for Behaviors of Practitioners at Medical Institutions", provide education on professional ethics and legal disciplines for medical personnel, so as to raise the ethos of the profession and morale of the doctors. They will strengthen mass health education, spread health knowledge and improve people's health literacy. They will establish the system of publicizing the service hospitals' institutional administrative procedures and information, by setting complaint boxes, opening hotlines and web-mails, and other variety of forms of communication, so as to unblock channels for complaints and reports, actively accept supervision by citizens, and continuously improve their work.

10. Establishing a good image of the profession. Practitioners must show good work ethics, good service and spirit of dedication in providing humanized services and humanistic care for women and children. Institutions will find and publicize excellent model

practitioners, strengthen publicity on model professionals and their devotion, hard work, and dedication, especially those who serve at the grass-root level, at ethnic minority areas and remote areas, so as to show health workers serving the women and children and transmit positive energy through these good images.

Text 6

Keynote Speech by Consul General Liu Yongfeng at the International Women's Forum Chinese New Year Dinner

8 February 2011

Respected guests,

Good evening.

I am honored to have been invited to this evening's gathering, particularly in the company of accomplished women.

I am especially pleased that the International Women's Forum has chosen to celebrate the Chinese New Year. There is perhaps no greater sign of friendship than to share each other's special occasions. I would like to take this opportunity to tell you about women in modern China.

As recent as the beginning of the last century, in China, as it was in the West, men dominated the society and women were subordinates. Women had almost no voice in the society and did not have rights or privileges. Perhaps the most infamous symbol of the oppression of Chinese women, foot-binding, went on until the beginning of the 20th century. My own grandmother was subjected to the agony and humiliation of foot-binding.

What is encouraging is that China's Xinhai Revolution of 1911 has overthrown the feudal emperor system. After 1949, Chinese government took a series of measures for promotion and protection of the equality between man and woman.

1) The Chinese Constitution provides equal legal rights for men and women. Laws and regulations have been enacted to protect this equality in all areas of life, including ownership of property, inheritance, marriage and divorce, and educational opportunities.

2) Our government has set up committees and departments to promote and protect women's rights. For examples, the promotion of women health and income equality, which are perhaps the two most important women issues, are made the mandates of certain departments in our government: The Department of Community Health and Maternal &

Child Health Care of the Ministry of Health is in charge of the promotion of women health. And the Department of Labor and Wages of the Ministry of Labor and Social Security is in charge of the promotion of income equality. As well, non-governmental organizations (NGOs) have been formed to further equality for women. As early as 1949, the All-China Women's Federation was established to promote the advancement of Chinese women of all ethnic groups in all walks of life and gender equality. In recent years, committees and associations have been formed, such as, the Women Worker's Committee of the All-China Federation of Trade Unions, the China Women Entrepreneurs Association, China Women Judges Association, Society of Chinese Women Doctors, and many more, all working to ensure that the rights of women are protected in their special areas. There are also about 27,000 women and children's rights protection agencies in China, all working towards the goal of achieving and protecting women's rights.

In fact, there is one women organization, almost within each independent enterprise or public institution and any level government department. We also have a women working group in our Consulate General in Calgary. And the chair of the group, Ms. Yan, is just sitting over there.

What have the joint efforts of government and civilians achieved in the last sixty years for gender equality in China?

First, women's status in modern Chinese society has improved quite dramatically. According to last year's statistics, 99.54% of all school-age girls have access to elementary education, and women represents 49.86% of the student population in advanced education. Considering only 48.47% of the population in China is female, it indicates that the ratio of women students in the women population is higher than its counterpart. It is quite an achievement! Women account for 45.4% of China's employed population and women officials account for over 40% of all government officials. The mortality rate of women giving birth in China had dropped from 15 per thousand in the 1950s to about 0.5 per thousand by 2003.

Second, views about women have changed. Although traditionally, Chinese families favored sons over daughters, in modern Chinese society, dedication and devotion of families and their resources are lavished on daughters as much as sons. The percentage of women in advanced education is proof of this change in attitude. And if you look around you in your daily life, you will find just as many Chinese female foreign students in Calgary as there are male. Girls are encouraged to participate and excel in academic research sports, artistic endeavors, and all other areas of achievements.

Many women in modern urban China are well-educated, confident, assertive, career-minded, and well-paid. They are doctors, lawyers, judges, entrepreneurs, and even astronauts. Every year, in the past ten years, there is at least one woman within the Top 10 on the Forbes' China Rich List!

In modern China, men are no longer assumed to be superior to women. In many instances, wives or girlfriends, are now the higher-income earning partners, and are treated as equals. In modern China, women do not take their husbands' last names after marriage, and sometimes, children even take their mothers' last names, and not their fathers! Marriage is now a choice, and not a "must" for modern Chinese women.

But of course, despite all the improvements and advances made in women's rights, as in elsewhere in the world, gender inequality still exists in China, particularly in rural China. In rural China, many women are still earning substantially less than their male counterparts. They are still relegated to the traditional roles of serving the families and being subservient to men.

But change is coming. I am very hopeful, as I am sure you all are, that gender equality is achievable. It is just a long and difficult road. And we must not give up. We have already made significant changes, we just need to persevere.

With organizations, such as the International Women's Forum, offering a global stage to meet and connect, providing the support and network for women around the world, I believe that we will be able to bring out our potential to continue to make great contributions to better the lives of women around the world.

There is a Chinese saying: "Women can hold up half the sky." Let us just hope that our counterpart is holding up the other half.

Thank you for this wonderful opportunity for me to meet all of you and to share my thoughts with you this evening. I hope we can continue to exchange ideas Finally, wish you and your families good health, happiness, success and prosperity in the year of rabbit. Thank you.

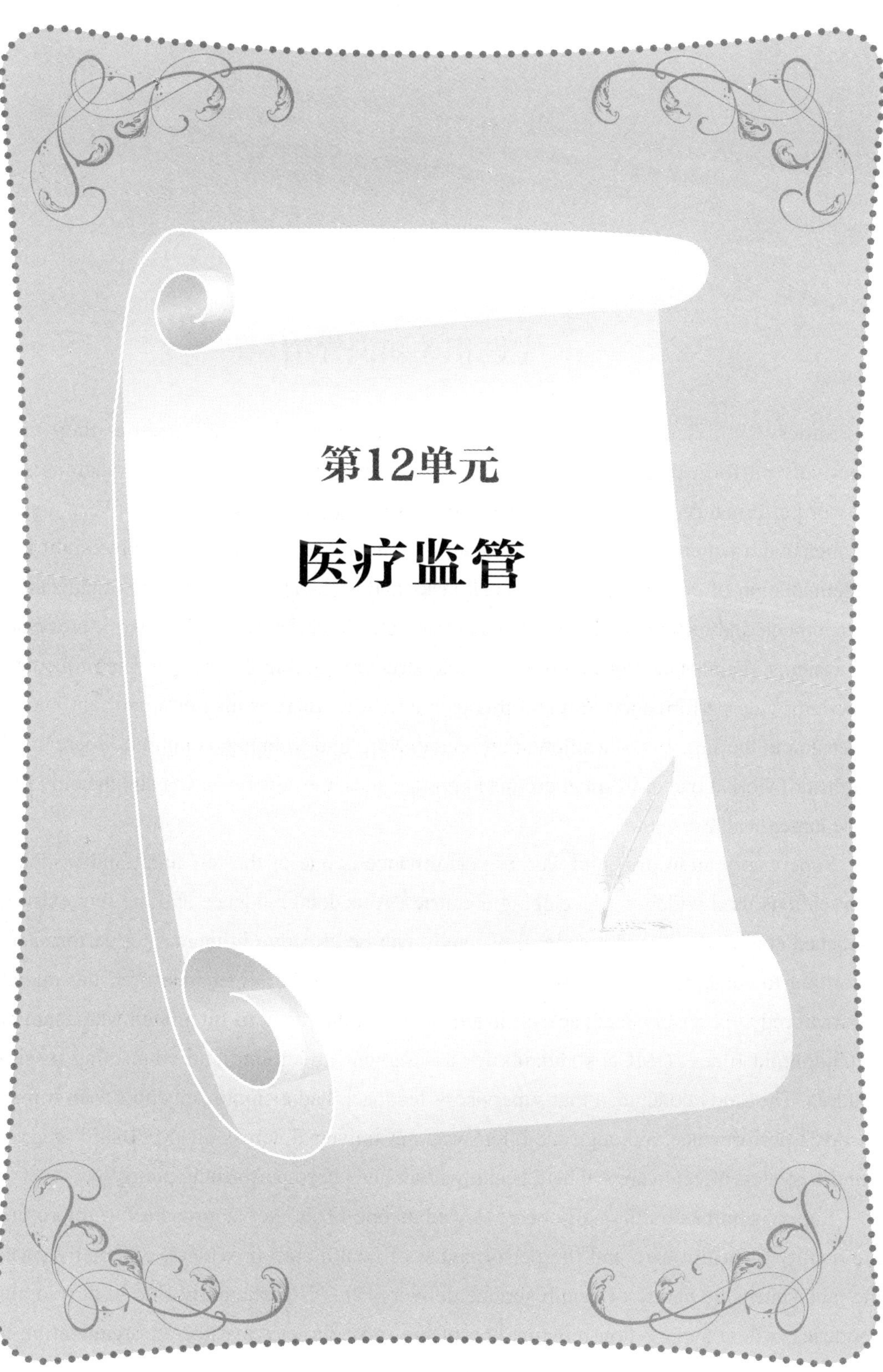

第12单元

医疗监管

一、主题相关知识介绍

Supervision is the process of directing and supporting staff so that they may effectively perform their duties. Supervision may include periodic events, such as site visits or performance reviews, but it also refers to the ongoing relationship between a staff member and a supervisor. In the health care setting, supervision includes oversight and implementation of clinical and non-clinical tasks and activities that affect the organization, management, and technical delivery of health services, including control of work processes and systems, maintenance of facilities and infrastructure, and monitoring and improvement of system-wide performance. Beyond this technical role, there is also an important human dimension to the supervisor-health worker relationship. In developing countries, where many health staff work alone or in small groups in remote sites, the supervisor may be the only link to the larger health system.

Supervisory audit of health worker performance is one of the few audit and feedback interventions used widely in developing countries. Anecdotal evidence and the few existing published studies suggest that supervisory audit can be effective in increasing performance according to standards. A Quality Assurance Project study in Niger measured the impact of structured supervisory feedback on health worker adherence to Integrated Management of Childhood Illness (IMCI) standards for assessment, treatment, and counseling of sick children. The study concluded that supervisory feedback had a significant short-term impact on IMCI performance, although the effect was not universal across all IMCI skill areas: it had the greatest effect in areas where health workers had been performing poorly.

Supervision has traditionally been viewed as one of the key approaches to improving the quality of health care and the performance of health care providers, especially given the labor-intensive nature of health service delivery. This is particularly true in developing countries, where supervision remains one of the most direct ways for an organization to affect what its staff does. At the same time, disappointment that the "promise" of supervision is frequently not realized or sustained is pervasive. USAID and its cooperating agencies have invested significant resources to strengthen supervision systems in developing countries through supervisor training and supervisory tools and checklists, yet interventions to strengthen supervision systems have often faltered after the pilot phase or have failed to demonstrate results independent of other efforts to improve service delivery.

International health agencies have reached consensus in recent years about the key functions of supervision: setting objectives, providing training and guidance, monitoring and evaluating performance, providing feedback, motivating staff, and providing support to solve problems. At the same time, a growing body of experience from different settings suggests that expanding the realm of how supervision functions can be performed—with ways of doing supervision that involve health workers themselves, peers, and even communities—may broaden and enhance supervision. Evidence suggests that these alternative approaches achieve better health worker performance and outcomes than traditional supervisory approaches, and some evidence indicates that these approaches may be more sustainable.

Source: United States Agency for International Development: Health Care Improvement Project. *Supervision*. http://www.hciproject.org/improvement_tools/improvement_methods/approaches/supervision.

二、技巧指导：数字转换

由于中文数字与英文数字在位数上的表达有不一样的地方，因此数字的翻译一直是口译中的难点。在记录上，英文数字表达是从右往左，三位数用一个逗号分开，比如：1,745,809,371,676,720。这意味着每一组数字都有个位、十位、百位。从右往左，每个逗号要涉及的位数分别是hundred，thousand，million，billion，trillion。综合起来，在读数时，每一组数都要用到个位、十位与百位，大的数字则需加用大一级的量词。以上文中的这个数字为例：

676,720
读为：six hundred (hun), seventy-six thousand (ths), seven hundred and twenty
371,676,720
读为：3 hun 71 million(m), 6 hun 76 ths, 7 hun 20

809,371,676,720

读为：8 hun and 9 billion(bi), 3 hun 71 million(m), 6 hun 76 ths, 7 hun 20

745,809,371,676,720

读为：7 hun 45 trillion(tri), 8 hun and 9 billion(bi), 3 hun 71 million(m), 6 hun 76 ths, 7 hun 20

1,745,809,371,676,720

读为：1ths 7 hun 45 trillion(tri), 8 hun and 9 billion(bi), 3 hun 71 million(m), 6 hun 76 ths, 7 hun 20

中文的数字单位有个、十、百、千、万、亿，大数字是万和亿，从千位数以后就与英文的不一样了。翻译的方法是往左挪动一位小数点，这样就变成四位数一组（为了讲解清晰，这里用竖线表示）。在数字1,745,｜809,3｜71,67｜6,720中，竖线刚好隔开千位数、万位数、亿位数，万亿位数。读法是：

7167｜6720

读作：七千一百六十七万六千七百二十。竖线前面是以万为单位。

8093｜7167｜6720

读作：八千零九十三亿七千一百六十七万六千七百二十。竖线前面是亿位数。

1745｜8093｜7167｜6720

读作：一千七百四十五万亿八千零九十三亿七千一百六十七万六千七百二十。竖线前面是万亿位数。

反过来，在中译英的情况下，听到“八千零九十三亿 七千一百六十七万六千七百二十”。可以记成8093 7167 6720，从右至左三位打一逗号809,371,676,720直接读出。这样的方法能够使较长的数字得到准确记录和表达。

在不需要精确数字的情况下，上述数字可以做模糊处理，如记成809billion。

我们可以从表12-1中直观地看到两种表达法的不同。

表12-1　中、英文数字单位表达

中文的数字单位表达	英文的数字单位表达
1　个	one
10　十	ten
100　百	hundred
1,000　千	thousand

续表12-1

中文的数字单位表达	英文的数字单位表达
10,000 万	ten thousand
100,000 十万	hundred thousand
1,000,000 百万	million
10,000,000 千万	ten million
100,000,000 亿	hundred million
1,000,000,000 十亿	billion
10,000,000,000 百亿	ten billion
100,000,000,000 千亿	hundred billion
1,000,000,000,000 万亿	trillion
10,000,000,000,000 十万亿	ten trillion
100,000,000,000,000 百万亿	hundred trillion
1,000,000,000,000,000 千万亿	thousand trillion

表12-2 随机大数字英语读数与翻译练习

1,299,880,000	1 bn 2 hun 99 m 8 hun & 80 ths	12亿9千9百88万
542,830,000	5 hun 42 m 8 hun 30 ths	5亿4千2百83万
757,050,000	7 hun 57 m & 50 ths	7亿5千7百零5万
669,760,000	6 hun 69 m 7hun 60 ths	6亿6千9百76万
630,120,000	6 hun 30m 1 hun 20 ths	6 亿3千零12万
297,490,000	2 hun 97 m 4 hun 90 ths	2亿9千7百49万
921,840,000	9 hun 21 m 8 hun 40 ths	9亿2千1百84万
98,570,000	98 m 5 hun 70 ths	9千8百57万
159,300,000	1 hun 59 m 300 ths	1亿5千9百30万
8,320,000	8 m 3 hun 20 ths	8百32万
76,100,000	76 m 100 ths	7千6百10万
73,500,000,000	73 bi 500 m	735亿
27,800,000,000	27 bi 800 m	278亿
107,200,000,000	107 bi 200 m	1千零72亿
9,100,000,000	9 bi 100 m	91 亿
159,300,000	1 hun 59 m 300 ths	1亿5千9百30万
8,320,000	8 m 3 hun 20 ths	8百32万

续表12-2

76,100,000	76 m 100 ths	7千6百10万
73,500,000,000	73 bi 500 m	735亿
27,800,000,000	27 bi 800 m	278亿
107,200,000,000	107 bi 200 m	1千零72亿
124,900,000,000	124 bi 900 m	1千2百49亿
70,100,000,000	70 bi 100 m	701亿
44,700,000,000	44 bi 700 m	4百47亿
9,496,915,292	9 bi 496 m 915 ths 292	94亿9691万5292
68,345,529	68 m 345 ths 529	6千834万5529
9,565,260,821	9 bi 565 m 260 ths 821	95亿6526万零821
1,808,427,239	1 bi 808 m 427 ths 239	18亿零842万7239

表12-3　随机大数字汉语读数与翻译练习

32,896.03亿	3,289,603,000,000	(3 tri 2 hun 89 bn 6 hun & 3 m)
3476.89亿	347689,000,000	(3 hun 47 bi 6 hun 89 m)
9856.25亿	985,625,000,000	(9 hun 85 bi 6 hun 25 m)
1487.77亿	1487,77,000,000	(1 hun 48 bi 7 hun 77 m)
8087.05亿	808,705,000,000	(8 hun & 8 bn 7 hun 5 m)
568.70亿	56,870,000,000	(56 bn 8 hun 70 m)
931.68亿	93,168,000,000	(93 bn 1 hun 68 m)
67.98亿	6,798,000,000	(6 bn 7 hun 98 m)
8.589亿	858,900,000	(8 hun 58 m 9 hun ths)
53.71亿	5,371,000,000	(5 bn 3 hun 71m)
6.891千万	68,910,000	(68 m 9 hun 10 ths)
5.384千万	53,840,000	(53 m 8 hun 40 ths)
6891万7348	68,917,348	(68 m 9 hun 17 ths 3 hun 48)
6384万4323	63,844,323	(63 m 8 hun 44 ths 3 hun 23)
2409万8453	24,098,453	(24 m 98 ths 4 hun 53)
98.365万	983,650	(9 hun 83 ths 6 hun 50)
52.021万	520,820	(5 hun 20 ths 8 hun 20)
32.876万	328,760	(3 hun 28 ths 7 hun 60)

表12-4 整数大数字翻译练习

1500万	15 m
3400万	34 m
4.5亿	450 m
8.8亿	880 m
47亿	4.7 bi
53亿	5.3 bi
960亿	96 bi
210亿	21 bi
4300亿	430 bi
9200亿	920 bi
67000亿	6.7 tri
78000亿	7.8 tri
130000亿	13 tri
460000亿	46 tri
170万亿	170 tri
250万亿	250 tri
3300万亿	3300 tri
6900万亿	6900 tri

表12-5 中英单位名称对照

Linear Measure长度	Square Measure面积	Cubic Measure体积
inch英寸	square inch平方英寸	cubic inch立方英寸
foot英尺	square foot平方英尺	cubic foot立方英尺
yard码	square yard平方码	cubic yard立方码
statute mile英里	square mile平方英里	
nautical mile海里	square millimeter (mm^2)平方毫米	cubic millimetres立方毫米
millimetres毫米	sq. centimetres平方厘米	cubic centimetres立方厘米
metre米	sq. decimetres平方分米	cubic metre立方米(m^3)
kilometres千米	sq. metre平方米	
	hectare公顷	
	acre英亩	

表12-6 容积单位

	British英制	American Dry美制干量	American Liquid美制液量
gram克	pint品脱	pint品脱	pint品脱
fluid oz.液量盎司	quart夸脱	quart夸脱	quart夸脱
	gallon加伦	peck配克	gallon加伦
litre升	peck配克	bushel蒲式耳	
hectolitres百升	bushel蒲式耳		
	quarter八蒲式耳		

表12-7 其他常用单位

Avoirdupois Weight 常衡	
grams 克	radian (rad) 弧度
kilogram 千克	degree (°) 度
grain 格令（谷）	Celsius 摄氏
dram 打兰	Fahrenheit (F) 华氏
pound 磅	million pascal (MPa) 百万帕斯卡
stone 英石	Joule (J) 焦耳
quarter 四分之一英担	kilowatt (kW) 千瓦
kilopound (kip) 千磅	volt (V) 伏（伏特）
ton (t) 吨	ampere (A) 安（安培）
pounds per square inch (psi) 磅/平方英寸	ohm (Ω) 欧（欧姆）
parts per million (ppm) 百万分之一	

附：部分常用单位及其缩写

BK (book) 本
BT (bottle) 瓶
BU (bucket) 桶
MO (month) 月
CA (catty) 斤
DZ (dozen) 打
EA (each) 每个
PR (pair) 对
BR (branch) 支
MH (man hour) 人工工时
BX (box) 盒
WK (week) 周
MT (metric ton) 公吨
PI (piece) 件
PK (package) 包
GP (group) 组

RL (roll) 卷
SH (sheet) 张
SL (slice)片
ST (set) 套
TU (tube) 管
VC (vehicle) 辆

三、词汇准备

Text 1

fraud 舞弊，欺诈
strike force 突击部队，警察快速行动部队
takedown （警方的）抓捕行动，临检，突检
Attorney General 司法部长
turn the tide on 扭转局势
law enforcement 执法，法律的实施
coordinate across agencies 跨机构协调
pool resources 汇总资源
Affordable Care Act 平价医疗法案
suspend 暂停，中止
medicare payments and reimbursements 医保支付和报账
credible 可信的
allegations of fraud 欺诈指控
submit fraudulent Medicare claims 提交欺诈性的医保索赔申请
providers and suppliers 医疗卫生服务机构和供应商
obstruct a fraud investigation 妨碍欺诈调查
predictive and data analytics 预测分析和数据分析科技
violate that trust 破坏信任
jail time 服刑时间
pocketbook 财政状况，财力，钱包
defraud 欺骗，诈骗

Acting Assistant Attorney General of the Criminal Division 分管司法部刑事司的代理助理司法部长

Text 2

Dr. Shin Young-soo, WHO Regional Director for the Western Pacific 世界卫生组织西太平洋区域主任申英秀博士

Health Technology Assessment International 卫生技术评估国际协会

National Evidence-based Healthcare Collaborating Agency and the Ministry of Health and Welfare of the Republic of Korea 韩国国家循证医疗卫生合作机构和韩国卫生福利部

customize 定制

lack access to 缺乏，不能获得

ad hoc 临时安排的，专门的

faulty assumption 错误的假设

advocacy 倡导

cost-effective 费用低廉的，低成本的

universal health coverage 医疗卫生服务覆盖全民

equitable 公平合理的，公正的，均等化的

access 获取途径

stepping stone 踏脚石，进身之阶

national planning 国家规划

systematic cost-containment process 系统化的成本控制流程

scrutiny 仔细检查，认真彻底的审查

commendable 值得表扬的，值得称赞的

build capacity 能力建设

stakeholder 利益相关者

regulatory authorities 监管机构

priority-setting 决定轻重缓急

convening power 召集能力，召开会议的权力

roundtable 圆桌会议

infant mortality 婴儿死亡率

at the operational level 操作层面的

scale up 扩大规模

Text 3

The Rt Hon Jeremy Hunt MP，Minister of the Department of Health 英国卫生部部长杰里米·亨特议员阁下

NHS (National Health Service) 英国国民医疗保健系统
Health Secretary 卫生大臣
campaigner （尤指政治或社会变革的）运动领导者
in the wake of 紧跟在……之后，紧接着
lapse 疏忽，失误，过失
grim 严酷的，严厉的，冷酷的
fatalism 宿命论，宿命主义
statistics 统计数据，统计资料
blunt 使减弱，使降低效应，使（尖端、刃）变钝
uncompromising determination 坚定的决心，不屈不挠的决心
incidents of harm 伤害事件
operating theatre 手术室
notes 病历
condition 疾病，病情
GP, general practitioner 全科医师；普通医生
be allergic to 对……过敏
drip 静脉滴注，输液
postbag 公众来信（寄给报纸、电视台、网站、要人等）
Royal College of Surgeons 皇家外科医学院
green 不成熟的，缺乏经验的
patently 毫无疑问，显然，明显地
never events 从来不会发生的事件，绝不事件
under-reporting 低报（报告的数字比实际情况低），报告不足
foreign objects 异物，外来异物
swab 棉签
surgical instrument 手术器械，手术用具
wrong site surgery 错误部位手术，开错刀
implants 植入物
prosthesis 假体（如假肢、假眼或假牙），复数为prostheses

Text 4

Acting Assistant Attorney General 代理助理司法部长
Justice Department's Criminal Division 司法部刑事司
Inspector General 检察长

Deputy Administrator for Program Integrity of the Centers for Medicare and Medicaid Services 医疗补助和老年医疗保险服务中心分管程序廉正的副主任

alleged participation in 涉嫌参与

billing 收费

fraudulent 欺骗的，欺诈的

unlicensed 未经授权的，没有执照的

illicit financial gain 非法经济利益

integrity 完好，完整

Health Care Fraud Prevention and Enforcement Action Team (HEAT) 医疗保健欺诈预防和执法行动小组

groundbreaking 全新的，开创性的，突破性的

initiative 倡议

leverage 施加影响力

bolster 改善，加强

yield extraordinary results 取得非凡的成果

fiscal year 会计年度，财政年度

U.S. Treasury 美国财政部

Medicare Trust Fund 老年医保信托基金

deter 制止，威慑

would-be criminal 潜在的罪犯

bill something to someone 给……开账单，把账单开给……

home health service 家庭健康服务

providers 医疗卫生服务提供机构

backfill 回填（用挖出的材料重新填回洞穴）

deficit reduction plan 削减赤字计划

slate 安排，预定，计划

hold... accountable 让……（对自己的决定、行为）负责任

execute search warrant 执行搜查令

Text 5

全国药物政策与基本药物制度工作会议 National Drug Policy and Essential Drugs System Work Conference

政府办基层医疗卫生机构 public primary health care institution

新疆生产建设兵团 Xinjiang Production and Construction Corps

采购机制 procurement mechanism

招采合一 one institution taking charge of both tender offer and procurement

量价挂钩 adjusting the price according to the quantity of purchase

双信封制 two-envelope system for tender bidding

集中支付 direct payment to the supplier

全程监控 close monitoring of the whole process

基层和二三级医院 primary, secondary and tertiary-level hospitals

村卫生室 village clinics

《国家基本药物目录（基层部分）》 *National Essential Drugs Inventory* (*Primary Health Care*)

临床应用指南和处方集 national clinical guidelines and formulary

可负担性 affordability

筹资机制 fund-raising mechanism

报销 reimbursement

质量监管 quality control

以药补医 the mechanism of doctors supplementing their incomes with the drugs they prescribe

药品加成政策 drug mark-up policy

优化重组 optimized restructuring

零差率销售 make drugs available at wholesale price

压缩药品虚高价格 mark-down of overpriced drugs

Text 6

三好一满意 Good Service, Good Quality, Good Medical Ethics and High Satisfaction

创先争优 strive for excellent performance

新型农村合作医疗制度 New Rural Health Care Cooperative System

新农合参合率 enrollment in the New Rural Health Care Cooperative System

突发公共卫生事件 public health emergency event

中医药 traditional Chinese medicine

保基本、强基层、建机制 ensure basic health insurance coverage, strengthen the grassroots, and formulate new mechanism

基本医疗保障制度 basic health insurance

筹资标准 fund-raising standards

农民受益水平 coverage level of farmers' benefits

门诊医疗费用统筹 a health insurance plan that covers outpatient medical expenses

门诊补偿 reimbursement rate of outpatient medical expenses

重大疾病保障 health insurance plan that covers major diseases

护理服务 nursing care

便民门诊 walk-in clinic

先诊疗、后结算 treatment first, and settlement of accounts at a later time

薄弱地区 underserved areas

专科医疗服务 specialist care

基层首诊、分级医疗、双向转诊、急慢分治 initial diagnosis at primary-care institutions, multi-tiered medical service, two-way referral, and separate treatment of acute and chronic conditions

医师多点执业 the system for doctors to practice at multiple sites

四、摘要练习

请听下面英语语篇，第一篇用源语言复述此段主要信息逻辑点及层次，第二篇用译入语复述此段主要信息逻辑点及层次。注意信息点之间的逻辑联系。

Text 1

Medicare Fraud Strike Force Takedown Press Conference

Kathleen Sebelius, Secretary of the Department of Health and Human Services (HHS), U.S.

Washington, DC, USA

14 May 2013

Thank you, Attorney General Holder. Today's takedown is the latest sign we're turning the tide on Medicare fraud with greater collaboration and a stronger commitment than ever before.

Attorney General Holder just described how our law enforcement measures have increased anti-fraud prosecutions and led to record recoveries. We've done so by coordinating across agencies. We've pooled resources and shared the tools at our disposal.

And this takedown clearly shows that the Affordable Care Act is one of the best tools we have to preserve Medicare and protect the tens of millions of Americans who rely on it each day.

One of the most important ways the law made a difference in these cases is by expanding our authority to suspend Medicare payments and reimbursements when fraud is suspected—to better preserve the system and save taxpayer dollars.

Because of the law, we can now suspend Medicare payments and reimbursements when there are credible allegations of fraud. It's a broader authority that helps us aggressively suspend payments and get results faster than in the past.

And the power to suspend payments is just one of the many common sense measures in the Affordable Care Act that make it harder for criminals to submit fraudulent Medicare claims and get paid in the first place.

We're able to stop criminals earlier through license checks and unannounced site visits that screen providers and suppliers who pose a high risk of fraud and abuse. The law increases penalties for Medicare fraud—criminals now face tougher sentences and longer jail time for fraud and for obstructing a fraud investigation.

And the law supports our other tools that use advanced technology, like predictive and data analytics, to better identify where Medicare fraud and abuse is happening the most.

It's clear that the Affordable Care Act safeguards Medicare as the sacred trust and guarantee that it is to our seniors who have spent a lifetime paying into it.

And while we know the range of ways criminals seek to violate that trust and shatter that guarantee, the takedown shows the range of ways we're fighting back—and beating them.

Today's announcement is yet another great result of a partnership that's protecting the health of our seniors and families, and the pocketbooks of American taxpayers.

And we're sending a strong, clear message to anyone seeking to defraud Medicare: You will get caught and you will pay the price. We will protect a sacred trust and an earned guarantee.

I'll stop there and turn it over to Acting Assistant Attorney General of the Criminal Division, Mythili Raman, who will provide more details on the takedown.

复述要点提示（主要信息逻辑点及层次）

Theme:

Affordable Care Act makes it possible for the takedown of Medicare fraud to happen and will effectively safeguard the interests of Americans who rely on Medicare.

Three keynotes of the speech:

1. The takedown is a cooperative effort of the Department of Justice and the Department of Health and Human Services. The two departments have pooled resources and shared tools they have access to.

2. Senior citizens have spent their life paying into Medicare. They should get the guarantee they deserve.

3. Affordable Care Act gives the two departments more power to stop Medicare fraud and better protect the people who rely on Medicare.

- The law gives the power to suspend Medicare payment and reimbursements when there are credible allegations of fraud.
- It also provides other measures to prevent criminals from submitting fraudulent Medicare claims and get payment.
- The law gives the power to make license checks and unannounced site visits, which will help identify health care providers and suppliers who might be involved in Medicare fraud and abuse.
- The law increases penalty for Medicare fraud. Medicare fraud criminals now face tougher sentences and longer jail time.
- The law supports the use of other advanced tools. For example, predictive and analytical tools can be used to find where Medicare fraud and abuse happen the most often.

Text 2

Congratulatory Remarks by Dr. Shin Young-soo, WHO Regional Director for the Western Pacific, at the 10th Annual Meeting of Health Technology Assessment International: "Evidence, Values, and Decision-Making: Science or Art?"

COEX Convention Center, Seoul, Republic of Korea

17 June 2013

Distinguished participants,
Honourable guests,
Ladies and gentlemen,

It is an honour to speak here at the 10th Annual Meeting of Health Technology Assessment International.

I would like to congratulate Health Technology Assessment International, the National Evidence-based Healthcare Collaborating Agency and the Ministry of Health and Welfare of the Republic of Korea for putting together this meeting.

In all, some 750 participants have come from more than 60 countries for this 10th anniversary meeting.

I am especially delighted to be invited to address this group because Health Technology Assessment is increasingly important to our work at WHO.

And its role will become more important in the future as we further customize our efforts to the needs of individual Member States.

In every country, the demand for health care and expenditures on health are increasing. Effective health technologies have been a foundation of many major health gains in recent history.

Unfortunately, government and donor resources are sometimes spent on expensive technologies that benefit few people—while millions lack access to basic, inexpensive lifesaving technologies.

Sometimes the decision to procure technologies can be ad hoc or based on faulty assumptions—more the result of advocacy than science.

To avoid such situations, we must support policy-makers with the evidence they need to select cost-effective and efficient health technologies and interventions.

Attaining universal health coverage requires strong, efficient and well-managed health systems that ensure equitable access.

Access to medicines and health technologies are at the heart of this approach.

But we know we cannot do it all.

Difficult decisions must be made.

Our challenge is to spend more wisely—to provide adequate quality services to as many people as possible with the limited resources at hand.

Health technology assessment—or HTA, as it is known—is an increasingly useful tool in making these tough choices.

HTA can help policy-makers direct resources to the most cost-effective interventions.

By helping define the best interventions, health technology assessment supports the development of universal health coverage.

HTA directly supports policy-makers working to improve access, quality and coverage of health care—the three stepping stones to universal health coverage.

One of the most inspiring developments I have seen as Regional Director for the

Western Pacific has been the incorporation of universal health coverage by countries into their national planning.

We must make certain, however, that this commitment does not fade.

Universal health coverage cannot become something that we keep moving toward but never reach.

Today HTA is applied primarily in high-income countries. However, there is a great need for HTA in low-and middle-income countries.

Where resources are tighter, buying decisions should be tougher. A systematic cost-containment process should be part of this increased scrutiny.

A number of HTA models have been developed around the world over the past decade. Many of you here have helped develop one or more of them.

You even may have played a role in convincing decision-makers to set up legal frameworks and integrate HTA in health-financing decisions.

Your work deserves praise. You have contributed to more equitable and fair allocation of resources and improved access.

But capacity needs to be developed further in many lower income countries in order to ensure the sustainability of universal health coverage.

To that end, many of you here have been actively promoting Health Technology Assessment.

You have done a commendable job of collaborating to build capacity in Europe, Asia, Latin America and other parts of the world.

Now more than ever, we need greater technical cooperation between all stakeholders. This critical link will allow us to strengthen regulatory authorities and improve the HTA-regulatory interface.

In the coming years, WHO will continue to expand its support for priority-setting and rationalizing investments in technologies.

To do this well, we need to focus on reducing waste as we improve quality and efficiency.

Increasingly, we need to sharpen strategies to move away from wasteful technologies—and redirect limited resources to more cost-effective interventions.

This is a critical task and a challenge for all countries as we move ahead with HTA implementation.

For years WHO has been working with international organizations and WHO collaborating centres.

We continue to actively extend collaboration with HTA organizations at the global, regional and national levels.

As always, WHO is ready to support and use its convening power to increase the role of health technology assessment in the decision-making process.

In fact, yesterday I convened an informal roundtable with global leaders and HTA experts. This meeting was short but productive.

As you know, WHO is the world's leading public health authority with many programmes, addressing everything from infant mortality to healthy aging.

As such, we have the power to bring all the parties to the table. But the solutions and follow through must come from you—the experts at the operational level.

I am eager to hear more about your work to help ensure value for money when investing in health technologies.

Working together, we can scale up support for Member States in their drive to build better health systems that serve all their people.

Thank you.

复述要点提示（主要信息逻辑点及层次）

主题：

卫生技术评估，即HTA，帮助政策制定者更好地做出决策，将有限的资源用于最具成本效益比的卫生技术，从而给更多人提供高质量服务，并实现医疗卫生服务覆盖全民。

背景：

卫生技术评估国际组织的第10届年会在韩国首尔举行，世界卫生组织西太平洋区域主任申英秀博士应邀发表开幕致辞。

四个要点：

1. 对与会者的介绍

参会人员约750名，来自60多个国家，参会人员中很多人是卫生技术评估的专家，对卫生技术评估工作做出大量贡献。例如：

●协助决策者做出购买卫生技术的相关决定；

●开发不同HTA模型；

●参与说服决策者设立法律框架，将HTA融入卫生筹资决策；

●他们的工作促进了卫生资源的均等化、公正的分配，改善了卫生服务的获取途径；

●努力推广卫生技术评估。

2. HTA的重要性

世界各国卫生服务的需求在增加，对健康的支出也在增加，有效的卫生技术可以帮助实现重大健康收益。

但是有关采购卫生技术的决策往往不科学，政府购买昂贵的技术，但结果受益人少。更重要的问题——实现全民卫生服务覆盖，没有得到解决。仍然有许多人缺乏基本的、廉价的卫生技术的获取途径。

HTA为决策者提供所需证据，更好地选择低成本高效益和高效率的医疗技术和干预方式。

3. HTA的作用

目前世界面临的挑战是要更明智地使用经费：以有限的可使用资源，为尽可能多的人提供充足的优质服务。在这方面，HTA可以发挥最大作用，帮助决策者将资源用于最具成本效益的干预措施。

HTA帮助决策者选择最佳干预方式，改善卫生服务的获取途径、质量和覆盖面，从而实现全民卫生服务覆盖。

在资源紧张的情况下，对采购决策的审查也应更严格，审查应包括系统化的成本控制程序。

4. 未来的发展

应有更多利益相关者参与技术合作，加强HTA在监管中的作用。WHO会和HTA机构在各个层面上进行更多合作。WHO将协助促进HTA在决策过程中发挥作用。

五、英译汉练习

Text 3

The Silent Scandal of Patient Safety (Excerpt)

The Rt Hon Jeremy Hunt MP, Minister of the Department of Health
UCLH, London
21 June 2013

If we are to improve the silent scandal of patient safety across the NHS[1] we need a new culture of openness, transparency and accountability.

Florence Nightingale said, "The very first requirement in a hospital is that it should do the sick no harm."

The many dedicated doctors and nurses I have met as Health Secretary would all agree.

Thanks to their commitment, the Commonwealth Fund[2] consistently rates safety in the NHS ahead of France, Germany, Sweden, Norway and the US.

But is it as good as it should be? Julie Bailey, James Titcombe and other brave campaigners who have lost their loved ones know the answer to that question is unequivocally "No".

---

1 NHS (National Health Service)，即英国国民医疗保健系统，主要经费来源于税收，是英国社会福利制度中最重要的部分之一。英国所有的纳税人和在英国有居住权的人都享有免费使用该体系服务的权利。其服务原则是：不论个人收入如何，只根据个人的不同需要，为人们提供全面的、免费的医疗服务。

2 Commonwealth Fund，英联邦基金会。1918年安娜·哈克尼斯捐出私人财产1 000万美元成立了英联邦基金，并把“为人类的社会保障做点事”作为基金会的宗旨。自1918年以来，基金会的工作一直都是把“让人们生活更健康”作为中心，同时帮助特殊群体解决被众人忽略的问题。20世纪20年代以后，基金会重点发展了儿童领域和日渐凸现的社区公共卫生领域。20年代晚期至40年代，基金会帮助乡村医院开展建设，使这些地区的医疗护理设备达到高标准。

In the wake of Mid Staffs[1], Morecambe Bay[2] and many other shocking lapses in care, we must ask ourselves whether we, along with other countries, have become so numbed to the inevitability of patient harm that we accept the unacceptable.

That grim fatalism about the statistics has blunted the anger that we should feel about every single individual we let down, anger that should be the fuel of an uncompromising determination to put things right.

It is time for a major rethink.

The NHS sees getting on for 3 million people every week. On the basis of the statistics we have, around 0.4% of those ended up with incidents of harm. 0.003% ended with a person's death.

This is a tiny proportion of the total number of people treated. But even those figures amount to nearly half a million people harmed unnecessarily every year. And 3,000 people who lost their lives last year—not despite our best efforts, but because of failures in our efforts. That's more than 8 patients dying needlessly every single day in our wards and operating theatres.

Like the woman who tragically died because her notes were mixed up with someone else, so she ended up with 8 different doctors prescribing 25 different drugs—including many for a condition she didn't have.

Or the woman who died shortly after being prescribed penicillin by a GP, even though the GP had been told she was allergic to it.

Or the 95 year old lady who starved to death because her drip was not fitted properly and over an entire week—the last week of her life—nobody checked to see if it was working.

All stories I have received in the last couple of months in my postbag.

I will never forget the first time I met Professor Norman Williams, President of the Royal College of Surgeons. I was a rather green Health Secretary with no medical background. At that meeting, he told me about something I had never heard of before—the concept of "never events," events so totally unacceptable and patently avoidable that they

---

1 Mid Staffs指英国斯塔福德郡医院丑闻（Stafford Hospital scandal）。英国政府2010年2月公布的一份调查报告显示，斯塔福德郡医院2005年至2009年存在严重玩忽职守行为，许多病人因得不到应有治疗而使病情加重甚至死亡。该医院为公立医院，由中斯塔福德郡NHS信托基金会（Mid Staffordshire NHS Foundation Trust）管理。

2 Morecambe Bay，莫克姆湾拾贝惨案。莫克姆湾是位于英国西北部兰开夏郡的一个小海湾，距英国兰开斯特市约10公里，一向以风急浪高、多流沙著称，因盛产鸟蛤而闻名。2004年2月5日晚，30多名劳工在莫克姆海滩拾贝时被突然上涨的海潮围困，其中23人丧生。随后的消息证实，这23名年龄在18岁到45岁的遇难者都是非法移民。

should simply never happen.

So I looked up the figures.

In 2011/12, there were 326 never events—although international studies suggest there is likely to be significant under-reporting. But the ones we know about include 161 people with foreign objects left in their bodies, like swabs or surgical instruments; 70 people suffering wrong site surgery, where the wrong part of the body or even the wrong patient was operated on; and 41 people given incorrect implants or prostheses.

Put another way—every other day we leave a foreign object in someone's body, every week we operate on the wrong part of someone's body, and every fortnight we insert the wrong implant.

This is the silent scandal of our NHS.

Text 4

Attorney General Eric Holder Speaks at the Medicare Fraud Strike Force Press Conference

14 May 2013

Good afternoon—and thank you all for being here. Today, I'm joined by Secretary [Kathleen] Sebelius, of the Department of Health and Human Services; Acting Assistant Attorney General [Mythili] Raman, of the Justice Department's Criminal Division; Assistant Director [Ron] Hosko, of the FBI; Inspector General [Daniel] Levinson, of the HHS Office of Inspector General; and Dr. [Peter] Budetti, Deputy Administrator for Program Integrity of the Centers for Medicare and Medicaid Services—in announcing the latest steps forward in the federal government's ongoing efforts to combat fraud and abuse in our health-care systems.

As part of a coordinated, nationwide takedown—the sixth that the Medicare Fraud Strike Force and its partners have conducted—this afternoon, we announce charges against 89 defendants in eight different cities for their alleged participation in fraud schemes to submit more than $220 million in false billings to Medicare. These defendants are accused of a variety of crimes involving the fraudulent use of Medicare information obtained illegally from elderly or low-income individuals; the submission of false billings for treatments that were never provided, or were performed by unlicensed individuals; and a range of other schemes that placed the safety of innocent people at risk in order to achieve illicit financial gain.

The Departments of Justice and Health and Human Services—working alongside federal, state, and local partners—will not tolerate such activities. We will use every appropriate tool and available resource to find, stop, and punish those who seek to take advantage of their fellow citizens. And our commitment to protecting the American people from all forms of health-care fraud, safeguarding taxpayer resources, and ensuring the integrity of essential health-care programs—such as Medicare and Medicaid—has never been stronger.

Four years ago this month, this commitment drove us to launch a new, joint initiative known as the Health Care Fraud Prevention and Enforcement Action Team—or, HEAT. As a result of this groundbreaking initiative, we've leveraged the strength of key federal, state, and local partnerships in order to take our comprehensive fight against health-care fraud to a new level. Through the enhanced efforts of our criminal Medicare Fraud Strike Force, we've bolstered our ability to identify and shut down fraud schemes across the country. And this work has yielded extraordinary results.

As a result of Strike Force operations conducted since 2007, we've filed charges against more than 1,500 individuals in connection with schemes involving over $5 billion in false billings. Over the last three fiscal years, for every dollar we've spent fighting against health-care fraud, we've returned an average of nearly eight dollars to the U.S. Treasury, the Medicare Trust Fund, and others. And our actions have helped to deter other would-be criminals from even attempting to defraud Medicare.

For example, after the Strike Force targeted group psychotherapy fraud in Detroit, we've seen amounts billed to Medicare for this type of treatment drop by more than 70 percent since January 2011. Just two years after Strike Force operations in Miami identified and targeted widespread fraud in the home health industry—and launched an initiative that led to numerous arrests and lengthy prison sentences—Medicare billings for home health services in the State of Florida dropped by more than $1 billion. And payments to providers fell by roughly $500 million.

We can all be proud of this remarkable progress. We should be encouraged by the significant actions we announce today. But we cannot yet be satisfied.

Unfortunately, our ability to keep building on this work, to backfill critical positions, and to strengthen Strike Force operations is being negatively impacted by sequestration[1]—which, earlier this year, cut over $1.6 billion from the Justice Department's budget for Fiscal Year 2013. Unless Congress adopts a balanced deficit reduction plan and stops the reductions currently slated for 2014, I fear that our capacity to protect the American people from health-care fraud, to safeguard vital programs and precious resources, and to hold criminals accountable—will be further reduced.

Allowing these cuts would be both unwise and unacceptable. Despite recent achievements, our work is far from over. Significant challenges lie ahead. And that's why we must remain steadfast in our determination to strengthen current efforts—and keep fighting to make the positive difference our citizens need and deserve.

I'd like to thank each of the approximately 400 law enforcement officials who made arrests, executed search warrants, and otherwise participated in the investigative and enforcement actions that made today's announcement possible. At this time, I'd like to turn things over to another key leader of this work—my good friend, Secretary Kathleen Sebelius—who will provide additional details.

1 sequestration或sequester，美国自动减支制度，指将自动生效的一系列联邦支出削减措施，属于2011年美国《预算控制法案》的规定内容。该法案规定，民主党和共和党的议员将组成一个减赤“超级委员会”，负责拟定十年内削减1.2万亿美元预算的具体方案，否则2013年初将启动自动减支机制。根据自动减支机制要求，美国将在9年内总体削减支出1.2万亿美元。

六、汉译英练习

Text 5

中华人民共和国卫生部尹力副部长在全国药物政策与基本药物制度[1]工作会议上的讲话

2012年7月3日

2009年3月，中央启动了新一轮深化医药卫生体制改革，明确将初步建立基本药物制度作为五项重点改革任务之一。三年来，在各级党委、政府的坚强领导下，卫生部门加强与有关部门的协调配合，加快工作进度，不断完善政策，改革体制机制，在基本药物制度建设和药物政策研究方面做了大量工作，取得明显成效。

（一）基本药物制度覆盖全部政府办基层医疗卫生机构。根据中央统一部署，到2010年2月底，全国各省（区、市）选择30%左右的政府办基层医疗卫生机构先行实施基本药物制度；到2010年底，基本药物制度覆盖全国60%左右的地区；2011年7月，各省（区、市）和新疆生产建设兵团提前实现了基本药物制度在所有政府办基层医疗卫生机构全覆盖的目标。

（二）构建新的基本药物采购机制。在总结地方做法并参照国际经验的基础上，2010年11月，国务院办公厅印发了《建立和规范政府办基层医疗卫生机构基本药物采购机制的指导意见》，要求建立以招采合一、量价挂钩、双信封制[2]、集中支付、全程监控[3]等为核心内容的基本药物采购新机制。目前，各省（区、市）都建立了政府主导的省级非营利性药品集中采购平台，多数省份已完成基本药物集中采购工作。河南、山东等一些省份还将非政府办基层医疗卫生机构纳入基本药物集中采购范围。

（三）推动基层医疗卫生机构综合改革。为配合和支持基本药物制度建设，各

---

1 中国国家基本药物制度是对基本药物目录制定、生产供应、采购配送、合理使用、价格管理、支付报销、质量监管、监测评价等多个环节实施有效管理的制度。国家基本医药制度可以改善目前的药品供应保障体系，保障人民群众的安全用药。国家将基本药物全部纳入基本医疗保障药品目录，报销比例明显高于非基本药物，降低个人自付比例，用经济手段引导广大群众首先使用基本药物。主要先由基层医疗机构开始执行。

2 双信封评标法是指投标人将投标报价和工程量清单单独密封在一个报价信封中，其他商务和技术文件密封在另外一个信封中，分两次开标的评标方法。

3 全程监控指药物采购从招标到付款整个过程所有环节的监控。

地开展了基层医疗卫生机构综合改革，积极推动人事制度、收入分配、绩效管理等机制改革，以投入换新机制，以新机制促发展、增活力。基层医疗卫生机构服务效率不断提高，服务能力显著增强。2011年，基层医疗卫生机构总诊疗人次比2009年增加了12.2%。

（四）基本药物制度有序拓展延伸。按照乡村医疗卫生机构联动、政府和非政府办医疗卫生机构联动、基层和二三级医院联动的工作思路，有序推进基本药物制度建设。各地按照国务院办公厅下发的《关于进一步加强乡村医生队伍建设的指导意见》要求，克服体制性障碍，推进村卫生室实施基本药物制度，重庆、山西等一些省份已率先实现村卫生室全覆盖。浙江、河南等13个省份结合推进公立医院改革，规定了本省二级以上公立医院配备使用基本药物品种和金额的比例，促进基本药物在不同医疗机构间的优先、合理使用。

（五）初步形成基本药物制度政策框架。在中央医改方针政策的总体框架下，由各有关部门组建了国家基本药物制度工作委员会，负责解决建立国家基本药物制度过程中各个环节的相关政策问题。2009年8月，颁布了2009年版《国家基本药物目录（基层部分）》，制定和发行了国家基本药物临床应用指南和处方集。同时，参照世界卫生组织以基本药物制度为核心的国家药物政策思路，协调有关地方和专业机构，启动并开展了涵盖基本药物遴选、药品可负担性、筹资机制、供应保障、质量监管、合理使用、监测评估等方面的研究，并提出了一系列政策建议。在此基础上，卫生部与有关部门研究制定了基本药物生产供应、定价、报销、质量监管等方面的政策措施，初步构建形成了基本药物制度框架。

总结基本药物制度实施三年来的成效，主要表现在五个方面：一是促进了基本药物的合理使用和足量供应。基层医务人员用药行为更加规范合理，减少了药品滥用，加强了药品质量的全程监管，保证了药品质量和用药安全。二是改革了基层医疗卫生机构“以药补医”机制。全面取消延续了半个多世纪的药品加成政策，同步推进基层综合改革，促进了基层运行新机制的建立。三是促进了药品生产流通企业优化重组。通过实施新的基本药物招标采购机制，带动了药品生产、流通、定价、使用、监管等各个环节的改革，推动了药品生产流通领域的结构调整、优化整合，促进了医药产业发展和科研水平的提升。四是患者用药负担大为减轻。通过零差率销售、压缩药品虚高价格等多种措施，基本药物在基层的销售价格较制度实施前平均下降约30%，有效控制了医药费用的不合理增长。五是培养和造就了一支管理人才队伍。卫生部和省级卫生行政部门建立了药物政策和基本药物制度管理机构，加强了管理人员队伍建设，开展了相关政策和业务培训，行业指导能力、服务水平和监管能力不断提升，保障了重点、难点工作的顺利开展。

Text 6

卫生部部长陈竺、党组书记张茅致2012年新年贺词

2011年12月31日

值此2012年新年即将来临之际，我们谨代表卫生部向全国卫生工作者致以新年的祝福和诚挚的问候！向关心、支持卫生事业发展的各级党委政府及有关部门，向社会各界、新闻媒体和广大人民群众表示衷心的感谢！

2011年，全国卫生系统以科学发展观为指导，群策群力，锐意进取，攻坚克难，谋全局、抓改革、促发展，大力推进深化医药卫生体制改革，深入开展以“三好一满意”[1]为实践载体的创先争优活动，各项卫生工作取得积极进展。

2011年，新型农村合作医疗制度进一步巩固完善，新农合参合率达97%。国家基本药物制度初步建立，政府办基层医疗卫生机构全面实施基本药物制度，群众用药负担明显减轻。覆盖城乡的基层医疗卫生服务体系不断健全，以全科医生为重点的基层卫生人才队伍建设逐步加强。公共卫生服务能力稳步提高，农村居民、困难群体和特殊群体得到重点保障。公立医院改革试点积极推进，便民惠民措施全面推开。

2011年，重大疾病防控工作得到加强，有效应对各种突发公共卫生事件。医疗质量安全和医疗服务监管进一步强化，医疗费用控制取得初步成效。食品安全、卫生监督和药品监管工作不断加强。有利于发挥中医药特色的体制、机制建设和投入政策逐步推进。卫生人才队伍建设、科技创新、信息化建设等支撑体系得到加强。

成绩来之不易，挑战依然严峻。2012年，我们将在党中央、国务院的坚强领导下，紧紧依靠全国卫生系统广大干部职工，团结奋斗，开拓创新，勇于担当，做好“十二五”期间卫生改革发展各项工作，促进医药卫生事业持续健康发展，提供群众满意的医疗卫生服务。

新的一年，深化医改进入攻坚阶段。全国卫生系统要进一步提高科学发展卫生事业的能力和水平，继续按照党中央、国务院对深化医改的部署和保基本、强基层、建机制的要求，在健全基本医疗保障制度、巩固完善国家基本药物制度和积极推进公立医院改革等方面实现重点突破。

新的一年，我们将认真总结新农合实施十周年来的经验，提高新农合筹资标准和农民受益水平。普遍开展门诊医疗费用统筹，逐步提高门诊补偿水平。提高新农

1 “三好一满意”是指：服务好、质量好、医德好、群众满意。为了落实深化医药卫生体制改革工作要求，深入开展创先争优活动，加强行业作风建设，卫生部决定在全国医疗卫生系统开展“三好一满意”活动。

合基金统筹层次[1]，以省为单位全面推开重大疾病保障工作。继续推进基层医疗卫生机构综合改革。巩固完善国家基本药物制度，扩大实施范围，确保群众基本用药。系统总结公立医院改革试点工作中取得的经验，以改革“以药补医”机制为关键环节，开展县级医院综合改革试点。继续推行优质护理服务、预约诊疗、便民门诊等便民惠民措施，优化就诊环境和流程，稳步推进“先诊疗、后结算”模式，控制医疗费用不合理增长。

新的一年，我们将加强医疗服务管理，保障医疗安全。进一步加大医疗机构设置规划管理力度，明确公立医院功能定位，优化公立医院布局结构，重点加强薄弱地区及专科医疗服务能力建设。支持社会资本开办医疗机构。加快建立公立医院与基层医疗卫生机构分工合作机制，逐步实现基层首诊、分级医疗、双向转诊、急慢分治的格局。完善公立医院人事和收入分配制度，继续推进医师多点执业，提高医务人员待遇水平，营造良好的医疗执业环境，充分调动医务人员积极性。

新的一年，我们将全面推进基本公共卫生服务逐步均等化，继续做好卫生应急、疾病防控和妇幼卫生工作；依法加强食品安全工作，强化卫生监督；完善药品科学监管体系，维护公众用药安全；发挥中医药特色和优势，不断提高中医药服务水平；深入开展创先争优活动，严肃查处商业贿赂案件和损害群众利益的不正之风问题，开创卫生改革发展新局面，努力缓解群众“看病难、看病贵”，以优异成绩迎接党的十八大胜利召开。祝大家新年愉快，身体健康，工作顺利，万事如意！

资料来源：

Text 1 http://www.justice.gov/opa/gallery/health-care-fraud-takedown-press-conference

Text 2 http://www.wpro.who.int/regional_director/speeches/2013/coex-korea-17jun2013/en/

Text 3 https://www.gov.uk/government/speeches/the-silent-scandal-of-patient-safety

Text 4 http://www.justice.gov/opa/speech/attorney-general-eric-holder-speaks-medicare-fraud-strike-force-press-conference-0

Text 5 http://www.moh.gov.cn/mohzcfgs/s6774/201208/55640.shtml

Text 6 http://news.cntv.cn/china/20111231/118672.shtml

1 提高新农合基金统筹层次：新农合原本以县、市、区为统筹单位，但低层次统筹导致新农合基金抗风险能力弱，区域间补偿政策不一致，影响了农村居民享受新农合制度的公平性，2012年开始开展新农合市级统筹工作，扩大基金规模，在市州范围内统一政策，提高参合农民的受益程度，巩固农民参合积极性。

参考答案

四、摘要练习

Text 1

医疗保险制度欺诈突击小组临检行动新闻发布会

美国卫生和公共服务部（HHS）凯瑟琳·西贝利厄斯部长
美国华盛顿特区
2013年5月14日

谢谢你，霍尔德司法部长。今天的临检行动是政府的最新姿态，为了扭转医疗保险欺诈行为的局势，我们将进行更多合作，做出比以往任何时候都更强有力的承诺。

霍尔德司法部长只是描述了我们如何通过执法措施增加了防欺诈起诉，并创纪录地追回款项。我们完成这些工作是通过跨机构协调，我们汇集资源，并共享可以使用的工具。

此次临检行动清楚地表明，平价医疗法案是我们维持医疗保险，保护数以千万计每天依靠它的美国人的最佳工具之一。

在这些情况下，平价医疗法案产生影响最重要的方法之一是扩大我们的权力，当怀疑欺诈时，暂停医保支付和报销，从而更好地维护医保系统，并为纳税人省钱。

由于法律规定，在出现可信的欺诈指控时，我们可以暂停医保支付和报销。平价医疗法案赋予我们更广泛的权力，帮助我们积极实施暂停付款，并比过去更快地得到结果。

暂停支付的权力仅仅是平价医疗法案许多常识性措施中的一项，这些措施使违法犯罪者难以提交欺诈性的医保索赔申请，并获得赔付。

通过许可证检查和现场突击检查，甄别医疗卫生服务机构和供应商，找出其中存在欺诈和滥用高风险的机构和供应商，这样我们能够更早地制止违法犯罪者。平价医疗法案增加了对医疗保险欺诈行为的处罚——若进行欺诈和妨碍欺诈调查，犯罪分子现在面临更严厉的刑罚和更久的服刑时间。

平价医疗法案支持我们使用其他工具，这些工具采用先进科技，例如预测分析和数据分析科技等，帮助我们更好地找出医疗保险欺诈和滥用发生最多的地方。

很明显平价医疗法案保障了医保对老年人所代表的神圣信任和保障，他们终生为医保支付费用。

尽管我们知道犯罪分子尽其所能寻找破坏信任、粉碎保证的方式，临检行动显示了我们反击、打败他们的各种办法。

今天的公告是合作关系的又一项重要结果，通过这个合作关系，我们保护老年人和家庭的健康，保护美国纳税人的荷包。

我们发出了一个强烈和清晰的信息，告诉任何试图进行医保欺诈的人：你会被逮住，你将为此付出代价。我们将保护医保的神圣信任和人们应得的保障。

我就讲这么多，下面交给代理助理司法部长迈西丽·拉曼，她负责分管司法部刑事司，她将提供更多临检行动的细节。

Text 2

世界卫生组织西太平洋区域主任申英秀博士在卫生技术评估国际协会第10届年会“证据、价值观、决策：科学还是艺术？”上的祝词

韩国首尔会展中心

2013年6月17日

尊敬的与会者，

尊贵的来宾们，

女士们、先生们：

很荣幸在卫生技术评估国际协会第10届年会上发言。

我想祝贺卫生技术评估国际协会、韩国国家循证医疗卫生合作机构和韩国卫生福利部成功组织这次会议。

共有约750名来自60多个国家的人参加这次10周年的会议。

我特别高兴受到邀请来发表讲话，因为卫生技术评估对我们世卫组织的工作具有越来越重要的意义。

而且随着我们更进一步根据各个成员国的具体需求进行相应工作，卫生技术评估在未来将会发挥更加重要的作用。

每个国家对医疗卫生服务的需求和在健康方面的支出都在增加。有效的卫生技术在近代历史上为许多重大的健康收益奠定了基础。

不幸的是，政府和捐助者的资源有时花费在昂贵的技术上，却只有少数人受益，而数以百万计的人缺乏基本的、价格低廉的卫生技术的获取途径。

有时采购技术的决定只是临时性的或基于错误的假设，是倡导带来的结果，但

不是科学的决定。

为了避免这种情况，我们必须支持决策者，为他们提供需要的证据，帮助他们更好地选择低成本、高效益、高效率的医疗技术和干预方式。

实现医疗卫生服务覆盖全民，需要强大、高效、管理良好、能保障获取途径均等化的医疗卫生系统。

其核心是药品和卫生技术的获取途径。

但我们知道，我们不可能做到面面俱到。

我们必须做出艰难的决定。

我们面临的挑战是如何更明智地使用经费：以有限的可用资源，为尽可能多的人提供足够的优质服务。

在做出这些艰难的抉择时，卫生技术评估——或简称为HTA——是一个越来越有用的工具。

HTA可以帮助决策者将资源用于最具成本效益的干预措施。

通过帮助确定最佳干预方式，卫生技术评估支持医疗卫生服务覆盖全民的发展。

HTA直接支持政策制定者改善获取途径、质量、卫生保健覆盖面的工作，这三项都是医疗卫生服务覆盖全民的必经步骤。

作为西太平洋区域主任，我所看到的最鼓舞人心的一项发展是，一些政府已将医疗卫生服务覆盖全民纳入国家规划。

然而，我们必须确保这一承诺不会湮没无闻。

医疗卫生服务覆盖全民不能成为我们一直努力但永远不能实现的目标。

今天HTA主要应用于高收入国家。然而，低收入和中等收入国家也对HTA有巨大需求。

在资源紧张的情况下，关于采购的决策会更困难，审查也应更严格，审查中应包括系统化的成本控制流程。

在过去的十年中，世界各地已开发出一些不同的HTA模型。你们当中许多人曾经参与一个或多个HTA模型的开发过程。

你们甚至可能还曾参与说服决策者设立法律框架，将HTA融入卫生筹资决策。

你们的工作值得赞扬，你们对均等化、公正分配资源和改善获取途径做出了贡献。

但许多低收入国家还有待进一步提高能力，以确保医疗卫生服务覆盖全民的可持续性。

为了实现这个目标，你们许多人一直在积极推广卫生技术评估。

在欧洲、亚洲、拉丁美洲和世界其他地区，你们已经完成了值得称道的工作，合作进行能力建设。

我们现在比以往任何时候都更需要所有利益相关者进行更多的技术合作。这个关键环节将使我们能够加强监管部门、改善HTA——监管界面。

在未来几年内，世卫组织将继续扩大支持，促进决定工作上的轻重缓急和对科技的合理化投入。

要做好这些工作，我们需要把重点放在提高质量和效率的同时减少浪费上。

我们有越来越多的需求，应当提升战略，摒弃造成浪费的技术，并把有限的资源重新转向用于更具成本效益的干预措施。

这是我们实施HTA的道路上，所有国家面临的一个重要的任务和挑战。

世界卫生组织多年来一直和其他国际组织、世卫组织合作性中心进行合作。

在全球、区域和国家层面，我们将继续积极扩大和HTA机构的合作。

与往常一样，世卫组织已做好准备提供支持和运用其号召力，以增强卫生技术评估在决策过程中的作用。

事实上，昨天我召集了一个非正式圆桌会议，全球领导人和HTA专家参加了会议。这次会议虽然简短，但很富有成效。

正如你们所知道的，世卫组织是世界领先的公共卫生权威，世卫组织有许多项目，解决从婴儿死亡率到老年健康等各种问题。

因此，我们有能力让所有相关方参与讨论。但解决方案及其贯彻实施必须来自你们——因为你们是操作层面的专家。

我渴望听到更多关于你们工作的介绍，了解你们怎样确保卫生技术上的投资物有所值。

通过合作，我们可以扩大对成员国的支持，帮助他们建立更好的卫生系统，为所有的人提供服务。

谢谢。

五、英译汉练习

Text 3

无声的病人安全丑闻（节选）

英国卫生部部长杰里米·亨特议员阁下
英国伦敦大学医院
2013年6月21日

如果要改善整个国民医疗保健系统，即NHS，应对无声的病人安全丑闻，我们需要一种新文化，具备公开性、透明度、问责制度。

弗罗伦斯·南丁格尔曾说过：“对医院的第一个要求是：对病人不造成危害。”

作为卫生大臣，我遇见过的许多富有奉献精神的医生和护士都会同意这个观点。

由于他们的努力，英联邦基金给NHS的安全评分始终领先于法国、德国、瑞典、挪威和美国。

但是，NHS是否达到应有的良好状态？朱莉·贝利、詹姆斯·蒂特科姆和其他失去了亲人的勇敢的活动家知道，这个问题的明确答案是“没有”。

继斯塔福德医院丑闻、莫克姆湾拾贝惨案和其他许多令人震惊的医疗过失事件之后，我们必须扪心自问，我们是否与其他国家一起，已经变得如此麻木，所以接受了病人伤害是不可避免的这样不可接受的态度。

这种关于数据的残酷宿命论减弱了我们的愤怒，让他人失望时我们不再那么愤怒，而正是这种愤怒刺激我们坚定决心，一定要纠正错误。

我们现在应当进行认真反思。

NHS每周为约300万人提供服务。根据我们手中的统计数据看，其中约0.4%的人最终发生伤害事故，0.003%以病人死亡结束。

就治疗病人的总数来看，这个比例很低。但即使是这些数字结果也会最终造成每年约50万人受到不必要的伤害。去年3 000人失去了生命，他们没有得到我们最大努力的帮助，我们工作中的失误导致他们的死亡。换算一下数字，这等于在我们的病房和手术室里，每一天有8例以上患者不必要地死亡。

例如有位妇女悲惨地死去，因为她的医疗记录与别人的混在一起，结果8个不同的医生给她开了25种不同的药物，其中许多药物治疗的是她没有的疾病。

另一位妇女使用青霉素后迅速死亡，她的全科医生在被告知她对青霉素过敏后，却仍然给她开了青霉素的处方。

还有一位95岁的女性病人被饿死，因为她的静脉注射用药没有正确实施，在她的生命的最后一周，整整一周期间，没有人检查过点滴是否正常。

所有这些故事都来自过去的几个月里我收到的公众来信。

我永远不会忘记第一次会见皇家外科医学院院长诺曼·威廉姆斯教授的情形。当时我是一个既没有医学背景，也没有什么经验的卫生大臣。在那次会议上，他告诉我一个我从来没有听说过的概念——“绝不事件”。这类事件完全不可接受，而且明显可以避免，因此它们本应该永远不会发生。

所以，我查找了相关数据。

在2011至2012年度，有326起“绝不事件”，但国际研究表明，很有可能很多事件没有被报告。但是，我们知道的“绝不事件”包括161人体内留有异物、棉签或手术器械等；70人发生手术部位错误，其中有些是错误的身体部位进行手术，有些甚至是错误的病人接受手术；41人接受错误的植入物或假体。

换句话说，每一天，我们会在一位病人的体内留下异物；每个星期，我们会在一位病人身上的错误部位进行手术；每隔一周，我们会给一个病人插入错误的植入物。

这就是我们NHS无声的丑闻。

Text 4

美国司法部长埃里克·霍尔德
在医疗保险制度欺诈突击小组临检行动新闻发布会上的讲话

2013年5月14日

下午好！谢谢大家出席今天的新闻发布会。今天，和我一起出席新闻发布会的还有卫生和公共服务部凯瑟琳·西贝利厄斯部长、分管司法部刑事司的代理助理司法部长迈西丽·拉曼、联邦调查局副局长罗恩·霍斯科、卫生和公共服务部检察长办公室的丹尼尔·莱文森检察长，以及医疗补助和医疗保险服务中心分管程序廉正的副主任彼得·布代蒂博士，我们将一起宣布联邦政府在打击医疗保健欺诈、滥用行为过程中采取的最新举措。

这次行动是一个全国范围内协调进行的临检行动，也是医疗保险欺诈突击小组及其合作伙伴已经进行的第六次行动。作为这次行动的一部分，今天下午，我们宣布对89名被告提出指控，他们涉嫌参与欺诈计划，向医疗保险申报超过2.2亿美元的虚假医疗费用。这些被告人被指控的各种犯罪涉及非法获取和冒用老年人、低收入个人的医保信息；通过凭空捏造治疗或由无执照的个人实施治疗，申报虚假医疗费用；以及为了牟取非法经济利益，实施一系列其他计划使无辜的人处于危险之中。

司法部、卫生与公共服务部、联邦、州和当地的合作伙伴一起合作，不会容忍这样的活动。我们将利用一切适当的工具和可用资源，发现、制止、惩罚那些企图欺骗他们的同胞的人。我们承诺保护美国人民免遭各种形式的医保欺诈，保护纳税人的资源，确保基本医疗保健服务的健全，例如医疗保险和医疗补助的完整性，我们的承诺从未如此强大。

四年前的这个月，这一承诺促使我们推出一项新的联合倡议，被称为医疗保健欺诈预防和执法行动小组，或简称HEAT。作为这一突破性举措的结果，我们已经利用联邦、州、当地合作伙伴的关键力量，将医疗保健欺诈的全面打击工作带到一个新的层面。通过医疗保险制度欺诈突击小组的加倍努力，我们已经增强了发现并关闭全国各地的欺诈计划的能力。这项工作已经取得了非凡的成果。

作为自2007年以来突击小组进行的行动的结果，我们已经对1 500多名个人提出控告，他们涉嫌申报超过50亿美元虚假费用。在过去三个财政年度，我们每用一美元打击医疗保健欺诈，就能平均为美国财政部、医保信托基金和其他机构收回近8美元。我们的行动有助于制止其他潜在的罪犯产生对医保进行欺诈的企图。

例如，在突击小组针对底特律的团体心理治疗欺诈采取行动后，我们看到自2011年1月起这种类型治疗的医疗费用金额减少了70%以上。突击小组在迈阿密发现家庭健康行业存在普遍欺诈行为，之后推出的举措导致无数的逮捕和长期监禁，仅仅两年后，佛罗里达州家庭健康服务的医疗账单减少超过10亿美元。对医疗服务机构的支付减少了5亿美元。

我们都应当为这一显著进步感到自豪。我们应该为今天宣布的重大行动感到鼓舞振奋。但是，我们还不能就此满足。

不幸的是，我们在原有基础上加强工作的能力，回填关键岗位的能力，加强突击小组行动的能力受到了自动减支政策产生的负面影响。今年早些时候，根据这项政策，司法部2013财政年预算削减超过16亿美元。除非国会采取一个平衡的削减赤字计划，并停止目前计划的对2014年的削减，我担心，我们的能力将进一步减弱，包括保护美国人民免于医疗保健欺诈的危害、保障重要程序和宝贵的资源、追究罪犯责任的能力。

允许这些削减将是不明智的，也是不可接受的。尽管有最近取得的这些成就，我们的工作还远没有结束。前方还有重大挑战。这就是为什么我们必须保持决心，坚定不移地加强当前的努力，并坚持斗争，为我们的人民带来他们需要和应该得到的好的改变。

我想感谢近400名执法官员中的每一个人，由于他们实施逮捕、执行搜查令，并以其他方式参与调查和执法行动，今天的公告才能成为可能。至此，我想把话筒转交给这项工作的另一个主要领导，我的好朋友，凯瑟琳·西贝利厄斯部长，她将提供更多的细节。

六、汉译英练习

Text 5

Remarks by Yin Li, Chinese Vice Minister of Health, at the National Drug Policy and Essential Drugs System Work Conference

3 July 2012

In March, 2009, the Central Government launched a new round of campaign to deepen the health care system reform and explicitly defined the establishment of an essential drugs system as one of the five key tasks of the health care reform. For three years, under the strong leadership of Communist Party committees and governments at all levels, health departments strengthened coordination and cooperation with the departments concerned to accelerate the progress of health care reform, constantly improve the policy, and implement system and institutional reform. Much work has been done for the construction of the essential drugs system and drug policy research, resulting in remarkable achievements.

A. The essential drugs system has covered all public primary health care institutions. According to the coordinated arrangements of the central government, by the end of February 2010, all the provinces (autonomous regions and municipalities) across the country picked out about 30% of the public primary health care institutions and first implemented the essential drugs system in these institutions; by the end of 2010, the national essential drugs system covered about 60% of all the regions across the country; in July 2011, all the provinces (autonomous regions and municipalities) and Xinjiang Production and Construction Corps have reached the target of full coverage of the essential drugs system of all public primary health care institutions in advance.

B. We have built a new essential drugs procurement mechanism. After summing up the experience and lessons from different parts of the country and from other countries, on November, 2010, the State Council issued *Guidance for the Establishment and Regulation of the Essential Drugs Procurement Mechanisms of Public Primary Health Care Institutions*, demanding the establishment of a new mechanism for procurement of essential drugs centered on the following principles: one institution taking charge of both tender offer and procurement, adjusting the price according to the quantity of purchase, two-envelope system for tender bidding, direct payment to the supplier, close monitoring of the whole process, etc. Currently, all the provinces (autonomous regions and municipalities) have established a provincial government-led nonprofit centralized drug procurement platform. Most provinces have completed centralized procurement of essential drugs. Henan, Shandong and a few other provinces have also covered private primary health care institutions with the centralized procurement of essential drugs.

C. We have promoted the comprehensive reform of primary health care institutions. In order to support the construction of the essential drugs system, the local governments have carried out the comprehensive reform of primary health care institutions by actively promoting the reform of mechanisms, including the human resources system, income distribution, and performance management. They have increased input to developing new mechanisms and using new mechanisms to enhance development and vitality. The service efficiency of primary health care institutions has continuously been improved and the service capacity has also been significantly enhanced. In 2011, the total number of patient visits to primary health care institutions increased by 12.2% compared with that of 2009.

D. The essential drugs system has been expanded in a well-organized way. Following the guideline of coordinated action and linkage among rural health care institutions, between public and private health care institutions, and between primary and secondary and tertiary-level hospitals, the construction of the essential drugs system was carried out in a well-organized way. According to the requirement of the State Council's *Suggestions for Further Reinforcement of the Human Resources Development of Rural Doctors*, the local governments have overcome institutional barriers and promoted the implementation of the essential drugs system in village clinics. Chongqing, Shanxi and a number of other provinces were the first ones to have achieved full coverage of all village clinics. Zhejiang, Henan and 13 other provinces combined the reform of public hospitals with the implementation of the essential drugs system. They have issued requirements on the proportion of essential drugs used in secondary and tertiary-level public hospitals, as well as the ratio of the cost of essential drug in the total cost of drugs, promoting the prioritized and rational use of essential drugs in different medical institutions.

E. The policy framework of the essential drugs system has been formed initially. Working under the overall framework of health care reform policies of the central government, the departments concerned established the National Essential Drug System

Working Committee, which is responsible for dealing with the policy issues concerning the various aspects of the whole process of establishing the national essential drug system. The *2009 Edition of National Essential Drugs Inventory (Primary Health Care)* was issued in August, 2009. The national clinical guidelines and formulary of the essential drugs were developed and published. In addition, using as a reference the World Health Organization concept of a national drug policy focused on the essential drugs system, we have coordinated the local organizations and professional organizations concerned to initiate and conduct research on the selection of essential drugs, their affordability, financing mechanisms, the security of supply, quality control, rational use, and monitoring and evaluation. A series of policy recommendations have been made accordingly, on the basis of which, the Ministry of Health and the relevant departments developed policy and measures for the production and supply, pricing, reimbursement, and quality control of essential drugs. Consequently, the framework of the essential drugs system has been initially formed.

In conclusion, the outcomes of the essential drugs system after the implementation of the system started three years can be summed up in the following five aspects: Firstly, we have effectively promoted the rational use and adequate supply of the essential drugs. Grassroots health care workers are now using drugs in a more rational and standardized way, helping reduce drug abuse, strengthen the full-course supervision of drug quality, and ensure drug quality and drug safety. Secondly, we have reformed the mechanism of doctors supplementing their incomes with the drugs they prescribe in the primary health care institutions. We have completely abolished the drug mark-up policy that had been practiced for over half a century in China. In addition, we have simultaneously promoted comprehensive reform and the establishment of new operation mechanisms at the grassroots level. Thirdly, we have promoted the optimized restructuring of pharmaceutical production and distribution companies. The implementation of a new tender bidding mechanism of essential drugs has driven forward the reform of drug production, distribution, pricing, use, and regulation, promoted the structural adjustment, optimization and integration in the field of drug production and distribution, and enhanced the development of the pharmaceutical industry and scientific research. Fourthly, we have greatly reduced patients' financial burden caused by drug cost. Through measures such as making drugs available at wholesale price and mark-down of overpriced drugs, the price of the essential drugs available at primary health care institutions have been reduced by approximately 30% compared to their price before the essential drugs system was implemented. The unreasonable increase in the cost of health care has been effectively put under control. Fifthly, we have helped train a team of management professionals. The Ministry of Health and the provincial health care administrative departments have all established their respective drug policies and management agencies of the essential drugs system. We have reinforced the development of the management personnel and organized policy trainings and professional skills trainings. Throughout the health care sector, the guidance, service and regulatory capabilities have constantly been improving, ensuring the smooth implementation of the key and challenging tasks.

Text 6

Happy New Year Congratulatory Remarks by Chen Zhu, Minister of Health, and Zhang Mao, Secretary of CPC (Communist Party of China) Committee of the Ministry of Health, Government of China

31 December 2011

On this auspicious occasion when 2012, the New Year, is approaching, we would like to extend best wishes and sincere greetings for the New Year to all the health workers in China on behalf of the Ministry of Health! We sincerely appreciate the attention and support given to the development of the health care industry by governments and CPC committees at all levels and the departments concerned, people from various sectors of the society, the media and all the Chinese people!

In 2011, the national health care system used the scientific development concept as a guiding principle, worked hard together, remained determined to forge ahead to tackle tough problems, took a global perspective, focused on reform, and promoted development. We have vigorously promoted the further implementation of medical and health care system reform. We have reinforced our efforts in the striving-for-excellent-performance activities, which are conducted through the support of the "Good Service, Good Quality, Good Medical Ethics and High Satisfaction" activities. We have made positive progress in various aspects of health care.

In 2011, the New Rural Health Care Cooperative System was further consolidated and improved, with enrollment in the system reaching 97%. The National Essential Drugs System was initially established and has already covered all the government-run primary health care institutions, significantly reducing the burden caused by the cost of drugs. We have worked continuously to improve the urban and rural primary health care systems and reinforce the recruitment and training of highly-competent primary-care health workers, especially general practitioners. Public health service capacity has improved steadily. Rural residents, disadvantaged groups and special groups are receiving special protection. We have actively promoted the pilot projects of public hospital reform and fully implemented measures that will bring people convenience and benefits.

In 2011, we have reinforced our efforts in the prevention and control of major diseases and effectively responded to a variety of public health emergency events. The quality and safety of health care have been improved and the supervision of medical services has been further strengthened. Efforts to control health care costs have shown initial effect. Food safety, health care and drug supervision have been continuously strengthened. We have gradually implemented the construction of systems and mechanisms and input policies conducive to the full play of the characteristics of traditional Chinese medicine. Health care personnel recruitment and training, technology innovation, information technology and other support systems have been strengthened.

Even with the hard-won achievements, the challenges we face remain grim. In 2012, under the strong leadership of Central Committee of the Communist Party of China (CPC Central Committee) and the State Council, we will rely heavily on everyone working in the national health system and strive to complete all the tasks incorporated in the health care reform to be implemented during the 12th Five-Year Plan period through solidarity, hard work, innovation, courage and a strong sense of responsibility. We will also promote sustained and healthy development of the medical and health care sector, providing people with health services that meet their needs.

In the next year, the campaign to deepen the on-going health care reform has entered a crucial phase. The national health system will further enhance its capacity and competence for implementing scientific development in the health care sector. With continued effort to follow the CPC Central Committee and State Council's plan for deepening health care reform and requirement for ensuring basic health insurance coverage, strengthening the grassroots, and formulating new mechanism, we will strive for major breakthroughs to improve basic medical insurance coverage, reinforce and improve the national essential drugs system and actively promote the reform of public hospitals.

2012 will witness the 10th anniversary of the implementation of the new rural cooperative health care system. We will carefully sum up the experience and lessons accumulated over the course of the 10 years. We will raise the fund-raising standards of the new rural cooperative health care system and the coverage of the system. We will launch a health insurance plan to cover outpatient medical expenses throughout the country, and gradually increase the reimbursement rate of outpatient medical expenses. We will improve the overall coordination of the new rural cooperative health care funds and use cities, rather than counties, as the basic unit for overall coordination of funds. We will use provinces as individual units to fully implement the health insurance plan that covers major diseases. We will continue to promote the comprehensive reform of primary health care institutions. We will reinforce and improve the national essential drugs system and expand the scope of implementation to ensure that people have access to the basic drugs. We will make a systematic summary of the experience and lessons learned from pilot programs of public hospital reform. Relying on the key step of reforming the mechanism of doctors supplementing their incomes with the drugs they prescribe, we will carry out pilots of comprehensive reform of county hospitals. We will continue our efforts in providing high-quality nursing care, appointments with doctors, walk-in clinics and other measures that will bring people convenience and benefits. We will continue our efforts to optimize the environment and process for patients to see doctors and steadily carry out the model of "treatment first, and settlement of accounts at a later time" to curb the unreasonable increase of medical expenses.

In the next year, we will strengthen medical service management and ensure medical safety. We will further intensify efforts in the planning and managing medical institution set-up, defining the function of public hospitals, optimizing the layout and the structure of public hospitals, and focusing on strengthening capacity building in underserved areas and specialist care. We support using social capital to open medical institutions. We will accelerate the establishment of mechanisms for cooperation and division of labor between public hospitals and primary health care institutions, and gradually establish the pattern of initial diagnosis at primary-care institutions, multi-tiered medical service, two-way referral, and separate treatment of acute and chronic conditions. We will improve the human resources system and the income distribution system in public hospitals, continue to promote the system for doctors to practice at multiple sites, improve the salaries and benefits of medical workers, create a sound environment for medical practice, and fully stimulate the enthusiasm of the health workers.

In 2012, we will promote the gradual realization of equitable basic public health services in an all-round way, and continue to undertake our responsibilities for responding to emergency health events, disease prevention and control, and women and children's health; we will strengthen food safety and health supervision according to the law; we will improve the scientific drug regulatory system and ensure drug safety for the people; we will give full play to the characteristics and strengths of traditional Chinese medicine, and continuously improve traditional Chinese medical services; we will thoroughly implement the campaign to deliver excellent performance, severely punish business bribery cases and dishonest practices that damage the interests of people, create a new drive of reform and development of health care, strive to alleviate the problem of "difficult access to medical service and expensive medical bill", and welcome the opening of the 18th Congress of the CPC with outstanding achievements. I wish you all a happy New Year, good health, great success at work, and good luck!

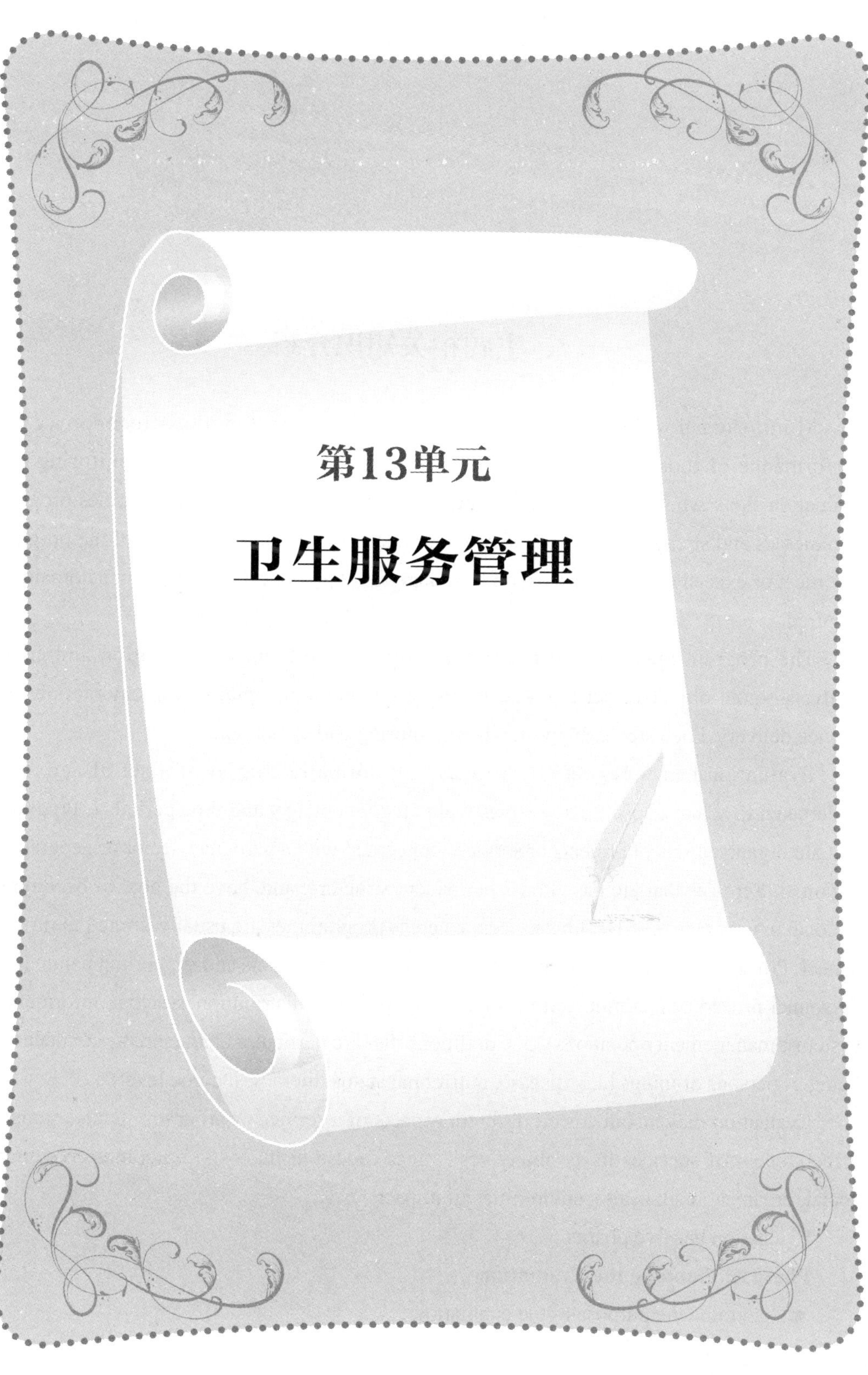

第13单元

卫生服务管理

一、主题相关知识介绍

Monitoring progress and evaluating results are key functions to improve the performance of those responsible for implementing health services. Monitoring and evaluation show whether a service/program is accomplishing its goals. It identifies program weaknesses and strengths, areas of the program that need revision, and areas of the program that meet or exceed expectations. To do this, analysis of any or all of a program's domains is required.

The program management cycle is as follows: problem identification and cause analysis→goal objective setting→designing implementation plan→implementation and service delivery. Each step is supported by monitoring and evaluation.

Evaluation can focus on: 1. Projects that normally consist of a set of activities undertaken to achieve specific objectives within a given budget and time period. 2. Programs that are organized sets of projects or services concerned with a particular sector or geographic region. 3. Services that are based on a permanent structure, and, have the goal of becoming, national in coverage, e.g. Health services, whereas programmes are usually limited in time or area. 4. Processes that are organizational operations of a continuous and supporting nature (e.g. personnel procedures, administrative support for projects, distribution systems, information systems, management operations). 5. Conditions that are particular characteristics or states of being of persons or things (e.g. disease, nutritional status, literacy, income level).

Evaluation may also focus on different aspects of a service or program: inputs; outputs; effectiveness of services in its objectives; effectiveness in its costs; outcomes;economic, social, organizational, health, environmental impacts.

Evaluation has five phases:

Phase A: Planning the Evaluation

- Determine the purpose of the evaluation.

● Decide on type of evaluation.

● Decide on who conducts evaluation (evaluation team).

● Review existing information in programme documents including monitoring information.

● List the relevant information sources.

● Describe the programme.

● Assess your own strengths and limitations.

Phase B: Selecting Appropriate Evaluation Methods

● Identify evaluation goals and objectives. (SMART)

● Formulate evaluation questions and sub-questions.

● Decide on the appropriate evaluation design.

● Identify measurement standards.

● Identify measurement indicators.

● Develop an evaluation schedule.

● Develop a budget for the evaluation.

Phase C: Collecting and Analysing Information

● Pre-test data collection instruments.

● Undertake data collection activities.

● Analyse data.

● Interpret the data.

● Develop data collection instruments.

Phase D: Reporting Findings

● Write the evaluation report.

● Decide on the method of sharing the evaluation results and on communication strategies.

● Share the draft report with stakeholders and revise as needed to be followed by follow up.

● Disseminate evaluation report.

Phase E: Implementing Evaluation

Recommendations

● Develop a new/revised implementation plan in partnership with stakeholders.

● Monitor the implementation of evaluation recommendations and report regularly on the implementation progress.

● Plan the next evaluation.

Source: "Monitoring and Evaluation of Health Services", Dr. Rasha Salama, PhD Public Health, Faculty of Medicine, Suez Canal University, Egypt.

二、技巧指导：口译临场应对策略

尽管译员在口译工作之前做了充分准备，但由于知识更新快、译员的知识结构存在局限，以及翻译过程中技巧掌控等因素的影响，加上口译的现场性、即时性和时限性，在实际口译工作中要达到出口成章的效果，出点问题在所难免。即使是基础扎实、经验丰富的译员，也都会碰见紧急情况。

上述紧急情况包括语言类紧急情况和与非语言类紧急情况。语言类紧急情况大致指遇到没有见过的词，对内容不熟悉而没有听懂，现场卡壳；非语言类紧急情况包括因为文化差异而不解其意、心理准备不充分而怯场、讲话者的发音不清晰或口音很重、各种原因造成的讲话者语速过快甚至话不得体等。

应对上述这些紧急情况需要做好三个方面的工作。一是做好平时的功课。平时在提高英文、中文语言能力的同时，还应重视自我思辨能力的培养，提高反应力。参加读书会、聆听演讲会、阅读演讲材料、参与辩论会、了解国家大事、广泛阅读等都是提高思辨能力的途径。阅读《中国日报》（*China Daily*）、《时代周刊》（*Time*）、《北京周报》（*Beijing Review*）、《上海日报》（*Shanghai Daily*）、《上海英文星报》（*Shanghai Star*）、《新闻周刊》（*Newsweek*）等外语刊物也是很好的途径。二是形成良好的译前准备习惯（"译前准备"一节有详述），提高猜测力和预测力，并做好充分的心理准备。三是临场情况处理。处理的方式有适当推迟翻译、鹦鹉学舌、沟通、与讲话人核实、补救、纠错、跳译或略译、情绪控制。

适当推迟翻译

有时候译员会因为讲话人语速太快、专注于文字而产生理解滞后，导致卡壳。此时，要稍微慢半拍，通过回忆上下文来整理思路，或根据上下文推测大意。

鹦鹉学舌

在对某个单词的意思完全没有任何印象，但却记住了该单词的发音的情况下，可以重复所听到的源语言中的发音，形成汉英夹杂表述，这样至少听众中的专业人员能够理解。

沟通

如果讲话人语速过快，译员可以与讲话人沟通，请求他为了演讲与翻译的效果而放慢语速。有的演讲人因紧张而语速加快，有的则是本来说话就快而含混不清。因此在提醒不奏效的情况下，译员必须自己稳住情绪，仔细听出段落大意，译出中心思想。若讲话人有较重的口音，译员最好能在口译之前与讲话人进行谈话或沟通，以熟悉其口音。在口音方面有困难的译员，平时必须训练自己听各个国家的英语讲话。临时去适应口音就难了。

与讲话人核实

在小型的不是非常正式的交替传译场合，有时可以请演讲者重复某个关键词，或解释某个词语的意思；有时可以与听众核实某个意思。但这种求助只能偶尔采用，因为这只是没有办法的办法。重复使用会让所有听众对译员失去信心，产生急躁情绪。在特别正式的场合此方式不适用。

补救

在自己发现漏译的情况下，一个办法是在进入下文的翻译时补救，或加以解释。在可能的情况下，可以直接将漏译的地方接上，也可以重新提及，例如可以用“关于……这一点”“刚才的问题是……”等补上漏译的内容。

纠错

发现自己译错时，如果是不影响大局的小错误，最好忽略，继续下面的翻译。如果错误大，影响前后逻辑意义，则需即刻纠正。可以告知听众遇到翻译问题，明确地说：“刚才×××点的翻译有误，现更正如下……”意识到大错而不纠正是不负责任的表现。漏译的处理与此大致相同。如果漏译的一句话无关紧要，那就不再处理；而如果漏译的是关键词语，在交传中可以在接下来的上下文中加进这个意思。这种情况，文字量要控制好，不能多也不能少，不能扩展原文而加上无关的内容。

跳译或略译

如果遇到个别不知道的词，在紧急情况下又不能拘泥于这一个词，注意力要马上转到整段话的逻辑结构上，听完整段后根据上下文猜出大意。在这种情况下会忽略掉个别不那么重要的词，但是不能影响大意。实际交传中也有讲话者说话拉拉杂杂，重点不突出，或一次性说太长而不给翻译应有时间的情况。这种情况下，也只能跳过一些无关紧要的信息，归纳总结段落大意。

情绪控制

在未听清或翻译出错的场合，译员都会有不同程度的心理波动，会分神而影响下文的翻译。所以译员必须学会控制情绪。要认识到，口译现场的特性要求译员只能全神贯注于不断需要翻译的话，因此译员没有任何时间去纠结于某一个没有听清的词语、某一句未能译出的话，没有时间去胆怯，责怪自己，或感到不好意思，因为这些都没有用，只能使情况更糟。在有内容听不懂的情况下，在情绪上译员必须当什么也没发生，只能忠于职责去完成未完成的任务，防止因为情绪而导致的进一步的错误，高度集中精力，不露声色地将翻译进行下去。

不可译性

不可译性（untranslatability）是指一种语言中的词语在另一语言中找不到对等词，通常这类词被附着了很多文化内涵。中文中有两类，一是概念名词，例如阴阳（Yin Yang）、八卦（Ba Gua）、五行（Wu Xing）；二是敬谦辞，例如“拜读”“大作”“鄙人”“寒舍”“拙文”“老朽”。这些词在英语中都难以找到对等词。在笔译中，这样的情况需要译者解释或处理。在口译场合，这样的词出现的机会不多。但出现了，还是要用笔译的原则处理，即加以解释。以“年糕”为例，译文用“Nian Gao”，解释可以是这样的：“A steamed pudding of glutinous rice in various shapes and flavors, traditionally wishing you happy growth and prosperity in the new year.”有时间还想多解释也是可以的。比如：“Nian”and“Gao”are homophones, meaning“year”and“higher”。像这样附有文化意义的中文菜肴还有很多，可采取上面这种“音译+食材+佐料+做法+附加解释”的方式处理。有一些词已经有了已经广为流传的译名，如wanton（云吞，即馄饨或抄手）、toufu（豆腐）、spring roll（春卷），这些词的译名就不能再生造了。

三、词汇准备

Text 1

coverage 覆盖，覆盖范围，覆盖面

MCA or MNCAH WHO’s Department of Maternal, Newborn, Child and Adolescent Health 世界卫生组织孕产妇、新生儿、儿童与青少年处

health service delivery 卫生服务，提供卫生服务

effective interventions 有效干预措施

disseminate results 传播效果

MDG Millennium Development Goals千年发展目标。MDG1：千年发展目标一；MDG4：千年发展目标四

Commission on Information and Accountability CIA 信息和问责委员会

determinants of health 健康决定因素

channels 渠道

MNCAH Household Survey 孕产妇、新生儿、儿童与青少年处住户调查

sub-national level 次国家级，国家二级

SARA Availability and Readiness Assessment 可用性和成熟度评估

The Health Facility Survey 卫生设施调查

Hospital Assessment Tool HAT 医院评估工具

Adolescent Friendly Health Services AFHS 青少年友好健康服务

Beyond the Numbers 超越数

WHO Near-Miss Approach 世界卫生组织临错方法（一种有效的干预措施，可降低已经存在的对孕产妇与新生儿健康的威胁、降低孕产妇和新生儿死亡率和发病率）

Text 2

Healthy Communities Program 健康社区计划，健康社区项目

CDC 疾病预防控制中心，疾控中心

water fluoridation 饮水氟化，加氟饮用水

incentive 动机，动因

"A Practitioner's Guide to Advancing Health Equity"《推动卫生公平性从业者指南》

Tobacco-Free Living Strategies 无烟草生活策略

The Health Metrics Network 卫生计量网络

countdown country 倒计时国家

Text 3

World Health Assembly 世界卫生大会

WHO Patron of Nursing and Midwifery 世卫组织护理和助产服务赞助人

tuberculosis 结核病

malaria 疟疾

respiratory infection 呼吸道感染

undernutrition 营养不足

morbidity 发病率
cardiovascular diseases 心血管疾病
diabetes 糖尿病
socioeconomic determinants 社会经济决定因素
rigorous appraisal 认真评估

Text 4

HHS Health and Human Services 卫生和福利部
Food and Drug Administration Safety and Innovation Act 美国食品和药品监督管理局安全和创新法案
culmination 顶点，高潮
generic drugs 通用药物
biosimilar biologics 生物仿制药物
Executive Order （美国总统颁布的具有法律效能的）行政命令
antibiotics 抗生素

Text 5

中国共产党中央委员会（党中央） CPC Central Committee
政务公开 make government affairs public
知情权 the right to be informed
参与权 the right to participate
监督权 the right to supervise
院务公开 hospital information release
《政府信息公开条例》 *The Regulations on Government Information Disclosure*
行风建设 development of industry morals
医政司 The Department of Medical Administration
监察局 The Supervisory Bureau
《院务公开目录（试行）》 *The Content of Hospital Information Release (the Trial Edition)*
《医院向内部职工公开的信息目录》 *The Content of Hospital Information Released to Employees*
《医疗机构院务公开监督考核办法（试行）》 *The Measures to Oversight and Evaluate Hospital Information Release in Healthcare Institutions (the Trial Edition)*
全国院务公开示范点 demonstration sites for the hospital information release in China

《关于做好深化医药卫生体制改革形势下院务公开工作的通知》 *Notice about Strengthening the Implementation of Hospital Information Release under the Circumstance of Medical and Healthcare System Reform*

Text 6

提高农村儿童白血病和儿童先天性心脏病医疗服务能力现场工作会议 The Field Work Meeting on Promoting the Rural Medical Service Capability of Treating Childhood Leukemia and Congenital Heart Disease

儿童白血病 childhood leukemia

先天性心脏病 congenital heart disease

集聚区 agglomeration

新型农村合作医疗 the New Rural Co-operative Medical System

城镇职工基本医疗保险 Basic Medical Insurance for Urban Workers

城镇居民基本医疗保险 Basic Medical Insurance for Urban Residents

基本药物制度 the essential medicine system

因病致贫 become poor because of illness

初筛 preliminary screening

四、摘要练习

请听下面英语语篇，第一篇用源语言复述此段主要信息逻辑点及层次，第二篇用译入语复述此段主要信息逻辑点及层次。注意信息点之间的逻辑联系。

Text 1

Monitoring and Evaluation
Focus on Coverage, Quality and Health Systems

WHO

WHO's Department of Maternal, Newborn, Child and Adolescent Health (MCA) supports countries to develop better monitoring and evaluation systems within the health sector to improve outcomes along the continuum of care for mothers, newborn infants, children and adolescents. Thus, within a health systems approach, MCA promotes improved monitoring of the quality of health service delivery as well as the coverage of effective interventions for improving maternal, newborn, child and adolescent health.

It does this in collaboration with partners to support countries to develop and implement national monitoring and evaluation plans, to analyse data, to report on and disseminate results. The current work of the MCA Department includes monitoring progress in countries towards achieving the Millennium Development Goals and supporting the work of the Commission on Information and Accountability.

WHO uses the following measurement framework developed by the Health Metrics Network to ensure comprehensive monitoring and evaluation of health and health system. It indicates three major measurement domains: determinants of health; health system; and health status. This framework is useful for illustrating these measurement activities which may be applied at global, regional, and national levels and at facility and community levels.

Examples of measurement activities undertaken include:

Determinants of Health

The MNCAH Household Survey collects data on the behaviours of caretakers that affect the use of maternal and child health interventions, and the behaviours of adolescents that affect their sexual and reproductive health outcomes. It also identifies "channels" and their functioning for the effective delivery health services for mothers and newborn infants, children and adolescents. This survey has been implemented in sub-national areas of 5 countries, where maternal, child and adolescent health interventions are in place.

Inputs to the Health System

The MNCAH Questionnaire collects health policy and systems related information that are critical for the implementation and improvement of the maternal, newborn, child and adolescent health agenda at global, regional and country level. The strategic information will inform MNCAH related policy and systems action and targeted response in countries. It also contributes to the updating of countdown country profiles and other processes as relevant.

Outputs of the Health System

At sub-national level, the MNCAH Household Survey and at national level, the Service Availability and Readiness Assessment (SARA) tool provide valuable data on service availability.

The Health Facility Survey for services delivered to improve child health measures quality of services at first level facilities and the Hospital Assessment Tool can be used in district hospitals. Quality assessment tools are available for determining if standards are being met for the delivery of Adolescent Friendly Health Services.

Approaches used in Beyond the Numbers and the WHO Near-Miss Approach go beyond just counting deaths to developing an understanding of why deaths and severe morbidity happen and how they can be averted.

Beyond the Numbers and Achievement of Outcomes

The MNCAH Household Survey provides sub-national data on the coverage of key interventions for maternal, newborn infants, children and adolescents.

MCA also monitors and evaluates achievement of outcomes through the compilation, syntheses and analyses of secondary data, providing information for action.

Health Status

MCA monitors and evaluates progress towards MDG4 through the assessment of trends in the distribution (including inequities) in under-five mortality at country, regional and global levels for informed action and changes in policies, strategies, and ultimately in health status. It also monitors the nutritional status of children under-five and evaluates trends towards the achievement of MDG1.

复述要点提示（主要信息逻辑点及层次）

MCA promotes improved monitoring of the quality of health service delivery and the coverage of effective interventions for improving maternal, newborn, child and adolescent health.

The way is collaboration with countries to have national monitoring and evaluation plans, and to analyse data, report on and disseminate results, such as monitoring progress in countries in achieving the MDG and supporting the work of CIA.

The measurement framework indicates three major measurement domains: determinants of health, health system, and health status. This framework is good for illustrating these measurement activities at global, regional, and national levels or at facility and community levels.

Examples of measurement activities are as follows:

In Determinants of Health, the MCA Household Survey collects data on both the caretakers' behaviors that affect maternal and child health interventions and the adolescents' behaviors that affect their sexual and reproductive health. The survey also identifies "channels" and their function for the effective delivery of health services.

In Inputs to the Health System, the Survey collects information on health policy and systems so as to inform MNCAH related policy, systems action, and targeted response to health agenda at global, regional and country levels. It updates countdown country profiles.

In Outputs of the Health System, the survey provides valuable data on service availability at sub-national level, while SARA's similar data are for the national level.

The Survey for services for child health measures service quality at first level facilities, and HAT in district hospitals. Quality assessment tools are for determining if standards are being met in delivering Adolescent Friendly Health Services.

Beyond the Numbers and the WHO Near-Miss Approach are for understanding the cause of deaths and severe morbidity MCA also monitors and evaluates outcomes through the compilation, syntheses and analyses of secondary data.

MCA also monitors and evaluates health status progress towards MDG4. It also evaluates trends towards the achievement of MDG1, and monitors the nutritional status of children under five.

Text 2

Advancing Health Equity: Community Strategies for Preventing Chronic Diseases (Excerpt & Adapted)

Centers for Disease Control and Prevention

Heart disease, cancer, diabetes, and stroke are the most common causes of illness, disability, and death affecting a growing number of Americans. Many of these chronic conditions tend to be more common, diagnosed later, and result in worse outcomes for particular individuals, such as people of color, people in low-income neighborhoods, and others whose life conditions place them at risk for poor health.

Despite decades of efforts to reduce and eliminate health disparities, they persist—and in some cases, they are widening among some population groups. Such disparities do not have a single cause. They are created and maintained through multiple, interconnected, and complex pathways. Some of the factors influencing health and contributing to health disparities include the following:

- Root causes or social determinants of health such as poverty, lack of education, racism, discrimination, and stigma.
- Environment and community conditions such as how a community looks (e.g., property neglect), what residents are exposed to (e.g., advertising, violence), and what resources are available there (e.g., transportation, grocery stores).

● Behavioral factors such as diet, tobacco use, and engagement in physical activity.

● Medical services such as the availability and quality of medical services.

While health disparities can be addressed at multiple levels, this resource focuses on policy, systems, and environmental improvement strategies designed to improve the places where people live, learn, work, and play. Many of the 20th and 21st century's greatest public health achievements (e.g., water fluoridation, motor vehicle safety, food safety) have relied on the use of laws, regulations, and environmental improvement strategies. Health practitioners play an important role in these improvements by engaging the community, identifying needs, conducting analyses, developing partnerships, as well as implementing and evaluating evidence-based interventions.

These intervention approaches are briefly described below:

● Policy improvements may include "a law, regulation, procedure, administrative action, incentive, or voluntary practice of governments and other institutions". Example: A voluntary school wellness policy that ensures food and beverage offerings meet certain standards.

● Systems improvements may include a "change that impacts all elements, including social norms of an organization, institution, or system". For example: The integration of tobacco screening and referral protocols into a hospital system.

● Environmental improvements may include changes to the physical, social, or economic environment. For example: A change to street infrastructure that enhances connectivity and promotes physical activity.

Such interventions have great potential to prevent and reduce health inequities, affect a large portion of a population, and can also be leveraged to address root causes, ensuring the greatest possible health impact is achieved over time. However, without careful design and implementation, such interventions may inadvertently widen health inequities. To maximize the health effects for all and reduce health inequities, it is important to consider the following:

● Different strategies require varying levels of individual or community effort and resources, which may affect who benefits and at what rate.

● Certain population groups may face barriers to or negative unintended consequences from certain strategies. Such barriers can limit the strategy's effect and worsen the disparity.

● Population groups experiencing health disparities have further to go to attain their full health potential, so even with equitable implementation, health effects may vary.

● Health equity should not only be considered when designing interventions. To help advance the goal, health equity should be considered in other aspects of public health practice (e.g., organizational capacity, partnerships, evaluation).

Our resource, "A Practitioner's Guide to Advancing Health Equity" provides lessons learned and practices from the field, as well as from the existing evidence-base. This resource offers ideas on how to maximize the effects of several policy, systems, and environmental improvement strategies with a goal to reduce health inequities and advance health equity. Additionally, the resource will help communities incorporate the concept of health equity into core components of public health practice such as organizational capacity, partnerships, community engagement, identifying health inequities, and evaluation.

This resource address health issues in four sections:

- Incorporating Health Equity into Foundational Skills of Public Health
- Maximizing Tobacco-Free Living Strategies to Advance Health Equity
- Maximizing Healthy Food and Beverage Strategies to Advance Health Equity
- Maximizing Active Living Strategies to Advance Health Equity

复述要点提示（主要信息逻辑点及层次）

心脏病、癌症、糖尿病、中风等常见病导致残疾和死亡，影响越来越多的美国人。在特定人群例如有色人种和低收入社区人群中，这些慢性病更为常见，往往诊断滞后，结果更糟，健康状况风险大。

尽管消除健康差距的努力已付出了几十年，但在某些人群中差距却在加大。导致差距的原因众多，错综复杂：

- 根本原因即社会原因是贫穷、缺乏教育、种族主义、歧视和耻辱感；
- 社区环境条件：如社区面貌（如物业状态不佳）、居民环境（如广告、暴力）、可用资源（如交通条件与药店）；
- 行为因素如饮食、吸烟、体力活动的参与；
- 是否可获得医疗服务及医疗服务质量。

作为多层次解决健康状况差异的办法之一，本资源聚焦于政策、系统和环境改进策略，改善人们的生活、学习、工作、娱乐环境。卫生工作者鼓励社区参与，识别需求，进行分析，建立合作伙伴关系，实施并评价循证干预。

干预方法包括：

- 政策改进：法律、法规、程序、行政行为、激励方法、自愿实施的政府和其他机构，例如确保学校食品和饮料产品符合标准；
- 系统改进：改进组织、制度、社会规范或制度，例如医院集成烟草筛查和转诊协议；
- 环境改善，改变自然、社会、经济环境，如改进街道基础设施，促进体育活动。

为了确保干预措施不会扩大健康不平等，要考虑：

- 战略的多样性、个体与群体的不同利益以及速度问题；
- 策略也会导致未预料到的后果，对某些人群产生负面影响而影响措施的实施；
- 即使实现公平健康原则，结果也会有所不同；
- 不但设计措施时要考虑健康公平的原则，也应同时从其他领域角度考虑此事（如组织能力、合作、评价方面）。

归纳起来，本资源的目的是：

- 将健康公平与公共卫生基础技能相结合；
- 通过全面实现无烟生活、健康食品、积极生活方式来推动健康公平。

五、英译汉练习

Text 3

Address by Her Royal Highness Princess Muna Al-Hussein at the 61st World Health Assembly (Excerpt)

Geneva, Switzerland

20 May 2008

Mr. President, Director-General, Ministers of Health, delegates, ladies and gentlemen,

May I congratulate the President of the Assembly for his election to this office and thank Dr. Chan for inviting me to participate in this prestigious annual gathering of the world's Ministers of Health and the delegates of WHO's Member States.

This is my second participation in the work of the World Health Assembly. The first was two years ago when I addressed Committee A in my capacity as WHO Patron of Nursing and Midwifery. I am therefore honoured to be here again to address this distinguished audience.

This year marks the 60th anniversary of the World Health Organization and I would like to congratulate WHO's Member States and the Secretariat on this occasion. This Organization has made immense strides in serving its Member States over the last six decades and its accomplishments are manifold. Indeed, I am proud to work closely with the

World Health Organization and privileged to continue to witness the excellent contribution WHO provides to the health sector, not only in my own country but in others. I am sure I convey the sentiments shared by all of you in confirming how crucial the work of the Organization is to world health and in expressing our appreciation of the dedication of its staff. This Organization belongs to you all and is governed by you all. As such, it is our collective responsibility to ensure that it is supported and enabled to work effectively in addressing the serious health challenges of the 21st century.

Ladies and gentlemen,

Today's world is facing very serious health problems despite the great advances in health and medical science, the remarkable achievements made in combating major diseases and health problems, and the overall rise in life expectancy.

Millions continue to die from preventable diseases like HIV/AIDS, tuberculosis, malaria and respiratory infection. Undernutrition is responsible for one third of all child deaths and contributes substantially to the global burden of disease. Morbidity, disability, and death from cardiovascular diseases, diabetes and cancer are also rapidly and persistently increasing across the globe.

What is also worrying and unacceptable is that the progress towards the health-related Millennium Development Goals is hampered in many countries. While some nations are on track, others are progressing too slowly, and some are even regressing. Resources allocated for health continue to remain limited, with 20% of the world's population suffering from poverty. The serious impact of climate change and the effects of increasing food prices are resulting in hunger and becoming even more serious as a global problem, with grave consequences on health. Conflicts and other crises continue to disrupt and strain health systems and have an enormously negative impact on health in many parts of the world including my own region.

The two natural disasters that recently hit both Myanmar and China have shocked the world. Only international solidarity and cooperation will help the two nations cope efficiently with the health consequences.

These are some examples of the complex challenges that countries, WHO and other health partners have to face at the turn of WHO's 60th anniversary. These challenges require a comprehensive approach to health, rather than emphasis on health care alone. They require solid commitment in addressing the socioeconomic determinants of health, stronger collaboration with nonhealth sectors, more effective and new alliances, closer coordination between global health partners, and considerably more effective health systems.

Mr. President, ladies and gentlemen,

I have come here today to share with you my conviction that the health workforce should be promoted to a much higher place on the agendas of ministers of health, leaders of the health professions, and other policy makers. Time has repeatedly shown that the key determining factor for human resources development in many countries has been the level of commitment among those in the highest level of leadership in governments and in ministries of health and education.

It has been made clear that when there is political commitment, the whole process of development is facilitated and targets are met. Strengthened human resources for health is the basis of improved health care and is a prerequisite for a more effective primary health care.

In my address to Committee A two years ago, I highlighted the urgent need for a critical review of the human resources situation with respect to planning, development and management. Planning should take into account monitoring of supply and demand, improving recruitment, retention, deployment, and examining working patterns.

How can we attempt to strengthen health systems without addressing the human resources crisis? Indeed, failure to develop and implement effective strategies and plans will seriously impair any initiative to reinforce primary health care and the achievement of national health goals. In many countries, a start can and must be made by making a rigorous appraisal of the current state of human resource development in terms of personnel policies, capacity, training, and management of performance.

I very much look forward to the follow up of *The World Health Report 2006* and to more progress made in strengthening the health workforce. No investment is better than investing in health and education. This is true for all countries without any exception, and I am confident that investing in the health workforce will yield the highest return.

Your Excellencies, distinguished delegates,

You have great opportunities to further increase investment in health development. Together with the World Health Organization, other UN agencies and main stakeholders in global health, you can play a major part in joined efforts to make this world a better place—a place where populations can enjoy their fundamental rights to better health and live in harmony and security.

Thank you.

Text 4

Statement from HHS Secretary Kathleen Sebelius on the Signing of the Food and Drug Administration Safety and Innovation Act

9 July 2012

Today, the President signed into law S.3187, the "Food and Drug Administration Safety and Innovation Act." This legislation, which passed both the House and Senate with overwhelming bipartisan majorities, will help speed safe and effective medical products to patients and maintain our Nation's role as a leader in biomedical innovation.

S.3187 is the culmination of the work of the administration and Congress, in partnership with patients, the pharmaceutical and medical device industries, the clinical community, and other stakeholders, to provide the Food and Drug Administration with the tools needed to continue to bring drugs and devices to market safely and quickly and promote innovation in the biomedical industry, and to help secure the jobs supported by drug and device development.

This legislation will drive timely review of new innovator drugs and medical devices, implement the program proposed in the 2013 President's Budget to accelerate approval of lower-cost generic drugs, and fund the new approval pathway for biosimilar biologics created by the Affordable Care Act. These new programs are important to increasing patient access to affordable medicines.

S.3187 also enhances the tools available to the FDA to combat drug shortages by requiring manufacturers of certain drugs to notify the FDA when they experience circumstances that could lead to a potential drug shortage. This is consistent with the administration's request to Congress to complement the actions directed by the 2011 Executive Order to address this significant public health issue.

Provisions in the legislation also will help enhance the safety of the drug supply chain in an increasingly globalized market, increase incentives for the development of new antibiotics, renew mechanisms to ensure that children's medicines are appropriately tested and labeled, and expedite the development and review of certain drugs for the treatment of serious or life-threatening diseases and conditions.

While enactment of S.3187 marks an important moment for innovators across industry, research and clinical care settings, its most important beneficiaries are the patients and families that will be helped by the next generation of affordable medical products this bill will help to foster.

六、汉译英练习

Text 5

关于确定第二批公立医院改革国家联系试点城市及有关工作的通知

国家卫生计划委

2014年4月28日

各省、自治区、直辖市及计划单列市、新疆生产建设兵团卫生计生委（卫生厅局）、财政（务）厅（局）、医改领导小组办公室：

为全面贯彻党的十八大和十八届三中全会精神，落实2014年《政府工作报告》中“扩大城市公立医院综合改革试点”的任务要求，按照扩大城市公立医院改革试点范围，每个省份有一个国家联系试点城市和地方党委政府重视、部门协同配合、工作基础较好、有一定的代表性等原则，同时兼顾各省申报试点城市时的优先排序，我们确定了天津市等17个城市为第二批公立医院改革国家联系试点城市（见附件1）。根据国务院医改领导小组第2次全体会议的部署，经商中央编办、国家发展改革委、人力资源社会保障部，现将第二批公立医院改革国家联系试点城市名单印发你们，并就试点工作提出如下要求。

一、充分认识推进公立医院改革的重要意义，加强对改革试点的领导。推进公立医院改革是贯彻落实十八届三中全会精神和政府工作报告的客观要求，是建立符合国情、惠及全民的中国特色基本医疗卫生制度的重要环节，是用中国式办法破解医改难题的必然举措。各国家联系试点城市人民政府要充分认识公立医院改革的重要性、艰巨性和复杂性，进一步增强改革的机遇意识、责任意识、紧迫意识，健全工作机制，落实工作保障，更加主动、积极地开展改革试点。各级医改领导小组要切实加强对试点的指导和支持。卫生计生（卫生）、财政等有关部门要凝聚共识，协同配合，形成合力。

二、科学制订公立医院改革试点实施方案，强化责任落实。各地要按照《国务院关于印发“十二五”期间深化医药卫生体制改革规划暨实施方案的通知》（国发〔2012〕11号）和原卫生部等5部门《关于公立医院改革试点的指导意见》（卫医管发〔2010〕20号）的要求，在深入调研、精心测算、充分协商、科学论证的基础上，制订路线清晰、措施具体、任务明确、分工细致的试点实施方案。实施方案要注重系统性、整体性和协同性，着力创新体制机制，统筹推进综合改革；要注重针对性和可操作性，聚焦解决当地公立医院存在的突出问题，力求在关键环节有所突破。各地要围绕试点实施方案，进一步分解任务、明确分工，建立问责机制，做到早部署、早开展、早落实。试点城市范围内县级（二级）以上公立医院都要开展综合改革。

三、加强督导考核，扎实推进公立医院改革试点工作。各地要认真组织开展摸底调查，为今后开展试点评估工作提供基线数据。加强对试点情况的监测，收集相关数据并定期上报，及时研究解决改革过程中遇到的问题和困难，不断总结经验，完善政策措施。在试点过程中取得的重大进展和重要经验，遇到的重要情况和重大问题，请及时向国家卫生计生委等部门上报。要加强对改革试点的督查考核，对于未按要求开展综合改革的试点城市，将取消试点资格，并相应扣回中央财政补助资金。

四、做好宣传培训，营造公立医院改革的良好社会环境。加强政策解读，做好有关部门管理人员和试点医院院长的培训，增强对政策的把握理解，提高推进改革的管理能力。积极做好有关改革内容的宣传解释和舆论引导工作，宣传公立医院改革的方针政策、重要部署以及各地推进改革的新举措、新进展、新成效。加强舆情监测，及时向公众解疑释惑，合理引导社会预期，让群众了解改革、理解改革、支持改革、参与改革。

请各国家联系试点城市抓紧制订试点实施方案，由省级医改领导小组审核后组织实施，报国家卫生计生委备案。为加强中央和地方的沟通联系，请将省级分管公立医院改革试点的政府领导、省级有关部门试点工作负责同志和联络员信息以及试点城市分管公立医院改革试点工作的市政府领导、市级有关部门试点工作负责同志和联络员信息（见附件2）于5月30日前报送国家卫生计生委。

Text 6

四川省人民政府陈保明副秘书长在卫生部提高农村儿童白血病和儿童先天性心脏病医疗服务能力现场工作会议上的致辞

尊敬的陈竺部长，各位领导、各位代表，同志们：

下午好！

今天，卫生部在我省召开提高农村儿童白血病和儿童先天性心脏病医疗服务能力现场工作会议，这是对我省工作的巨大鼓励和鞭策，也为我们提供了学习、提高的难得机会。我谨代表四川省人民政府向来川的各位代表表示热烈欢迎！对本次会议的召开表示衷心祝贺！

四川是西部大开发的重要省份之一，全省辖21个市（州），181个县（市、区），有8 800多万人口，面积48.5万平方公里，居住着50多个民族，是全国第二大藏区，最大的彝族集聚区，唯一的羌族集聚区。2009年全省生产总值14 000多亿元，经济总量居全国省（区、市）第9位。

"5·12"汶川特大地震发生以来，在党中央、国务院的坚强领导下，在卫生部及国家有关部委、各兄弟省（区、市）和社会各界的大力支持下，我省灾后恢复重建工作取得了重大的成果。今年将基本完成灾后恢复重建任务，灾区基本经济条件和经济社会发展水平总体达到或超过灾前水平。

近年来，在卫生部和陈竺部长的关心支持下，我省以深化医药卫生体制改革为契机，卫生事业得到长足发展：以新型农村合作医疗、城镇职工基本医疗和城镇居民基本医疗保险为主体的多种形式的医疗保障体系初步建立，参保人数达到了8 200多万人，基本覆盖城乡居民；30%的政府举办的城市社区卫生服务机构和基层医疗卫生机构基本药物制度扎实推进，群众就医费用下降达30%以上；城乡基层医疗卫生服务体系进一步健全，人民群众的就医环境不断改善；基本公共卫生服务均等化逐步推进，9大类基本公共卫生服务惠及城乡；公立医院改革试点顺利启动。

儿童白血病和儿童先心病是严重危害部分儿童身体健康的重大疾病之一，具有治疗难度大、治疗费用高、对儿童危害大等特点。提高对农村儿童白血病和儿童先心病的医疗保障水平，是减轻农民重大疾病医疗负担的有效途径，也是缓解农村家庭因病致贫、因病返贫的重要举措，更是一项体现党和政府执政为民、促进社会和谐的民生民心工程。四川省委、省政府高度重视提高农村儿童白血病和儿童先心病的医疗保障水平工作，按照卫生部的统一部署，于今年初积极探索开展此项工作。通过深入调研、精确测算，我省试点工作顺利推进，确定了试点地区，明确了纳入试点工作的疾病种类，核定了补偿标准，选定了初筛和定点救治的医疗机构。这项工作是一项创新性工作，还处于摸索阶段，我们决心通过极大的努力，建立起我省提高农村居民重大疾病医疗保障水平的长效机制和稳定的资金机制。同时，也希望得到卫生部一如既往的关心和支持，我们深信，这次现场经验交流会在四川召开，对我省提高农村儿童白血病和儿童先天性心脏病医疗服务能力，乃至整个卫生事业的发展，无疑是一个有力的推动和促进。

感谢卫生部和各兄弟省、区、市一直以来对四川卫生事业的关心和支持，最后，预祝卫生部提高农村儿童白血病和儿童先天性心脏病医疗服务能力现场工作会议取得圆满成功。谢谢大家。

资料来源：

Text 1 http://www.who.int/maternal_child_adolescent/planning/monitoring/en/#

Text 2 http://www.cdc.gov/nccdphp/dch/pdfs/health-equity-guide/Health-Equity-Guide-intro.pdf

Text 3 http://www.hhs.gov/secretary/about/speeches/sp20120423.html

Text 4 http://www.hhs.gov/news/press/2012pres/07/20120709b.html

Text 5

中文

http://www.nhfpc.gov.cn/tigs/s3581/201405/e16bc82c70594c26902454fc97c7ec76.shtml

英文

http://en.nhfpc.gov.cn/2014-06/25/content_17614921_4.htm

Text 6 httpcn.nhfpc.90v.cn/2014-06/09/c.45809.htm://live.people.com.cn/note.php?id=823100624145024_ctdzb_001

参考答案

四、摘要练习

Text 1

监测和评价

世界卫生组织

以覆盖范围、质量和卫生系统为重点

世界卫生组织孕产妇、新生儿、儿童和青少年健康部（MCA）支持各国在卫生系统开发更好的监测和评价系统，以改善在持续照顾、新生婴儿、儿童和青少年方面的情况。因此，通过健康系统方法，MCA促进改善监测健康服务质量的监测，孕产妇、新生儿、儿童及少年健康的有效干预覆盖面。

它与合作伙伴合作，支持各国制定并实施国家监测和评估计划，分析数据、报告和传播效果。MCA部门目前的工作包括监测各国实现千年发展目标的进展，以及支持信息与问责委员会的工作。

世界卫生组织使用卫生计量网络的测量框架来保证综合监测、健康评估以及健康系统。有三个主要测量领域：健康决定因素、卫生系统、健康状况。此框架用于说明测量活动可以应用于全球、区域及国家层面，也可用于设施和社区层面。

测量活动的例子包括：

健康决定因素

孕产妇、新生儿、儿童与青少年处（MNCAH）住户调查收集行为数据，对象是影响妇幼保健干预措施运用的健康服务人员以及影响自己生殖与性健康的青少年。此调查也为孕产妇、新生儿、儿童和青少年寻找并确定“渠道”，提供有效的健康服务。这项调查已经在5个国家以内孕产妇、儿童和青少年健康干预措施已到位的地区实施。

向卫生系统反馈数据信息

MNCAH问卷收集卫生政策和系统相关信息，这些数据对于在全球、地区及国家层面实施和完善孕产妇、新生儿、儿童和青少年健康计划至关重要。这些战略性信息将知会MNCAH相关政策、系统行为及各国有针对性的应对系统，也有助于更新倒计时国家的相关情况和相关过程。

卫生系统的数据输出

孕产妇、新生儿、儿童与青少年处（MNCAH）住户统计调查在次国家级层面上提供有关服务可获得性的宝贵数据；而服务可获得性与就绪性评估（SARA）在国家级层面上提供服务可获得性的宝贵数据。

卫生设施调查为已实施的改善儿童健康服务而设立，测量一级设施的服务质量；医院评估工具则可用于区级医院。已提供质量评估工具，用于测定青少年友好医疗服务是否达标。

超越数法和世界卫生组织临错方法不仅仅以只计算死亡人数的方式来理解死亡及严重并发症发生的原因及避免手段。

超越数方法取得的成果

MNCAH家庭调查针对孕产妇、新生儿、儿童和青少年的覆盖面问题提供次国家级数据。

MCA还通过汇集、合并整理与分析二级数据，监测和评估所取得的成果，同时为行动提供信息。

健康状况

在国家、地区与全球层面，MCA通过评估5岁以下儿童的死亡率分布趋势（包括不平等趋势）来监测和评价千年发展目标四的进展情况，以便在充分了解情况的基础上采取行动，改变政策和策略及最终改变健康状况。此举措同时监测5岁以下儿童的营养状况，并评价千年发展目标一的实现情况。

Text 2

促进健康公平：预防慢性病的社区战略（节选并改编）

美国疾病控制与预防中心

心脏病、癌症、糖尿病、中风等常见病导致残疾和死亡，影响越来越多的美国人。在特定人群中，例如有色人种和低收入社区人群中，这些慢性病更为常见，往往诊断滞后，结果更糟。另有其他人群，生活状况将他们置于健康风险之中。

尽管消除健康差距的努力已付出了几十年，但差距一直存在，并在某些人群中加大。导致差距的绝不是一个单一原因，其形成的原因路径众多、错综复杂。影响健康、造成健康差距的因素有以下这些：

● 根本原因，即社会原因，是贫穷、缺乏教育、种族主义、歧视和耻辱感；

● 社区环境条件原因，例如社区面貌（物业状态不佳）、居民环境（广告、暴力）、资源条件（例如交通条件与药店）；

● 行为因素如饮食、吸烟、体育活动的参与；

● 是否可获得医疗服务和医疗服务质量。

作为多层次解决健康差异的办法之一，本资源聚焦于政策、系统和环境改进策略，以改善人们的生活、学习、工作与娱乐环境。20世纪与21世纪许多最伟大的公共卫生成就（例如在水中加氟、机动车辆安全、食品安全）都依赖于实施法律、法规和环境改善策略。卫生工作者为实现这些成就发挥了重要作用，他们鼓励社区参与，识别需求，进行分析，建立合作伙伴关系，实施并评价循证干预措施。

简要介绍以下干预方法：

● 政策改进，包括法律、法规、程序、行政行为、激励方法、自愿实施的政府和其他机构，例如确保学校食品和饮料产品符合标准的学校健康自愿参与政策；

● 系统改进，包括影响所有因素的改进措施，包括组织、机构与系统之中的社会规范，例如将烟草筛查和转诊协议合并进医院系统；

● 环境改善，包括改变自然、社会、经济环境，例如改进街道基础设施、加强凝聚力、促进体育活动。

这种干预措施具有很大的潜力，可以预防并减少健康事业的不公平现象，影响很大一部分人；也可以发挥其杠杆作用，处理根源性原因，保证在一段时间里达到健康影响的最大化。然而，如果没有精心的设计和实施，这种干预可能会在不经意间扩大健康事业的不公平。为了达到健康影响的最大化，减少健康事业的不公平现象，考虑以下几点很重要：

●战略的多样性要求不同层面上个人和社区的努力，以及资源共享。这些因素会影响利益以及速度问题；

●某些策略也会导致未预料到的后果，给某些人群造成障碍，进而影响措施的实施，扩大并恶化差距；

●健康状况存在差距的人群需要有进一步去实现健康的潜力，所以即使公平地实施健康策略，健康的结果也会有所不同；

●不但设计干预措施时要考虑健康公平原则，为了推进并实现目标，也应同时从健康事业的其他领域角度考虑此事（例如组织能力、合作、评价方面）。

本资源，“推进卫生公平从业者指南”，提供从该领域及现有询证中得到的经验教训和实践经验。本资源提供了关于如何达到实施若干政策、制度和环境改善策略的最佳效果，减少健康不公平现象、推进健康公平的理念和构想。此外，本资源将帮助社区将健康公平的概念纳入公共卫生实践的核心组成部分，例如组织能力、合作伙伴、社区参与、确认卫生不平等现象及评价。

本资源分四个部分讨论健康问题：

●将健康公平与公共卫生基础技能相结合；

●无烟草生活最大化战略以推进健康公平；

●健康食品及饮料最大化战略以推进健康公平；

●积极生活最大化战略以推进健康公平。

五、英译汉练习

Text 3

穆娜·侯赛因公主殿下在第61届世界卫生大会上的致辞

瑞士日内瓦

2008年5月20日

主席先生，总干事，各位卫生部长，各位代表，女士们、先生们：

我谨祝贺大会主席的当选，并感谢陈博士邀请我来参加这个享有盛誉的年度聚会，加入世界各国的卫生部长和世卫组织成员代表之列。

这是我第二次参加世界卫生大会。第一次是在两年前，我是以世卫组织护理和助产服务赞助人的身份，在甲委员会发言。因此我很荣幸再次在这里向尊敬的各位讲话。

今年是世界卫生组织成立60周年。借此机会，我要向世卫组织各成员和秘书处表示祝贺！在过去的60年里，世卫组织在为成员服务方面取得了巨大进步，并且其取得的成就处处彰显。的确，我非常自豪可以与世界卫生组织紧密合作，有幸继续目睹世卫组织对卫生部门做出的卓越贡献，不仅仅是在我自己的国家，其他国家同样如此。我相信，我表达的情感各位也深有同感，认同这个组织对世界卫生而言是多么的至关重要，也表达我们对其职员所做奉献的感激之情。这个组织属于你们大家，由你们大家共同管理。正因如此，我们负有的共同责任是保证对该组织提供支持，使其具备能力能够有效应对21世纪面临的严峻卫生挑战。

女士们、先生们，

尽管我们在卫生和医学科学方面取得了很大进展，在应对主要疾病和卫生问题方面取得了引人瞩目的成绩，并且期望寿命总体上有所上升，今天的世界仍然面临着十分严峻的卫生问题。

数百万计的人仍死于本可预防的疾病，例如艾滋病、结核病、疟疾和呼吸道感染。营养不足导致的儿童死亡占所有死亡儿童的三分之一，也大大加重了全球疾病负担。心血管疾病、糖尿病和癌症的发病率及其造成的残疾和死亡也在全球范围内快速、持续增长。

同样令人担忧和不可接受的是，在迈向与卫生相关的千年发展目标方面，许多国家遇到了阻碍。一些国家进展良好，一些国家进展极其缓慢，有些国家甚至出现了倒退。由于20%的世界人口还在贫困中挣扎，卫生方面的资源分配仍然有限。气候变化和粮食价格的不断上涨带来了严重影响，引起饥荒，成为一个更为严重的全球问题，这给卫生带来了重大影响。冲突和其他危机继续干扰卫生体系，对其施压，对世界诸多地区的卫生工作带来了巨大负面影响，这也包括我所在的地区。

最近发生在缅甸和中国的两个自然灾害震惊了世界。只有国家间的团结和合作可以帮助这两个国家有效应对灾害所带来的卫生后果。

在世卫组织成立60周年的转折之际，这些不过是复杂挑战中的几个例证，需要各个国家、世界卫生组织和其他卫生领域合作伙伴加以面对。这些挑战要求有一个针对卫生的综合方法来应对，而不仅是单单强调卫生保健。还要求有实实在在的承诺，以解决健康的社会经济决定因素，有与非卫生部门更强的合作，有更为有效和新型的联盟，有全球卫生合作伙伴间更为良好的协调，以及更加有效的卫生体系。

主席先生，女士们、先生们，

我今天来到这里，是要与各位分享我的信念。这就是，卫生人力问题，应该在各位卫生部长、卫生行业领导和其他决策者的日程上，被提到一个更高的位置。时间已经反复证明，在许多国家，发展人力资源的关键因素在于政府、卫生部和教育部最高层领导的承诺水平。

很明显，一旦有了政治承诺，整个发展过程就能得到促进，目标就能得到实现。强化后的卫生人力资源，是改善卫生保健的基础，是更为有效的初级卫生保健工作的前提。两年前我在甲委员会发言，强调了严格审评人力资源状况的迫切性，这涉及人力资源的规划、发展和管理。规划应该考虑到监测需求和供给情况，改进招聘、留用和部署，以及审查工作方式等。

不解决人力资源危机，我们怎么可能加强卫生体系？事实上，开发和执行人力资源的有效战略和计划的失败，将严重影响任何强化初级卫生保健的行动和实现国家卫生目标。在许多国家，对当前人力资源状况进行认真评估是可能和必需的起点，包括人事政策、能力、培训以及业绩管理等。

我极其盼望看到《2006年世界卫生报告》的后续工作，看到在加强卫生工作人员队伍上取得更多的进展。最佳投资莫过于对卫生和教育的投资。这对所有国家都如是，没有例外。我相信，对卫生人力的投资，回报最为丰厚。

诸位阁下、尊敬的代表，

你们面临进一步提高对卫生发展投资的大好机会。与世界卫生组织、其他联合国机构以及全球卫生主要利益攸关方一道，你们可以在共同行动中发挥重要作用，使这个世界成为更加美好的地方。在这里，各种人群可以享有更加健康的基本权利，生活在和谐与安全之中。

谢谢各位！

Text 4

美国卫生和福利部部长凯瑟琳·西贝利厄斯
在美国食品和药品监督管理局安全和创新法案签署仪式上的讲话

2012年7月9日

今天，总统先生正式将美国食品和药品监督管理局安全和创新法案签入第S.3187号法律。该项法案获得了参众两院两党中大多数人的支持，将为病患提供更加安全、有效的医疗产品，维护我国在生物医学创新中的领先地位。

第S.3198号法案是政府和国会与病人、医药和医疗器械行业、临床领域及其他利益相关者合作的一个巅峰。让食品和药品监督管理局能够继续安全、快速地为市场引入新的药品和设备，推动生物医学行业的创新，保护医药及医药设备相关领域就业机会。

此项法案能促进我们及时地回顾创新型药品及医疗设备，实施2013总统预算中提议的项目，加快核准低成本通用药物，为平价医疗法案中所设立的生物仿制药物审批新路径提供资金支持。上述项目能够让病患获得更多实惠的药品。

通过要求特定药品生产商在面临潜在的药物短缺情境时告知食品和药品监督管理局，第S.3198号法案也提高了食品和药品监督管理局应对药物短缺的能力。这正符合食品和药品监督管理局解决这一公共卫生问题的要求，是国会对2011总统行政命令行动的一次补充。

在市场日益全球化的情景之下，法案条款将有助于增强药物供应链的安全性，推动新抗生素的研发，促进体制更新，保证儿童用药试验得当、标注准确，加快重大疾病治疗药物的研发，缩短此类药物复审周期。

尽管第S.3187号法案的颁布对行业创新者、医学研究和临床护理领域而言都意义重大，但是法案最大的受益人，却是那些受益于该法案所产生的下一代平价医药产品的病患及家庭。

六、汉译英练习

Text 5

Notice on Determining the Second Batch of Pilot Cities for National Public Hospital Reform and Other Related Work

National Health and Family Planning Commission

Ministry of Finance

28 April 2014

Health and family planning departments in provinces, autonomous regions and municipalities directly under the central government; municipalities with independent planning status; Xinjiang Production and Construction Corps; finance departments at various levels; and the State Council Leading Group Office of the Health Care System:

We have settled on 17 pilot cities, including Tianjin, for public hospital reform to fully implement the spirit of the 18th CPC National Congress and the third plenary session of the 18th CPC Central Committee and follow the government's call for expanding comprehensive public hospital reform in cities. Every province will have a pilot city where the local government will pay great attention to medical reform and work towards certain achievements. The relevant departments will be well coordinated. These cities reflect the general medical situation in their province. In accordance with deployments at the second plenary session of the State Council Leading Group Office of the Health Care System—and approved by the State Commission Office for Public Sector Reform, the National Development and Reform Commission, and Ministry of Human Resources and Social Security—we now issue the list of the second-batch pilot cities and requirements:

1. Fully understand the importance of advancing public hospital reform and strengthen guidance for reform.

Promoting public hospital reform is necessary in carrying out the spirit of the third plenary session of the 18th CPC Central Committee and the government work report. It is also a key link in establishing a basic medical and health care system with Chinese characteristics that can benefit the public at large. It is an inevitable move for China to break through its medical reform problems. Pilot city governments should fully recognize the importance, difficulties and complexity of public hospital reform; enhance the awareness of opportunity, responsibility and urgency; and improve work mechanisms to actively carry out pilot reform. The leading group for medical reform at various levels shall strengthen guidance and support for the pilot city. The health and family planning, as well as finance, departments should form a consensus and join forces through coordination and cooperation.

2. Make scientific implementation plan for public hospital reform and strengthen responsibility implementation.

Regions at various levels should follow the State Council's notice No 11 in 2012 on deepening the planning and implantation of medical and health care reform and the guidance No. 20 in 2010 on public hospital pilot reform issued by five government departments to clarify reform routes, concrete measures, unequivocal tasks and division of work. Plan implementation has to be systematic, holistic and collaborative; focus on innovation system mechanisms; promote comprehensive reform; be pertinent and practicable to solve prominent problems in local public hospitals; and strive for a breakthrough in key links. Regions at various levels should revolve around the pilot implementation plan, further break down tasks, clarify individual responsibilities, and establish an accountability mechanism for early deployment and implementation. Public hospitals in pilot cities at or above the county level (level 2) should all carry out comprehensive reform.

3. Strengthen supervision and inspection and steadily proceed with the public hospital reform work.

Regions at various levels should carefully carry out surveys at the grassroots level to provide baseline data for future evaluation work, strengthen pilot reform monitoring, regularly collect and report related data, study and resolve problems and difficulties in the process of reform, and continuously sum up experiences to improve policies and measures. Pilot cities should make timely reports on significant progress and important experience, as well as major situations and problems to the National Health and Family Planning Commission and other departments. The cities should also strengthen pilot reform supervision and evaluation. Pilot cities that fail to deliver comprehensive reform will be disqualified and must return subsidy funds from the central government.

4. Properly conduct publicity and training work, and create a good social environment of public hospital reform.

The cities will strengthen policy interpretation, provide training for relevant management personnel and heads of pilot hospitals, strengthen policy understanding, and improve management to push ahead reform. The pilot cities will actively publicize and explain reform content and guide public opinion. They will also promote public hospital reform policy; important deployments; and new measures, progress and achievements made in pilot cities across the country. Pilot cities will strengthen public opinion surveillance; answer public questions in time; guide social expectations; and help the public learn, understand, support and participate in the reform.

Pilot cities should formulate implantation plans in short order. They should carry them out after being approved by the provincial leading group of medical reform. They should also file the plan with the National Health and Family Planning Commission on record.

To strengthen communication between central and local governments, please send the National Health and Family Planning Commission information on government leaders at provincial or municipal levels in charge of local public hospital reform, as well as head or liaison officials from relevant provincial or municipal departments before May 30.

Text 6

Speech by Chen Baoming, Deputy Secretary General of Sichuan Provincial People's Government, at the MOH Field Work Meeting on Promoting the Rural Medical Service Capability of Treating Childhood Leukemia and Congenital Heart Disease

Distinguished Minister, Mr. Chen Zhu, respectable leaders, dear representatives and comrades:

Good afternoon!

Today, the Ministry of Health holds the Field Work Meeting on Promoting the Rural Medical Service Capability of Treating Childhood Leukemia and Congenital Heart Disease in Sichuan Province, which is a great encouragement and impetus for us. This meeting also provides us a rare opportunity to learn and improve ourselves. On behalf of the Sichuan Provincial People's Government, I would like to extend my warm welcome to all the representatives and heartfelt congratulations on the convening of this meeting.

Sichuan is one of the most important provinces in the national strategy of Going West. The province governs 21 cities (prefectures), 181 counties (cities, districts). The province has more than 88 million population, covering an area of 485,000 square kilometers, accommodating more than 50 nationalities. Sichuan province is the second largest Tibetan area, the largest agglomeration of the Yi ethnic group, and the only agglomeration of the Qiang ethnic group. In 2009, the GDP in Sichuan Province reached 1.4 trillion Yuan, with its economic aggregate ranking 9th in the country.

Since the devastating Wenchuan 5/12 earthquake, with the guide of the CPC Central Committee and the State Council, with the support of the MOH, other relevant ministries, provinces (districts, cities), and all society sectors, Sichuan has made great achievement in the post-disaster reconstruction. The reconstruction work is expected to be done this year, and the basic economic conditions and the economic and social development level in disaster strike areas will reach or surpass pre-disaster levels.

In recent years, with the care and support of the MOH and its minister Chen Zhu, taking the opportunity of deepening the medical and healthcare system reform, Sichuan Province has made a headway in the cause of healthcare. We have initiatively established the healthcare insurance system with various forms, which is centered on the New Rural Co-operative Medical system, Basic Medical Insurance for Urban workers, and Basic Medical Insurance for Urban Residents. More than 82 million people have joined the insurance system, covering almost all the rural and urban residents. 30% urban community health service institutions and grassroots medical service institutions set up by the government have steadily pushed forward the essential medicine system, bringing a more than 30% decrease of medical treatment fees. The urban and rural grassroots medical and healthcare system has been further improved, as well as the environment for the general public to get medical services. The equalization of basic public health services has been gradually promoted. Nine basic public healthcare services have brought benefits to rural and urban areas, and the pilot project of public hospital reform has been launched.

Childhood leukemia and congenital heart disease are two of the most serious diseases that damage some children's health. These two diseases are featured with great difficulty and high price in treatment, and huge damage to children. To average up the medical insurance level for rural children's leukemia and congenital heart disease is an effective measure to ease farmers' burden of treating major diseases. It's also an important measure to prevent rural families from becoming poor because of illness. Demonstrating the Party's and the government's commitment to administrate for the people and promote social harmony, this project is one that concerns the general public's interests and welcomed by the people. The Sichuan Provincial Committee of CPC and the provincial government attach great importance to improving the medical insurance level for rural children's leukemia and congenital heart disease. According to the unified planning of the MOH, Sichuan has actively carried out the project at the beginning of this year. Through thorough investigation and survey, we have propelled the pilot work, selected pilot areas, and specified diseases which should be included in the pilot work. We have evaluated and verified the compensation standard, and chosen the medical institutions for preliminary screening and targeted treatment. This is an innovative work which is still in the stage of exploration. Through vigorous efforts, we determined to establish a long-term mechanism and a steady funding mechanism to improve the medical insurance level for major diseases among rural residents. Simultaneously, we hope that we can receive care and support from the MOH as always. We firmly believe that this field experience exchange meeting held in Sichuan Province will be a powerful boost and impetus for the development of the medical service capability of treating leukemia and congenital heart disease in rural areas. And even it will push forward the development of health services.

We appreciate the care and support rendered by other brother provinces, districts and cities to the healthcare cause in Sichuan province. At last, wish the Field Work Meeting a complete succuss. Thank you.

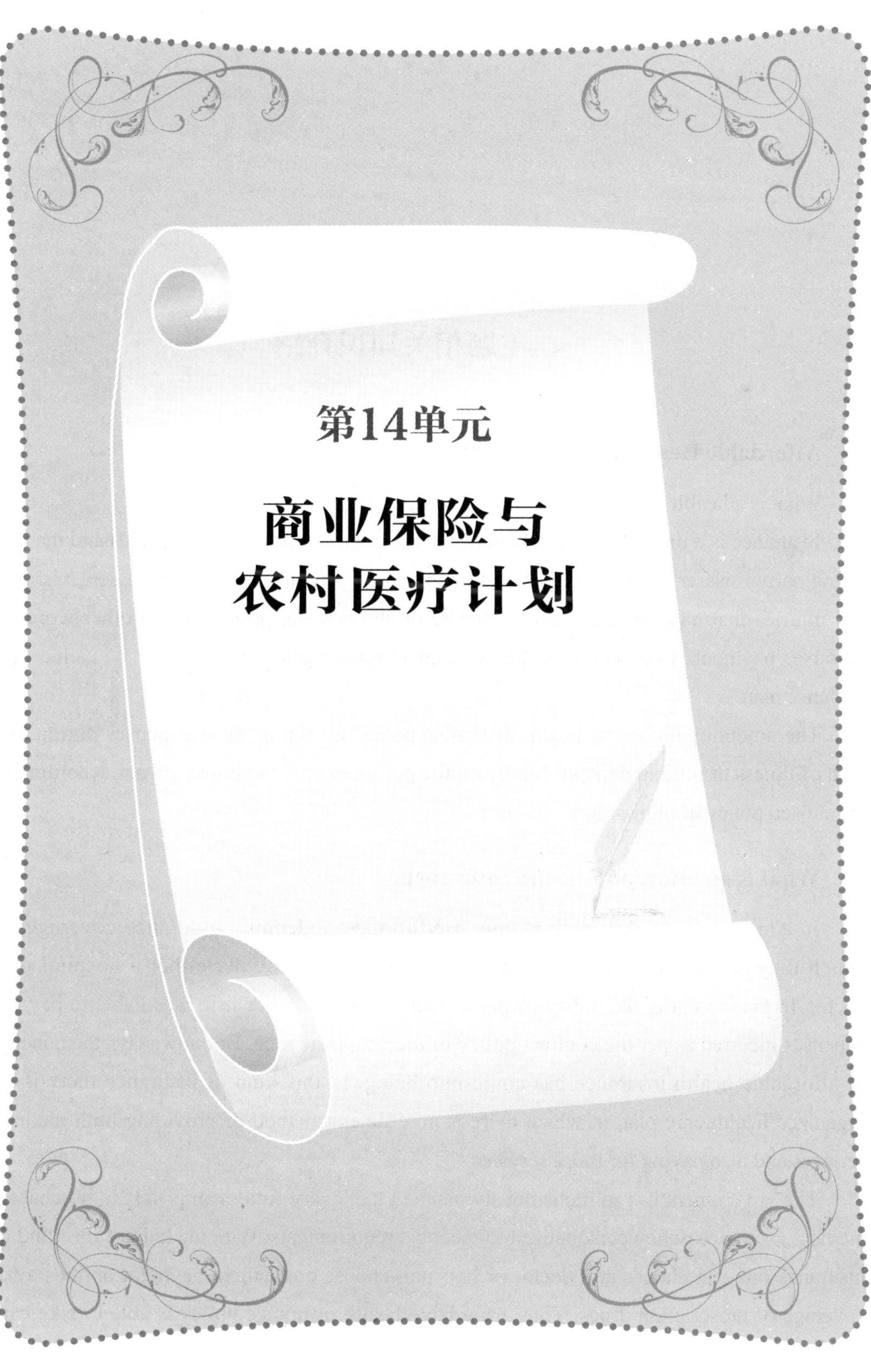

第14单元

商业保险与农村医疗计划

一、主题相关知识介绍

Affordable Health Insurance Policy

What is a health insurance and how it works?

Insurance is a mutual negotiation between the owner of the policy (insured) and the risk taking party (insurer), to wrap the cost of treatment for any unanticipated illnesses, mishaps, and injuries that happen to a person after he or she buy the policy. So, in other words it promises payments to a person in the event of illness or grievance and can be called as a "defense plan".

The amount paid by the health insurance policy for the medical expenses during any kind of illness or mishap depends totally on the premium paid the policy owner according to the chosen policy of high or low premiums.

What is an affordable health insurance?

In America few years back people used to have indemnity assurance coverage, in which they can avail facility from any medical service provider either a hospital or a doctor. In that scenario, the policy owner as well as the insurance firm was liable to pay the expenses incurred as per the contract policy of medical insurance. But nowadays the concept of affordable health insurance has come into being. In this kind of insurance there is an organized health care plan in which there is an efficient method of providing both medical services and also paying for those services.

The government has so meticulously planned that every American is able to purchase a medical insurance policy personalized to meet his requirements. With the help of this kind of insurance one can choose any doctor or hospital, choose convenient payment options avail coverage of prescription drugs. Thus, affordable health insurance policy is able to take care of expenses such as price of drugs, examinations, doctor's fees, charges of hospital room, surgeries sometimes even emergency surgeries and haulage, etc.

How and why affordable health insurance helps?

According to the survey in the year 2004 in USA, it was reported that 245.3 million people had health insurance coverage. So one can anticipate how far the number has increased till now. But still 45.8 million lived did not have health insurance in the same year.

Case study and statistics for affordable health insurance policy.

Let us see why personal and affordable health insurance is all the more important in a country.

In our country and most of the developing countries very less is expensed on the growth of medical and health sector because the basic developmental and infrastructural needs drag the attention due to which the government hospitals are deficiently facilitated particularly for any advanced treatments.

Hardly 2% of the GDP is spent on the health in our country.

In such a scenario with the help of health insurance one can avail the benefit from the insurance firms as per his financial capabilities.

So health insurance in India is being warmly welcomed by the citizens, senior citizens of the country.

Developed countries spend as much as 6% to 8% of their GDP on health area.

Nowadays, some of the highly regarded companies offer health insurance assistance to their employee. Some countries offer free health insurance to their citizens. In India railways and army employees of the central government are provided health benefits to almost 20 million people in our country.

Affordable Health Insurance cover should be able to take care of costs such as cost of drugs, investigations, surgical procedures, doctor's fees, cost of hospital room and sometimes even emergency transportation.

Insurance industry in India has witnessed a sea of change since the opening of the sector for private participation. Most of these insurance companies have appointed Third Party Administrator thus landing into the concept of "Reinsurance".

The introduction of this concept of reinsurance is profitable for both the insured and the insurer. While the insurers are gained by reduction in their payable amount at the same time the insured is happy by superior medical facility.

二、技巧指导：跨文化交际意识

在社会生活中，涉及跨文化交际的口译场合有很多，比如学术交流，中外合作，政府外事活动，跨境旅游，独资、合资公司工作，跨境贸易往来，体育赛事，音乐会，会展等。作为口译译员，必须有跨文化交际意识，将自己定位到沟通的桥梁上。

既然在跨文化交际中持不同语言、有不同文化背景的人们要沟通，交际的双方只有使用同一种语言才能达到目的。使用同一种语言时，必然有一方要用母语，另一方用习得语。在有口译译员的场合，译员本身便要在母语与习得语之间转换。转换之中，难免有误。在这种情况下，作为准译员的我们应该知道，交际之中经常会产生的语义误解除了出自语言本身，还会出自语言背后的文化习惯。比如，中国人习惯关心他人的冷暖，会说“你穿多了/少了”，因此会提醒“加/减一件衣服吧”。西方人也许不会把这样的提醒看成关心，反而有可能觉得干涉了个人自由。再举一个例子：一次在一个连续一周的讲习班里，一位老师因胃肠性感冒一天没有露面，再出现时，中方老师们都主动询问病情，并劝其继续休息；而外方老师则没有询问，因为在他们眼中，生病也是隐私，别人不主动说，就不好问。习俗没有对错，尊重是正确的选择。

也有观念上的差异导致的信息接受障碍。比如，没有读过《圣经》，中国学生翻译西方人的圣诞演讲一类的讲稿就会漏译错译；而西方译员不读中国古代文学也翻译不好引经据典的中国领导讲话。对于中方译员来讲，中文的成语、谚语、典故的翻译方法也是必须平时积累的，既要学会翻译方法，也要背记译文。

在实际口译工作之时，除了需要平时积累文化与习俗知识以利于翻译本身以外，还需要礼仪知识来指导译员的行为规范。从礼仪的角度看，不同的人种之间完全能够感受到相同的行为正能量。跨文化交际中有“谦逊”的文化特征，因此通行的国际礼仪有几个主要原则：（1）信守承诺（无论是信用还是守时）；（2）尊重隐私，不打听他人的政治主张、宗教信仰和私人生活等；（3）尊重他人，热情有度，矜持有范；（4）自信而不自傲，谦恭有度；（5）女士优先。

除此之外，还有下面一些细节需要注意。

称呼

英语国家的职位称呼没有中文繁杂，如“李秘书”“张经理”“王科长”“赵店长”“孙木匠”基本上不用于口头称呼人，只会偶尔出现在他人的口头描述中；而在书信交往时，称谓上加上姓氏则比较常见。因此，无论是在正式场合还是非正式的口头交际场合，“先生、夫人、女士、小姐”已经是尊称了。例如Mr. Wood，

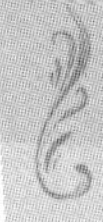

Mrs. Wood，Ms. Wang，Miss Zhao。对法官、律师、教授、医生，可以在这些称谓之前加上姓氏，例如Judge Temple，Attorney Hanks，Dr. White，Professor Brown，Doctor Lock等；也可以单独使用，与中文一样。军人的称谓与此相同，可以用军衔、姓或名加军衔，译成中文可用军衔加“阁下”或“先生”。例如General（将军阁下），Colonel Gray（格雷上校），Major（少校先生）。

在特别正式的场合，部长以上的官员可用“阁下”称呼。例如“总统阁下”“主席先生阁下”“总理阁下”“大使先生阁下”“部长阁下”等。君主制国家的国王和皇后有“陛下”之称，亲王、王子、公主有“殿下”之称。公爵、侯爵、伯爵、子爵、男爵等人被称为“阁下”。

介绍

介绍他人的时候应将年纪轻、身份低的介绍给年纪大、身份高的，把男士介绍给女士。介绍的内容为姓名、身份、就职单位等。被别人介绍时，应该回应“您好”。如果站的地方没有障碍物，应该站起来应答以示尊敬。

握手

礼节性地握手时，一般是身份高的人、主办方、年长者、妇女先伸手，身份低的人、年轻人、访问方待对方伸手再握手。另外，无论是见面、祝贺，还是感谢，握手的时候应该微微有点力度，以示真诚，同时双目注视对方并微笑致意。身份低的、年轻的与身份高的、年长的握手时身体应稍微前倾，用双手握住对方的手，以示尊敬。

打招呼

与认识的人或初识者在一个场合多次碰面或相遇，且距离较远时，应该点头致意或点头微笑。两人侧身而过时，有必要轻轻说一声“Hi”或道声“您好”。

交谈

口译工作空隙之间所发生的交谈能够增进了解，融洽关系，在某种意义上是工作的延续。因此在交谈时应该注意别人的感受。具体表现在：

● 谈别人感兴趣的话题。

● 用委婉的表达方式，观点不同也不争执。

● 说话顾及在座所有人，不忽视任何人，除非是私聊的场合，在多人的场合窃窃私语不合时宜。

● 声音不高不低，语速不快不慢，语调和缓不急躁。

●专心聆听，在别人说完之前，不打断、不急于插话或另起话题。不得已要插话之前要先说“对不起，我插一句”。即使别人谈你已熟知或完全陌生、不感兴趣的话题，也不能表现出不耐烦。积极的沟通不是急于表达自己，而是通过聆听和回应首先了解他人，再做出适宜的回应。与人谈话时不断地打电话、看手机也是不礼貌的。离开时要打招呼，不能拔腿就走。

●礼貌地适当提问，既是尊重他人，也能获得知识和信息。

●慎用夸张的表情或手势。在非正式场合常有的如转笔杆、掸灰尘、压指节、整理头发等行为都不合时宜。

●保持社交距离。与日常生活不同，在正式的跨文化交际场合，社交的空间距离一般需要保持一米左右。

●事先了解他人的宗教禁忌是一种礼貌。

接收名片

在翻译工作中需要译员递出名片的场合不多，也因为工作为服务性质，主动索要他人的名片不合礼仪。但译员有时也会跟随所服务的对象接收他人出于礼貌递过来的名片。这时应该稍稍躬身，用双手接过名片，微笑着道声谢谢。时间充足的话，还应当着对方的面阅读名片，然后郑重地放在自己随身携带的文件夹或包中。工作紧张时可以握在手中，但不可以随手塞在什么地方。需要回赠的时候，也要稍微躬身，双手握着名片的上方递出，让对方能够正对文字，并同时说“请您多关照”等谦语。

着装

在工作场合中，译员不是事件的主体，而是事件进行的协助者，因此着装需要收敛，只能穿庄重的服装。男性只能穿衬衫、西服等，休闲款式如圆领衫、牛仔裤、运动装是不正式的；女性也应穿西服裙或长裤，除了休闲服装之外，旗袍和其他紧身服装也不合适。在颜色方面，鲜艳的颜色和花衣服都不合适，应该选择色彩柔和的颜色，比如米色、灰色、浅蓝色、浅绿色、豆沙色等。白色和黑色都比较抢眼，应该让给服务对象用。

告别

交谈之中提前离开，或结束交谈离开之时，应告知对方。工作结束时，对别人在工作中给予的帮助，即使是举手之劳，有机会也应表示感谢。

三、词汇准备

Text 1

New Rural Cooperative Medical Scheme (NRCMS) 新型农村合作医疗
universal coverage 全覆盖
pilot programs 试点项目
targeted population 目标人群
per capita cost of the insurance package 人均保险费用
hospitalization compensation 住院补偿
reimbursement for hospitalization costs 住院费用报销
comprehensive institutional framework 综合机构框架
operational mechanism 运行机制
insurance agencies 保险代理公司
designated hospitals 指定医院
separating supervision from operation, and separating government administration from medical institutions 监管与操作分离，政府与医疗机构分离
all-in-one-card pilot program 一卡通试点项目
crystallization 具体化

Text 2

a point of service plan 服务点计划
Health Maintenance Organization (HMO) 健康维护组织
fee-for-service 一次一付的按服务付服务费
policyholder 投保人，保险单持有人
The Association of British Insurers 英国保险协会
Critical Illness 重症
Financial Services Authority 金融服务管理局
recurring 复发
cosmetic surgery 整容手术
Health Insurance Portability and Accountability Act 《健康保险携带和责任法案》

Text 3

New Rural Cooperative Medical Scheme (NRCMS) 新型农村合作医疗（新农合）

new round 新一轮
the three-tier rural health service delivery system 农村三级卫生服务体系
county-level hospitals 县级医院
township health care facilities 乡镇卫生院
village clinics 村卫生室
primary health care 初级卫生保健
health inspection 健康检查
county maternal and children's hospitals 县妇幼卫生院
allocate 分配
person-times 人次
general practitioners (GP) 全科医生
licensed practitioners 执业医师
the Urban Employees' Basic Medical Insurance Scheme 城镇职工基本医疗保险
the Urban Resident's Basic Medical Insurance Scheme 城镇居民基本医疗保险
non-working urban residents 非在职城镇居民
congenital heart disease 先天性心脏病
acute leukemia 急性白血病
reimburse 报销
pilot diseases 试点病种
Medical Financial Assistance 医疗救助
end-stage renal disease 终末期肾脏疾病
hemophilia 血友病
chronic myeloid leukemia (CML) 慢性粒细胞白血病
cleft lip and palate 唇腭裂
esophagus cancer 食道癌
gastric cancer 胃癌
type I diabetes Ⅰ型糖尿病
hyperthyroidism 甲状腺功能亢进症
cerebral infarction 脑梗死
acute myocardial infarction 急性心肌梗死
colon cancer 结肠癌
rectal cancer 直肠癌
screening 筛查
folic acid supplements 叶酸补充剂

Text 4

multilevel 多层次
reimburse 报销
phenylketonuria 苯丙酮尿症
congenital hypospadias 先天性尿道下裂
commission 正式委托
trans-provincial 跨省的

Text 5

商业医疗保险 commercial medical insurance
赢利性 profit earning
保障金额 premium
保险代理公司 Insurance Proxy Companies
保险经纪公司 Insurance Broker Companies
非定额补偿 non-quota compensation
意外伤害 accidental injury
附加责任 additional responsibility
终止 terminate

Text 6

中国医师协会健康管理与健康保险专委会 (HMO) Professional Committee of Health Management & Health Insurance of Chinese Medical Doctor Association (HMO-CHINA)

慈铭健康体检管理集团 Ciming Health Checkup Management Group

卫生行政和保监主管部门 Health Executive Department and the Insurance Regulatory Department

中国医师协会 CMDA (Chinese Medical Doctor Association)

生力军 the new force

保监会 CIRC (China Insurance Regulatory Commission)

人保健康 PICC Health Insurance Company Limited

平安健康 Ping An Insurance (Group) Company of China, Ltd

逡巡踟蹰 hesitate to move forward

病根 the root cause

职业资格评审 the examination of the professional qualification

晋升机制 the promotion mechanism

核保核赔 underwriting and claim settlement

中央财经大学保险学院 the Insurance Institution at the Central University of Finance and Economics

中国保监会政研室 the Political Survey Office of the CIRC

执业资格审核注册 the examination and registration of the qualification

职称评定晋升 the professional-title evaluation and promote

四、摘要练习

请听下面英语语篇，第一篇用源语言复述此段主要信息逻辑点及层次，第二篇用译入语复述此段主要信息逻辑点及层次。注意信息点之间的逻辑联系。

Text 1

The Development of China's New Rural Cooperative Medical Scheme

2012 marks the tenth anniversary of the implementation of the New Rural Cooperative Medical Scheme (NRCMS). Over the past decade, with Party Committees and governments at all levels attaching great importance to NRCMS and under their strong leadership, relevant departments have given full cooperation and farmers have actively participated in the scheme. Therefore, NRCMS has made solid progress and remarkable achievements.

First, NRCMS has almost realized universal coverage with the participation remaining stable at a high level. Since the pilot programs in 2003, NRCMS has achieved a comprehensive coverage in 2008. The participation number has grown steadily every year, from 80 million in the early stage of the pilot programs to 812 million by the end of June 2012, with over 95% of the targeted population covered.

Second, the financing continues to grow and the protection level improves gradually. The per capita cost of the insurance package increased from 30 Yuan in 2003 to 250 Yuan in 2011. In 2011, 1.315 billion person-times benefited from NRCMS with average hospitalization compensation amounting to 1,894 Yuan. In 2012, the reimbursement for hospitalization costs will reach around 75%, with an annual payment ceiling of no less than 8 times of farmer's per capita net income (no less than 60,000 Yuan).

Third, a comprehensive institutional framework and operational mechanism is established in line with China's national conditions, i.e. led by the government; in the charge of health departments; supported by relevant sectors; operated by the insurance agencies; with services provided by the health institutions; participated by farmers and transparent reimbursement of the medial costs. NRCMS is co-financed by individual contributions, farmers' cooperatives and both central and local governments, with families participating on a voluntary basis. The coordinated compensation focuses on reimbursement for hospitalization costs and gradually expands to out-patient care. In 2011, over 90% of areas carried out out-patient compensation which benefited the farmers in a wider range. The insured farmers can choose independently the designated hospitals for treatment and get real-time reimbursement. In 2011, over 2/3 of provinces (autonomous regions or municipalities) adopted real-time reimbursement in their designated provincial and municipal hospitals. The funds are operated in closed-end mechanism and supervised by multi-sectors. In 2011, over 80% of areas carried out various payment reforms, which supported NRCMS to effectively control the medical costs. Commercial insurance agencies are encouraged to involve in the operation of NRCMS, which explores the operational mechanism of "separating supervision from operation, and separating government administration from medical institutions".

In the next stage, integrating with the overall arrangements for deepening the reform by the central government, we will press ahead in the following aspects:

First, the financing for NRCMS should grow in a steady pace. The fund pooled per capita will reach 300 Yuan by 2012. By 2015, government subsidies will reach 360 Yuan per person per year. The individual contribution will grow as appropriate. A financing mechanism that suits the economic development in China will be gradually established.

Second, the NRCMS should be meticulously managed, including strict utilization of the funds and enhancing supervision on designated hospitals. Real-time reimbursement should be established in designated provincial and municipal hospitals as well as village clinics across the country. Reimbursement for medical costs outside of one's registered province should be gradually realized. The information engineering of NRCMS should be accelerated, in combination with distributing the health cards for the residents, in order to press ahead the all-in-one-card pilot program. The information systems of NRCMS and related schemes such as the medical assistance scheme should be better synchronized, to provide one-stop real-time compensation service.

Third, the pilot program of compensation for major diseases should be promoted, including 20 diseases such as child leukemia, lung cancer etc. The Guiding Opinions on the Supplementary Insurance of Major Diseases for Urban and Rural Residents collectively issued by six ministries should be implemented. Supplementary Insurance should be well connected with NRCMS policy on the benefits for major diseases and should cover the mentioned 20 major diseases as preference.

Fourth, NRCMS payment reforms should be accelerated, in terms of using pre-payment of total medical cost, disease-based payment, service unit-based payment and capitation to replace fee-for-service. The reforms aim to control medical costs, modify health service behaviors and enhance fund performance.

Fifth, the engagement of entrusted qualified commercial insurance agencies in the operation of NRCMS should be accelerated, so as to establish an operational mechanism that to some degree separates the management, operation and supervision of NRCMS.

Sixth, the experience of the last decade should be diligently studied to facilitate the formulation of the Regulations on Administration of New Rural Cooperative Medical Scheme. The administration of NRCMS should be legislated as soon as possible.

It has been proven that NRCMS, a suitable mechanism for rural China, is an important crystallization of basic medical insurance system for rural residents in current circumstances. In the last decade, NRCMS has grown up from a new born baby and is now playing a vital role for the health of the rural residents. As the competent authority of NRCMS, the Ministry of Health will collaborate with other related ministries to continue to promote its development and steadily improve rural residents' health status.

复述要点提示（主要信息逻辑点及层次）

New Rural Cooperative Medical Scheme (NRCMS) has made solid progress and remarkable achievements.

1. NRCMS has almost realized universal coverage with the participation remaining stable at a high level. The participation number rose from 80 million in the pilot programs to 812 million by the end of June 2012. 95% of the targeted population is covered.

2. The financing continues to grow and the protection level improves gradually. The per capita cost of the insurance package increased from 30 Yuan in 2003 to 250 Yuan in 2011. 2012 reimbursement for hospitalization costs will reach around 75%.

3. NRCMS has established a comprehensive institutional framework and operational mechanism, one including government leadership, health department's responsibility, supports from relevant sectors, insurance agency's operation, services by health institutions, and farmers' voluntary participation.

● For example, NRCMS is co-financed by individual contributions, farmers' cooperatives and the central government and local governments.

● The coordinated compensation focuses on reimbursement for hospitalization costs and gradually expands to out-patient care.

● The insured farmers can choose independently the designated hospitals for treatment and get real-time reimbursement.

● Commercial insurance agencies are encouraged to involve in the operation of NRCMS.

What will be done next?

1. Financial development. The fund pooled per capita will reach 300 Yuan by 2012. By 2015, government subsidies will reach 360 Yuan per person per year.

2. Strengthening of NRCMS management. It includes strict utilization of funds, supervision enhancement, establishment of Real-time reimbursement in all leveled hospitals, allopatry reimbursement, acceleration of information engineering, provision of the all-in-one-card pilot program and one-stop real-time compensation service.

3. Promoting the pilot program of compensation for major diseases by implementing "The Guiding Opinions on the Supplementary Insurance of Major Diseases for Urban and Rural Residents".

4. Accelerating NRCMS payment reforms in terms of using pre-payment of total medical cost, disease-based payment, service unit-based payment and capitation to replace fee-for-service.

5. Accelerating the engagement of entrusted qualified commercial insurance agencies in the operation of NRCMS.

6. Promoting legislation of the administration of NRCMS.

Text 2

Commercial Health Insurance

What Is Commercial Health Insurance?

In America, commercial health insurance is also known as private health insurance. Commercial health insurance is any type of health insurance that is not offered and managed by a government entity. Companies that sell this type of insurance are for-profit corporations, and offer their insurance services through group insurance plans as well as individual or personal plans. In all situations, a commercial insurance of this type is available only to those who are willing to pay premiums in exchange for the coverage.

Many people have access to commercial health insurance through an employer. Sometimes referred to as group insurance, employees who meet the employer's criteria in terms of hours worked, time with the company, and other factors may be enrolled into the program. Depending on the way that the insurance program is arranged, the employer may absorb the total cost of the monthly premium for each employee, or pay a percentage of the total premium. When that is the case, the employee pays for the remainder of the premium due via a payroll deduction that is withheld by the employer.

While there are a number of different formats for commercial health insurance, three models are the most common around the world. The most popular is known as a point of service plan. This type of insurance coverage allows the client to choose a primary care physician from the list provided by the insurance carrier. Using healthcare professionals that are considered to be in-network ensures that the provider covers a larger share of any medical expenses that qualify under the terms of the contract. Should the client choose to utilize a physician outside the provider's network, the benefits paid per medical incident are usually decreased.

Another popular option is known as the health maintenance organization, or HMO. As with the point of service approach, participants in an HMO choose a primary care physician from a listing supplied by the provider. In order to see a specialist, the primary care physician must officially refer the patient to that specialist. This type of plan rarely covers medical care provided by healthcare professionals outside the network, except under unusual circumstances.

Another option for commercial health insurance is the fee-for-service, or indemnity model. This type of program covers a specific listing of healthcare procedures. Clients can see any physician or specialist they wish, without any decrease in benefits. Plans of this type may be very limited in scope, such as focusing on office visits and procedures that are done in the physician's office. Other indemnity plans are more comprehensive, and include coverage for hospital care related to conditions listed in the provisions of the contract.

When evaluating any type of commercial health insurance, it is important to make sure the plan will provide adequate coverage. This means reading the terms carefully as they related to routine checkups, outpatient procedures, hospital stays, mental health treatments, and the amounts of all applicable deductibles and co-payments. In addition, many people will want to include long-term care insurance in the coverage, as this can help alleviate financial hardship during an extended illness.

Do I Need Health Insurance?

The average wait for an outpatient appointment with the National Health Service in England is around seven weeks. Therefore, as a result many opt for a private health insurance policy, which covers the cost of private medical treatment in the case of curable or short-term medical conditions.

Health insurance provides the policyholder with the promise that treatment will be available as soon as they injure themselves or fall ill. The Association of British Insurers states: “Most people buy this type of insurance to gain the reassurance of knowing that treatment is available promptly, if they become ill or are injured.”

Private health insurance should not be seen as an alternative to the NHS, as private hospitals are generally not equipped for casualty situations. However, it will ensure that you get care more quickly.

Taking out a health insurance policy is a good idea as it can ease some of the common fears experienced by those who fall ill. For example there is no need to wait for a long time to find out what is wrong and patients will go straight on the waiting list for surgery if it is required.

So What Different Types of Health Insurance Exist in the UK?

There are many different plans available for health insurance in the UK.

Critical Illness—Critical illness insurance covers patients who are suddenly diagnosed with severe illness. They generally pay a tax-free lump sum of money that can be used by the patient according to their wishes. This money can be used for almost anything such as leisure or debt repayment.

Income Protection—Income protection insurance is important for self-employed people. In the UK should you become unable to work, you will receive £60.20 per week. Also the plan will pay up to 65% of your gross income should you find yourself unable to work due to sickness or an accident. The premium for this type of insurance is calculated depending on the type of work that you are involved in and how quickly you want benefits to pay. These benefit payments cease when you are fit enough to return to work.

The Health Trust Fund—This is a current policy designed to replace the traditional health insurance scheme. This type of plan takes advantage of trust fund laws in the UK that permit low cost cover, no excess payments, no automatic premium increases, comprehensive access to medical facilities and no age loading. However, the Financial Services Authority does not regulate health trust funds at this stage.

Cash Plans—This type of insurance is a low-cost plan that is put into place to provide cash for policyholder's medical expenses. These could include optical, dental or nursing benefits. This type of plan is available for both families and individuals.

However, it is important to bear in mind when choosing health insurance the pre-existing conditions and exclusions policy. Exclusions refer to conditions under which insurers will refuse to pay cover and sadly some of these exclusions exist in health insurance. These can include chronic, recurring or long-term conditions or diseases, cosmetic surgery and experimental treatments.

Pre-existing conditions refer to medical conditions that have been diagnosed or treated prior to joining a new health insurance plan. Commonly, the insurer will exclude cover for any condition that has existed in the last five years. Some insurers will make conditions eligible for cover when you are shown to be completely clear of the condition after your policy begins.

A law called the Health Insurance Portability and Accountability Act means that pre-existing conditions will be covered providing that you have been insured for twelve months previously, should you join a group plan through an employer.

复述要点提示（主要信息逻辑点及层次）

什么是商业健康保险？

在美国，商业健康保险也被称为私人健康保险，任何不由政府实体提供和管理的健康保险都是商业健康保险。出售这类保险的公司是以赢利为目的的，并通过团体保险提供保险服务计划，也提供个体和个人保险计划。在任何情况下，这种类型的商业保险只提供给那些愿意为健康保险覆盖支付保险费的人。

团体保险。员工在满足雇主制定的标准后，便可被纳入团体保险计划。雇主会视具体情况酌情为雇员全额或部分支付保险费。

世界各地最受欢迎的是“服务点计划”保险。客户可根据保险公司提供的名单选择医疗网络中的初级护理医师，并且能够得到比该合同份额更高的医疗费用。

另一种是健康维护组织（HMO）。参保人也在由供应商提供的名单上选择初级护理医师。如果见专科医生，初级保健医生必须向专科医生正式推荐病人。

另一种是一次一付的按服务付费。客户可以看任何医生或专家，并且受益方面没有任何减少。

在选择任何类型的商业健康保险时，都应确保保险计划能够提供足够的覆盖范围，因此要仔细阅读条款。

是否需要买健康险？

因为在英国等待国家医疗服务门诊预约的平均时间大约是7个星期，所以许多人选择私人健康保险。

健康保险公司向投保人承诺，一旦他们受伤或生病便可接受治疗。英国保险协会指出："大多数人购买这种保险是为了确保在生病或受伤的时候能及时得到治疗。"

办理健康保险可以减轻那些身患疾病的人的担忧。例如无须长时间等待来查病因；如果需要做手术，病人可以直接出现在等候表上。

英国不同类型的健康保险：

- 重大疾病保险，覆盖那些突然诊断出患有严重疾病的人。
- 收入保障保险，针对个体劳动者。如果生病或发生意外事故无法工作，该保险将支付高达你总收入的65%。
- 健康信托基金，这类保险利用英国的信托基金法，允许低成本保险，无超额支付，无自动保费增加，综合享有医疗设施且无年龄限制。
- 现金计划，低成本，为投保人的医疗费用提供现金的计划。

注意：

- 选择健康保险时要清楚投保前自己已患有的疾病和保险单不保的项目，因为慢性病、复发或长期疾病、整容手术和实验治疗不在保险范围内。
- 并非所有先前患有疾病的人都不能投保。并且投保人要有工作单位。

五、英译汉练习

Text 3

Rural Health Reform and Development in China

23 May 2012

Respected Assistant Director General Dr. Carissa F. Etienne,

Respected Secretary P. K. Pradhan,

Respected Dr. Jarvis Barbosa,

Ladies and Gentlemen,

Good afternoon! It was inspiring to listen to my colleagues' presentations on the rural health program in India and the family health program in Brazil. It is also my great pleasure to share with you China's experience in rural health reform and development.

China is a developing country with 1.37 billion people, over 60% of whom, or 850 million, live in rural areas.

The national condition of a big rural population and the gap between rural and urban areas in China makes it necessary to prioritize rural areas in its health policy. In April 2009, the Chinese government launched the new round of health care reform, making it an imperative to establish and improve the basic medical and health system for rural and urban residents, providing health services as public goods to the entire population, adding new meaning to the rural health reform and development in the new era.

Now I would like to update you on the results of this endeavor.

Ⅰ. Improving Three-Tier Rural Health Service Delivery System

The three-tier rural health service delivery system is composed of county-level hospitals, township health care facilities, and village clinics, providing the rural population with such services as prevention, primary health care, health inspection and health education. This network covers 2,856 counties across 31 provinces.

Since the launch of the health care reform, an earmarked 52 billion Yuan from the central governmental budget has been allocated to improve the rural health delivery system, including over 2,000 county hospitals and 25,000 village clinics. By the end of 2010, there were 6,400 county hospitals, over 1,500 county maternal and children's hospitals, nearly 1,700 county CDCs and over 1,500 county health inspection institutions in China. There were also

38,000 township hospitals, i.e. almost every township has one or more hospitals. There were 648,000 village clinics, covering 92.3% of all the villages. From 2006 to 2011, the number of visits to township hospitals and village clinics increased from 2.07 billion to 2.66 billion, an increase of 28.5%.

Ⅱ. Strengthening Rural Health Workforce

From 2004 to 2011, 2.26 billion Yuan was allocated from the central governmental budget to Mid-and-Western areas, providing 4.36 million person-times training among rural health professionals. The program of "Ten Thousand Medical Doctors Supporting Township Hospitals" was initiated in 2005, and 1.32 billion Yuan was allocated for the project of "Medical Institutions at and above Secondary Level Supporting Township Hospitals". So far the project has covered township hospitals in poverty-stricken areas in 21 provinces in central and western parts of China. 70,000 person-times of technical assistance have been provided there.

Strengthening health workforce with focus on training general practitioners has been one of several priorities in the past years. 36,000 rural health professionals have been trained to become GPs. Over 10,000 medical students have been enrolled without tuition fee on the condition that they promise to work in rural hospitals after graduation. Above 20,000 licensed physicians have been recruited at township hospitals.

By the end of 2010, there were nearly 1.6 million health workers in county hospitals, 1.2 million in township hospitals, about 1.3 health workers per thousand rural population at township level. Village clinics have 1.2 million health professionals, among whom over 1 million were village doctors and 173,000 were licensed practitioners or assistant licensed practitioners.

Ⅲ. Consolidating the New Rural Cooperative Medical Scheme (NRCMS)

China's basic health insurance system is composed of four parts: the Urban Employees' Basic Medical Insurance Scheme, the Urban Resident's Basic Medical Insurance Scheme, the New Rural Cooperative Medical Scheme and the Medical Financial Assistance Scheme, covering urban employees, non-working urban residents, rural residents and poverty-stricken people respectively.

NRCMS, a plan which provides coverage to rural residents, has played an essential role in reducing their financial burden, protecting them from falling into or back into poverty when being struck by catastrophic diseases, and improving their health. In the year 2011, the coverage has expanded to 832 million people, 97.5% of the rural population. So we can see basically this is universal coverage. The funding per person has increased from 30 Yuan in

2003 to 300 Yuan per person in 2012. Under the scheme, patients are reimbursed for about 75% of their inpatient expenditures and the annual reimbursement cap is no less than 60, 000 Yuan in 2012. The funding pool for the scheme has increased substantially from 4 billion Yuan in 2003 to 204.8 billion Yuan in 2011, out of which 77.2 billion Yuan are contributed by the central government. NRCMS has become the medical security scheme with the largest coverage in the world.

In June 2010, beginning with rural children's congenital heart disease and acute leukemia, we started a pilot program to improve the insurance level for catastrophic diseases for rural residents. NRCMS reimbursed 70% of the medical expenditures for the pilot diseases, and Medical Financial Assistance reimbursed another 20% for eligible patients. In 2011, another 6 catastrophic diseases, namely, end-stage renal disease, severe mental disease, breast cancer, cervical cancer, multi-drug resistant tuberculosis, opportunistic infections among HIV/AIDS patients, were included into the pilot program. In 2012, the insurance program for the above 8 diseases will be fully scaled up. Meanwhile, in 1/3 of the NRCMS covered areas, another 12 diseases, including hemophilia, chronic myeloid leukemia(CML), cleft lip and palate, lung cancer, esophagus cancer, gastric cancer, type I diabetes, hyperthyroidism, cerebral infarction, stroke, acute myocardial infarction, colon cancer and rectal cancer, will be included into the pilot program.

With NRCMS and improved health service delivery system, healthcare facilities are constructed or upgraded, and service capability of providers is enhanced in the rural areas and in particular remote areas, which leads to farmers' easier and more affordable access to medical and healthcare services.

From 2008 to 2011, the proportion of the rural households who had access to healthcare services within 15-minute walk climbed from 75.6% to 80.8%; the percentage of the out-of-pocket expenditure for rural residents dropped from 73.4% to 49.5%; the percentage of those who choose not to see a doctor when falling ill dropped from 12.4% to 6.1%.

IV. Providing Basic Public Health Services Across Rural Areas

Equitable access to basic public health services, a highlight of China's health care reform, provides institutional arrangements for its long-standing policy of putting prevention first. Currently, 41 basic public health programs under 10 categories are provided, as the government subsidy for basic public health services per person goes up from 15 Yuan in 2009 to 25 Yuan in 2011.

As a result, health development gap between rural and urban areas is narrowing and health indicators for rural residents are improving rapidly: for example, rural maternal mortality rate dropped from 36.1 to 26.5 per 100,000, which is exactly at the same level as in the cities; infant mortality rate dropped from 18.4‰ to 14.7‰.

In 2011 in rural areas, 62.6% residents had electronic health records; hospital delivery rate reached 96%; 8.84 million pregnant women received government subsidy for hospital delivery; 4 million women received cervical cancer screening; 400,000 women received breast cancer screening and 9.9 million women took free folic acid supplements.

Thanks to the strenuous efforts in the past few years, the health care reform has brought more tangible benefits to the people, improving their access to healthcare services and bringing down the out-of-pocket costs. This reflects that the target, direction and guidelines of the reform are in line with the law of health development, the specific national conditions of China and the aspirations of the people.

The objectives for the reform in the next few years are as follows: by 2015, China will provide more equitable access to basic healthcare services and improve the efficiency and quality of the healthcare services; while properly controlling the growth of total health expenditure, China will gradually enhance the share of government spending on health in the total fiscal expenditure to bring down the out-of-pocket expenditure for individuals to below 30%; the problem of inadequate and unaffordable healthcare services will be eased; average life expectancy will reach 74.5; infant mortality rate will be reduced to below 12‰, and maternal mortality rate below 22 per 100,000.

The Chinese government is committed to pushing forward the health care reform in rural areas through improving NRCMS, health infrastructure and health workforce, so as to achieve the goal of universal access to basic health care service. We will work unswervingly to overcome all difficulties and blaze a path of health development with Chinese characteristics!

I would like to thank WHO and the international community for your support.

Thank you!

Text 4

The Progress of the New Rural Cooperative Medical Scheme (NRCMS) in 2013 and Major Tasks in 2014

The Progress of the NRCMS in 2013

In 2013, the New Rural Cooperative Medical Scheme ran smoothly. Management and the overall system were improved, covering a large rural population that enjoyed more benefits, especially with a higher level of medical insurance for serious illnesses.

The financing and security level was improved, further benefiting rural residents. By 2013, a total of 802 million people nationwide were covered by the NRCMS, accounting for 99% of the whole population. Funds raised reached 370 Yuan ($59.45) per capita, increasing by 62 Yuan from the year before. The reimbursement rate for hospitalization expenses covered by relevant policies exceeded 75%, and the real compensation ratio continued to increase—nearly 80% at the town level, over 60% at the county level and over 50% at the clinic, benefiting about 1.94 billion people with a year-on-year growth of 11.3%.

A multilevel and multiform preliminary security mechanism for major illnesses has also been established. First, security mechanism for serious illness focusing on the type of disease was consolidated and improved. In 2013, two more diseases, childhood phenylketonuria and hypospadias, were included into the scope of medical insurance for major illnesses apart from 20 diseases such as childhood leukemia and congenital heart disease. About 1.99 million patients received reimbursements, and the real compensation ratio for 22 types of diseases reached 69%, largely reducing their financial burden. Second, the NHFPC actively encouraged buying major illness insurance by using the funds of the NRCMS. In 2013, about 28 provinces developed implementation plans for major illness insurance. Up to 1.23 million patients received compensation and further relieved their burden.

Management and services were also improved. First, management and service were further commissioned to the society, helping transform the functions of the government. Now, up to 24% of counties, districts or cities have commissioned commercial insurance companies to operate the NRCMS, the medical expenses reimbursement process was further facilitated. Rural residents participating in the new system in over 88% of areas nationwide are now able to get immediate reimbursement anywhere in their province. The national NRCMS information platform has connected with nine provincial platforms and several large medical institutions, which makes inspection of trans-provincial medical expenses possible and also paves the way for the pilot program of trans-provincial medical expenses reimbursement. Third, a reform in payment method has been deepened, covering over 80% of areas nationwide and helping curb soaring medical expenses to some extent.

Major Tasks of the NRCMS in 2014

According to the tasks of the health care reform, the NHFPC will continue to develop and improve the NRCMS on the basis of urban-rural overall development of medical insurance.

First, to further enhance the financing standards and security level of the NRCMS, maintain a participation rate of the NRCMS of above 95%, increase annual subsidies to 320 Yuan per capita, optimize and coordinate a compensation scheme, and keep the reimbursement rate for medical expenses covered by relevant policies at 75% and outpatient expenses at 50%.

Second, to improve the medical security mechanism for various major illness in the NRCMS, continue the security mechanism for 22 serious diseases including childhood leukemia, expand the security mechanism to more than half of the areas covered by the NRCMS, and take full advantage of the system based on types of disease and expenses. We should also establish a preliminary mechanism of disease emergency rescue and coordinate with basic medical security, serious illness insurance for urban-rural residents and medical assistance.

Third, to encourage more commercial insurance companies to operate the management and service of the NRCMS and serious illness insurance. We should improve the management and service and set up a multilevel security mechanism for serious illness by taking advantage of both the government and market.

Fourth, to accelerate the informationization construction of the NRCMS, improve the service of immediate reimbursement within a province, continue the construction of national and provincial information platforms, and expand to 15 provinces that can connect to national information platforms. We should also launch a pilot program of trans-provincial medical expenses checking and reimbursement.

Fifth, to strengthen delicacy management of the NRCMS, promote the reform of payment methods, curb soaring medical expenses and further benefit rural residents. We should regulate the utilization and management of the NRCMS fund to ensure its safety.

六、汉译英练习

Text 5

商业医疗保险

商业医疗保险是医疗保障体系的组成部分，单位和个人自愿参加。国家鼓励用人单位和个人参加商业医疗保险。商业医疗保险是由保险公司经营的营利性的医疗保障。消费者依一定数额交纳保险金，遇到重大疾病时，可以从保险公司获得一定数额的医疗费用。

商业医疗保险属于健康险。健康险不仅补偿疾病带给人们的直接经济损失，还可以补偿疾病带来的间接经济损失，且对分娩、伤残、死亡等也给予经济补偿。

目前的商业医疗保险最突出的问题是价格高，保障程度低。虽然医疗保险的投保价格超出百姓的承受能力，但经营此项业务的许多保险公司仍然亏本，这主要是由两种现象导致的：一是逆选择，即投保者在得知自己得病时才去投保，并以各种手段瞒过保险公司的检查，投保后保险公司不得不依照条款支付其医疗费用。二是道德风险，即病人和医院联合起来对付保险公司，采用小病大治、开空头医药费的方式，使保险公司支付高额费用。

我国医疗改革的目的是建立一个由基本医疗保险、用人单位补充保险、商业医疗保险三者共同支撑的健康保障体系。医改确定，单位为职工交纳其工资总额的6%作为统筹基金，职工看病所需费用超过本地年平均工资的10%的，统筹资金开始为职工支付费用，但最高支付限额控制在本地职工年平均工资的4倍左右。

投保渠道

1. 网上投保

随着互联网的发展，国内出现一批在线投保比价平台。消费者只要乐意，就可以在网上查到险种的基本内容，例如承保范围、保障金额、保费、时效。轻松填写一些基本资料，选择想要投保的险种就可以完成投保。

2. 代理人服务

虽然投保渠道越来越多，传统的代理人制度依然有它的优势。代理人对自家保险公司的产品非常了解，而且也有不少保险公司积极对自己的代理人进行财务规划

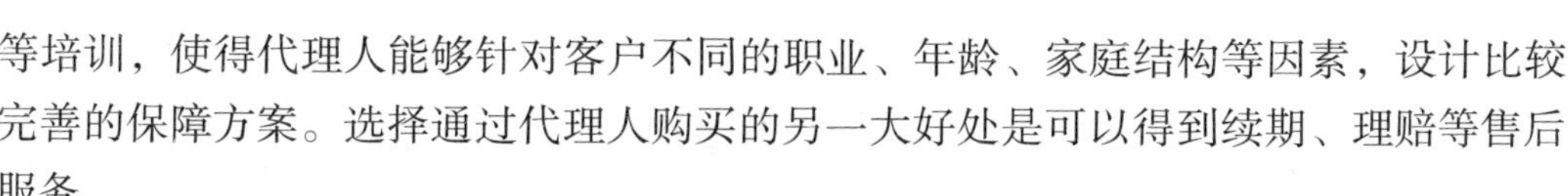

等培训，使得代理人能够针对客户不同的职业、年龄、家庭结构等因素，设计比较完善的保障方案。选择通过代理人购买的另一大好处是可以得到续期、理赔等售后服务。

3. 保险代理公司

如果说由于保险代理人只能推销自己公司的产品，其中不免存在言过其实、不够客观的方面，那么保险代理公司则可以推荐不同公司的险种，让消费者有个比较，也能比较客观地分析险种，更好地满足投保人需要。这种产品间的横向比较使投保人选择的范围更加广泛，这也是保险代理公司的最大优势。

4. 保险经纪公司

代理人是保险公司的代理人，代表保险公司的利益；而经纪人则是投保人的经纪人，考虑的是投保人的利益。保险经纪公司比代理人或保险代理公司更加客观，更有利于投保人找到合适的保险组合，而不受代理人或者代理公司偏好的误导。

5. 银行投保

通常在银行销售的保险是设计比较简单，消费者容易理解的储蓄、分红型保险，而需要仔细研究条款的健康险、长期寿险等产品，在银行柜台上很少见到。在银行买保险非常方便，只要当场签保险合同即可，在费率上通常会低一些。

二、医疗保险的特征

1. 实物补偿

这与许多人想象的现金补偿是完全不同的，参保人一定要知道，参加商业医疗保险后，只有在患病后需要到医院就医治疗才可享受商业医疗保险带来的利益。虽然商业医疗保险的目的是给予参保人员经济补偿，但却是以医疗服务的形式呈现给投保人员。也就是说，参保后，即便生病住院，得到的也不会是现金补偿，而是这些现金购买的医疗服务。这一点是大家首先一定要弄清楚的，因为这直接关系到个人利益如何实现。

2. 非定额补偿

这是商业医疗保险的又一个主要特征。参保人员患病后可享有到医院就医、享受医疗服务的待遇，其经济水平或者社会地位等因素不会对就医构成影响。但由于病种、病情的差异，每个患者所花费的金额是不相同的，因此获得的保险公司的补偿也并不相同。这一点，投保人也必须清楚，并非购买的保险价格越高，获得的补偿就越多，补偿金额是由病情决定，而非投保金额决定的。

三、保险种类

随着医疗体制改革的进行，各大保险公司的商业医疗保险险种也顺应形势，逐渐多了起来。那么，商业医疗保险究竟有哪几大类险种，它们各自保哪些，不保哪些，投保时有何具体规定？下面对医疗保险险种做了简要概括：

1. 普通医疗保险

该险种是医疗保险中保险责任最广泛的一种，负责被保险人因疾病和意外伤害支出的门诊医疗费和住院医疗费。普通医疗保险一般采用团体方式承保，或者作为个人长期寿险的附加责任承保，一般采用补偿方式给付医疗保险金，并规定每次最高限额。

2. 意外伤害医疗保险

该险种负责被保险人因遭受意外伤害支出的医疗费，作为意外伤害保险的附加责任。保险金额可以与基本险相同，也可以另外约定。一般采用补偿方式给付医疗保险金，不但要规定保险金额，即给付限额，还要规定治疗期限。

3. 住院医疗保险

该险种负责被保险人因疾病或意外伤害需要住院治疗时支出的医疗费，不负责被保险人的门诊医疗费，既可以采用补偿给付方式，也可以采用定额给付方式。

4. 手术医疗保险

该险种属于单项医疗保险，只负责被保险人因施行手术而支出的医疗费，不论是门诊手术治疗还是住院手术治疗。手术医疗保险可以单独承保，也可以作为意外保险或人寿保险的附加险承保。采用补偿方式给付手术医疗保险，只规定作为累计最高给付限额的保险金额，定额给付手术医疗保险，保险公司只按被保险人施行手术的种类定额给付医疗保险费。

5. 特种疾病保险

该险种以被保险人患特定疾病为保险事故。当被保险人被确诊为患某种特定疾病时，保险人按约定的金额给付保险金，以满足被保险人的经济需要。一份特种疾病保险的保单可以仅承保某一种特定疾病，也可以承保若干种特定疾病。可以单独投保，也可以作为人寿保险的附加险投保，一般采用定额给付方式，保险人按照保险金额一次性给付保险金，保险责任即终止。

Text 6

中国3 000亿健康保险亟待开发（节选）

为促进医疗与保险的共同合作与发展，中国医师协会健康管理与健康保险专委会（HMO）主办、慈铭健康体检管理集团承办的“第三届健康管理与健康保险国际高层研讨会”于2010年10月22日在沪举行。有关卫生行政和保监主管部门，中国医师协会领导及美国、加拿大、瑞士、新加坡等地的保险医学专家欢聚上海，与我国医疗保险精英共同交流医疗保险经验，为促进中国健康保险事业出谋划策。

中国健康保险潜力巨大前景广阔

根据与会外国专家报告中提供的数据，美国、加拿大、瑞士等西方发达国家健康保险年保费收入多年平均占到保险费总收入的25%～30%，与中国同处亚洲的新加坡该比例也达到了23%。显然，健康保险已经成为发达国家保险产品体系中的生力军。反观国内，保监会公布的保险业经营数据显示，2009年我国健康保险实现保费收入约574万，仅占当年原保险保费收入1 113.7万元的5.15%，与西方发达国家的差距竟达6倍。如果达到国际同等水平，意味着健康保险在中国存在着年总值高达3 000亿的巨大市场规模，其潜力和前景不可估量。

早在2002年，时任国务院副总理的温家宝就曾连续两次对商业健康险做出重要批示，希望结合社会医保大力发展商业健康保险。2005年前后中国保监会批准的人保健康、平安健康等5家专业健康保险公司也相继开业。时隔6年，在3 000亿诱人的奶酪前，中国健康保险逡巡踟蹰、步履蹒跚，内在原因值得深入探索研究。随着我国医药卫生体制深入改革，商业医疗保险在医改中的重要作用越来越受到政府主管部门的重视，卫生行政主管部门日前委托中国医师协会开展商业医疗保险为深化医改服务的调研，可以说是保险医学在我国现有体制下医疗与保险接合的新契机。

保险医学制度缺失是中国健康险发展的病根

参加“第三届健康管理与健康保险国际高层研讨会”的国内外专家同时指出，中国健康险目前纵然举步维艰，但市场潜力巨大，盈利只是时间问题，因为无论官方还是民间机构进行的保险需求调查，健康险都是排在第一位；其次，世界上已经有许多健康保险公司取得了成功，在西方发达国家，从综合性保险集团转型为专业健康保险公司的成功案例层出不穷。保险公司盈利的最大障碍是保险医学制度的缺失，具体表现在保险与医疗横向合作不充分，保险医师及专业培训、职业资格评审、晋升机制缺位，健康保险知识落伍等方面。

保险与医学结合已有近200年的历史，重大疾病保险的创意最先来自医生，而不是保险公司；健康管理理论和实务则最先由保险公司，而不是由医生创建。这充分说明医学是保险服务创新的工具和源泉。保险和医学的结合，有利于两者相得益彰共同发展壮大！

在这个领域里，目前我国还处于“参照国外标准”阶段，很多方面尚属空白，保险业在核保核赔过程中使用的技术手段不少都是国外的。其中一些引进的技术由于不适应中国国情，难免水土不服，未能给保险公司带来应有的经营效益，使我国的健康保险发展长期滞后。要想彻底改变这种局面，必须重视和加强我国保险医学的建设和研究。

今年年初中国医师协会健康管理与健康保险专委会总干事胡波、中央财经大学保险学院教授张国芳，应国际保险医学协会主席齐格弗里德·阿克曼的邀请，参加了国际保险医学会在南非开普敦召开的第23届年会。会后，胡总干事通过调研，提出了“关于建立和完善中国保险医学的几点建议”，受到了卫生行政和保险监管有关部门的充分重视和肯定。

中国保监会政研室蔡宇处长指出保险行业离不开保险医学的支撑，希望在专业协会和企业两个层面加强交流和沟通，促成更为广泛的有效合作。中国医师协会常务副会长杨镜表示，愿在保险医师专业人才培养、执业资格审核注册、职称评定晋升方面继续做出更多努力，以促进健康保险在中国的顺利发展。

资料来源：

Text 1 http://www.china.org.cn/china/2012-09/17/content_26545922.htm

Text 2 http://www.wisegeek.com/what-is-commercial-health-insurance.htm

http://www.onlyinsurance.com/Health-Insurance/Do-I-need-health-insurance.aspx

Text 3 http://www.who.int/pmnch/media/news/2012/wha_side_event_china_2012.pdf

Text 4 http://www.chinadaily.com.cn/m/chinahealth/2014-06/19/content_17559142.htm

Text 5 http://www.baike.com/wiki/%E5%95%86%E4%B8%9A%E5%8C%BB%E7%96%97%E4%BF%9D%E9%99%A9

Text 6 http://news.xinhuanet.com/health/2010-11/01/c_12725167.htm

参考答案

四、摘要练习

Text 1

中国新型农村合作医疗制度的发展

2012年是新型农村合作医疗制度（新农合）实施第十周年。过去十年来，各级党委和政府高度重视新型农村合作医疗制度，在他们的坚强领导下，有关部门通力合作，农民群众积极参与。因此，新型农村合作医疗取得了坚实的进步和显著的成就。

第一，由于参与人数稳定地保持在高水平之上，新型农村合作医疗制度实现了全面覆盖。自2003年的试点以来，新型农村合作医疗在2008年取得全面覆盖。参与人数逐年稳步增长，从试点初期的8 000万增长到2012年底的8.12亿，目标人群覆盖超过95%。

第二，融资持续增长，保护水平不断提高。保险计划的人均费用从2003年的30元增加至2011年的250元。2011年，13.15亿人次受益于新型农村合作医疗制度，平均住院补偿金额为1 894元。2012年，住院费用报销比例将达到75%左右，年最高支付限额不低于农民人均纯收入的8倍（不低于6万元）。

第三，建立了符合中国国情的、全面的机构框架和运行机制，即政府主导，卫生部门负责，有关部门支持，保险机构经营，医疗机构提供服务，农民参与，费用报销透明。新型农村合作医疗制度是由个人出资，农民合作，中央和地方政府拨款共同负担，同时家庭自愿参与。协调补偿侧重住院费用报销，并会逐渐扩大到门诊。2011年，试行门诊补偿的90%的地区在更广泛的领域使农民得到了实惠。参保农民可自主选择定点医院治疗并获得实时补偿。2011年，超过三分之二的省份（自治区、直辖市）在其指定的省级和市级医院采用实时补偿。资金运行机制采取封闭式管理，多部门监督。2011年，80%的地区进行了各种支付方式改革，支持了新型农村合作医疗，使其得以有效控制医疗费用。鼓励商业保险机构参与新农合的运行，探索“监管与操作相分离，政府行政与医疗机构相分离”的运行机制。

下一阶段，结合中央深化改革的总体部署，我们会继续在以下几个方面向前推进：

首先，新型农村合作医疗筹资应以稳定的速度增长。到2012年，新农合筹集的资金将达到人均300元。到2015年，政府补贴将达到每人每年360元。个人上交的资金将相应增长。将逐步建立一种适合中国经济发展的融资机制。

第二，新农合应得到精心管理，这包括严格使用基金及加强对定点医疗机构的监管。应在指定的省级医院、市级医院和遍布全国的乡村诊所建立实时补偿机制。应逐步实现医疗省外报销。应加速新农合信息工程，并为居民分发健康卡，推进一卡通试点项目。新型农村合作医疗的信息系统及相关方案，例如医疗援助计划，应该更好地同步进行，以便提供一站式服务的实时补偿。

第三，推进包括20种疾病如儿童白血病、肺癌等在内的重大疾病补偿试点方案。应当实施六部委共同发布的城市、农村居民重大疾病补充保险的指导意见。补充保险应与新农合政策关于重大疾病的福利妥善结合起来，应特别覆盖20种重大疾病。

第四，应加速改革新农合的支付方式，使用医疗总费用的预付款，按疾病支付，以按人付费取代按服务收费。改革的目的是控制医疗费用，改善卫生服务行为，提高资金绩效。

第五，加速受托的、具有资质的商业保险机构参与新型农村合作医疗的运行，从而建立一个在一定程度上与新农合的管理、运行及监管相分离的运行机制。

第六，应认真学习过去十年的经验，从而协助制定新型农村合作医疗的管理条例。应尽快为新型农村合作医疗的管理立法。

实践证明，新型农村合作医疗机制适合中国农村，在目前的情况下，是农村居民基本医疗保险制度的重要结晶。在过去的十年中，新型农村合作医疗已经成长起来，从一个新出世的婴儿成长到今天，已经在农村居民的健康问题上发挥了重要作用。卫生部作为新农合称职的主管部门，将会同有关部门一起继续推动新农合的发展，稳步提高农村居民的健康状况。

Text 2

商业健康保险

什么是商业健康保险？

在美国，商业健康保险也被称为私人健康保险，任何不由政府实体提供和管理的健康保险都是商业健康保险。出售这类保险的公司是以营利为目的的，并通过团体保险提供保险服务计划，也提供个体和个人保险计划。在所有情况下，这种类型的商业保险只提供给那些愿意为健康保险支付保险费的人。

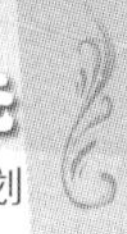

许多人通过雇主获取商业健康保险。这种保险有时被称为团体保险，员工满足雇主制定的标准，比如工作时间、在公司工作的时间长短以及其他因素，便可被纳入团体保险计划。根据保险计划的设置情况，雇主酌情或全额支付员工每月保费，或按百分比支付保费总额的一部分。如果是这种情况，雇主采用扣减工资的方式，用扣减的那一部分金额支付到期保费的剩余部分。

虽然商业健康保险有不同的形式，但世界各地最常见的有三种。最受欢迎的是被称为“服务点计划”的保险。这种类型的保险能够让客户选择初级护理医师，而医师名单由保险公司提供。使用医疗网络之中的医疗保健专业人员，能够确保保险公司覆盖比该合同份额更高的医疗费用。如果客户选择用保险公司网络之外的医生，保险公司为每笔医疗事件支付的费用通常会减少。

另一个流行的选择是众所周知的健康维护组织（HMO）。根据“服务点计划”，参加健康维护组织的人在保险公司提供的名单上选择初级护理医师。如果要看专科医生，初级保健医生必须向专科医生正式推荐病人。这种类型的计划很少涉及该医疗网络之外的医疗保健专业人员提供的服务，特殊情况除外。

商业健康保险的另一个选择是一次一付的按服务付费的模式，或者说赔偿模式。这种类型的保险覆盖一系列医疗程序的特别项目。客户可以看任何医生或专家，并且受益方面没有任何减少。这种类型的计划，其覆盖范围可能非常有限，例如注重到医生诊室就诊，在医生的诊室完成诊断过程。其他赔偿计划则更全面，能够覆盖保险合同规定的那些可以住院的疾病治疗。

在评估任何类型的商业健康保险时，确保保险计划能够提供足够的覆盖范围很重要。这意味着要仔细阅读条款，因为这些条款与例行检查、门诊治疗、住院治疗、精神病治疗，以及全部适用的免赔付金额和共付金额相关。此外，许多人需要将长期护理保险包括其中，因为这有助于缓解长期生病期间的财务困难。

我需要健康保险吗？

预约英国国民健康服务门诊的等待时间平均是7周左右。因此，许多人选择了私人健康保险，对于那些患可治疗疾病和有短期疾病的人来说，这种保险覆盖私人医疗费用。

健康保险向投保人提供服务，承诺他们一旦受伤或生病，就能立即获得治疗。英国保险协会称：“大多数人之所以购买这种保险，是为了确保自己在生病和受伤时可以获得及时治疗。”

私人健康保险不应被视为国民保健制度的替代品，因为私立医院一般都没有伤亡情况所需的设备。然而，它的确可以确保你迅速得到照顾。

获取健康保险是一个不错的主意，因为它可以缓解患者的部分恐惧心理。例如，不需要等待很长时间来找出到底哪里生了病，并且如果需要，患者可以直接被排到手术的等候名单之上。

那么，英国的健康保险有哪几种类型呢？

英国的健康保险有好几种不同的类型。

1. 危重病保险：危重病医疗保险覆盖那些突然被诊断出的严重疾病。保险公司会一次性支付一笔免税赔偿金给患者，患者可以随意使用这笔钱，将这笔钱用到几乎任何需要之处，例如用于休闲或偿还债务。

2. 收入保障保险：收入保障保险对于自由职业者而言非常重要。在英国，如果你无法工作，那么你可以每周拿到60.20英镑。如果你发现自己因疾病或意外事故而无法工作，此保险计划将支付高达你总收入65%的费用。这种类型的保险，是根据病人的职业类型以及支付的速度来计算保费的。病人病好后，能够回到工作岗位上时，保费给付便停止。

3. 健康信托基金：这是目前的一种保险形式，旨在取代传统的健康保险计划。这种保险方案利用了允许低成本覆盖、无超额支付、不自动增加保费、综合获取医疗设施、无年龄附加费用的英国信托基金法。不过，金融服务管理局目前尚未规范现阶段的卫生信托基金。

4. 现金计划保险：这是一种低成本的保险，为投保人的医疗费用提供现金，包含眼部护理、牙科护理以及护理等。家庭和个人都可以购买这种类型的保险。

然而，在选择健康保险时，需清楚地了解个人之前的疾病状况和责任免除的政策。责任免除指在一些条件之下，保险公司将拒绝支付持保人。遗憾的是，某些责任免除的情况的确存在于健康保险之中。责任免除可能包括慢性病、反复发作的疾病、长期不愈的疾病、整容手术和实验性的治疗。

之前的疾病状况指的是病患在加入一个新的健康保险计划之前就已经被诊断出患有某种疾病，或治疗过疾病。通常，保险公司会将过去五年里已经存在的任何疾病排除在保险覆盖范围之外。一些保险公司会在患者的保险计划已经开始后，在患者完全清楚自己的状况的条件下，设法使患者条件符合覆盖资格。

健康保险移动与责任法案规定，如果患者通过雇主参加团体保险，参保之前已经获得过12个月的保险，那么参保之前的疾病也会得到覆盖。

五、英译汉练习

Text 3

中国农村卫生改革与发展

2012年5月23日

尊敬的总干事助理卡瑞莎·福·艾蒂安博士，
尊敬的皮·克·普拉丹部长，
尊敬的贾维斯·巴博萨博士，
女士们、先生们：

下午好！听了我的同事们对印度农村健康项目和巴西的家庭健康计划的介绍，我感到很受鼓舞。我也非常高兴能有机会与大家分享中国农村卫生改革与发展的经验。

中国是一个拥有13.7亿人口的发展中国家。在中国，超过60%的人口，或者说8.5亿人生活在农村。

中国的国情是农村人口众多，城市和农村之间的差距大，因此非常需要优先考虑农村地区的健康政策。2009年4月，中国政府启动了新一轮的医疗改革，将建立和完善城乡居民的基本医疗卫生制度作为当务之急，将健康服务作为公共产品提供给全国所有居民，为新时期农村卫生改革与发展增加了新的意义。

现在我想讲讲这一努力带来的最新结果。

一、完善农村三级卫生服务体系

农村三级卫生服务体系由县级医院、乡镇卫生院和村卫生室组成，向农村人口提供预防、初级卫生保健、健康检查和健康教育等服务。这个卫生网络覆盖全国31个省份的2 856个县。

自医疗卫生体制改革启动以来，中央政府预算的520亿元专项资金已经被分配到改善农村医疗卫生服务系统之中，包括2 000多个县医院和25 000个村卫生室。截至2010年底，中国已经有6 400所县医院、1 500多个县妇幼卫生院、近1 700个县级疾病预防控制中心，以及1 500多个县卫生监督机构。还有38 000所乡镇卫生院，也就是说，几乎每个乡镇都有一个或多个医院。有648 000个村卫生室，覆盖了92.3%的村庄。从2006年到2011年，到乡镇卫生院和村卫生室看病的人从20.7亿人次增加到26.6亿人次，增加了28.5%。

二、加强农村卫生队伍建设

从2004年到2011年，中央政府预算的22.6亿元被分配到了中西部地区，提供了

436万人次的农村医务人员培训。2005年启动了“一万医生支持乡镇卫生院”项目，13.2亿元的资金被分配给“二级和二级以上的医疗机构支持乡镇卫生院”项目。到目前为止，项目已覆盖中国中西部21个省份贫困地区的乡镇卫生院，提供了7万人次的技术援助。

在过去的几年中，加强卫生人员的能力、培训全科医师一直是工作重点之一。我们已经培养了3.6万农村卫生技术人员成为全科医生，录取了超过1万名医学生，对他们免收学费，条件是承诺毕业后到农村医院工作去工作，招聘了2万多名执业医师充实到乡镇医院。

到2010年年底，县级医院已有近160万卫生人员，乡镇卫生院有120万卫生人员，乡镇农村人口中每千人就有约1.3名卫生工作者。村卫生室有卫生技术人员120万人，其中100多万是乡村医生，17.3万人是执业医师或助理执业医师。

三、巩固新型农村合作医疗（以下简称“新农合”）

中国的基本医疗保险制度由四部分组成：城镇职工基本医疗保险，城镇居民基本医疗保险制度，新型农村合作医疗制度，医疗救助方案。这四部分分别覆盖城镇职工、非在职城镇居民、农村居民、贫困人口。

新型农村合作医疗是一个为农村居民提供医疗保险的计划，在减少农村居民的财政负担、保护他们在被疾病袭击的灾难之中免于陷入贫困或因病返贫、改善他们的健康状况方面起到了关键的作用。2011年，新农合覆盖范围已扩大到8.32亿人，占农村人口的97.5%。所以我们可以说这基本上是全覆盖。给每个人的资金从2003年的30元人民币增加到2012年的300元。根据该计划，2012年患者的住院费用可报销75%，不低于6万元人民币。该计划筹措的资金大幅度增加，从2003年的40亿元人民币增长到2011年的2 048亿元人民币，其中772亿元来自中央政府。新型农村合作医疗制度已经成为世界上覆盖面最大的医疗保障方案。

2010年6月，我们由农村儿童先天性心脏病和急性白血病为起点，开始了一个试点项目，旨在提高农村居民重大疾病保障水平。新型农村合作医疗报销医疗费用的70%，对于符合条件的患者，医疗救助报销另外的20%。2011年，另外6种重疾，即终末期肾脏疾病、严重精神疾病、乳腺癌、宫颈癌、多药耐药结核、艾滋病毒/艾滋病患者机会性感染等，被纳入试点方案。2012年，对以上8种疾病的保险计划将进一步扩大。同时，在三分之一的新农合覆盖区域，另外12种疾病，包括血友病、慢性粒细胞白血病（CML）、唇腭裂、肺癌、食道癌、胃癌、I型糖尿病、甲状腺功能亢进症、脑梗死、中风、急性心肌梗死、结肠癌和直肠癌，将被纳入试点。

随着新型农村合作医疗的兴起和医疗卫生服务体系的改善，医疗保健设施得以建设和升级，农村，特别是边远地区的医疗机构的服务能力得到增强，农民看病更容易，并更能负担得起医疗保健服务。

从2008年到2011年，能够在15分钟内步行去获得医疗服务的农村家庭的比例从75.6%上升到80.8%。农村居民自行支付的比例从73.4%下降到49.5%，生病时选择不去看医生的人的比例从12.4%下降到6.1%。

四、在农村地区提供基本的公共卫生服务

基本公共卫生服务均等化是中国医疗改革的一个亮点。公共卫生服务为“以预防为主”这一长期的政策提供了机构安排。随着政府对每个人的补贴从2009年的15元上升到2011年的25元，目前已提供了10种类型之中的41个基本公共卫生项目。

取得的成果是，城市和农村之间的发展差距正在缩小，农村居民的健康指标迅速提高。例如农村孕产妇死亡率由36.1/10万下降到26.5/10万，与城市处在同一水平上；婴儿死亡率从18.4‰下降到14.7‰。

在农村，2011年有62.6%的居民建立了电子健康档案；住院分娩率达到96%，884万名孕妇获得政府住院分娩补贴，400万妇女接受了宫颈癌筛查，40万妇女接受了乳腺癌筛查，990万妇女获得了免费的叶酸补充剂。

由于过去几年的艰苦努力，医疗改革已经给人民带来更多实实在在的实惠，增加了他们获得医疗服务的途径，自付费用得到降低。这反映了改革的方向、目标、指导方针符合卫生发展法，符合中国具体国情和人民的愿望。

接下来的几年中改革目标如下：2015年，中国将提供更公平的获得基本医疗服务的途径，提高医疗服务的工作效率和质量；在稳妥控制卫生总费用增长的同时，中国将逐步提高政府卫生支出在财政总支出中的份额，目的是使个人支出降低到低于30%；医疗服务不足、价格过高的问题将得到缓解；人均寿命将达到74.5岁；婴儿死亡率将降低到12‰以下，孕产妇死亡率将低于22/10万。

中国政府通过完善新型农村合作医疗、改善卫生设施和卫生队伍，致力于推进农村地区医疗改革，实现人人享有基本医疗卫生服务的目标。我们将坚定不移地克服所有困难，走出一条具有中国特色的健康发展之路！

感谢世界卫生组织与国际社会对我们的支持。

谢谢大家！

Text 4

2013年新型农村合作医疗的进步和2014年的主要任务

2013年新型农村合作医疗的进步

2013年，新型农村合作医疗运行平稳。管理和整体系统得到改进，覆盖了大量的农村人口，使他们享受到更多的好处，特别是享受到更高水平的大病医疗保险。

融资和安全水平得到提高，进一步惠及农村居民。2013年，共有8.02亿人得到全国新型农村合作医疗的覆盖，占总人口的99%。筹集的人均资金达到370元（59.45美元），与去年相比增加了62元。由相关政策覆盖的住院费用报销率超过75%，实际补偿比例继续增加——乡镇增加近80%，县级增加60%多，村卫生室增加50%，惠及人群达到约19.4亿，同比增长11.3%。

重大疾病的多层次、多形式的初步安全机制也已建立。首先，以疾病类型为重点的大病安全保障机制得到巩固和提高。2013年，除了白血病、先天性心脏病等原来的20种疾病，儿童苯丙酮尿症和先天性尿道下裂这两种疾病也被纳入重大疾病医疗保险的范围。约199万患者得到了报销，并且这22种疾病的实际补偿比例达到69%，大大降低了他们的经济负担。第二，新型农村合作医疗积极鼓励利用新型农村合作医疗基金购买重大疾病保险。2013年，约28个省份建立了大病保险实施计划。高达123万患者得到补偿，进一步减轻了病患的负担。

管理与服务得到了改进。第一，管理和服务进一步委托给社会，帮助转变政府职能。现在，高达24%的县、区、城市已委托商业保险公司经营新型农村合作医疗，医疗费用报销流程也得到进一步改进。全国范围内参与新系统的农村居民达到88%，现在可以在其省内的任何地方得到即时报销。国家新农合信息平台与九个省级平台、多家大型医疗机构联网，使跨省医疗费用报销成为可能，也为跨省医疗费用报销试点铺平了道路。第三，支付方式的改革不断深化，覆盖全国80%以上的区域，并在一定程度上帮助遏制了医疗费用的飞涨。

2014新型农村合作医疗的主要任务

根据卫生保健改革的任务，国家卫生和计划生育委员会将在城乡统筹发展的基础上继续发展并完善新型农村合作医疗。

第一，进一步提高筹资标准和新农合的保障水平，将新型农村合作医疗的参与率保持在95%以上，将年度人均补贴增加到320元，优化和协调补偿方案，将相关政策覆盖的医疗费用报销率保持在75%，将门诊费用报销率保持在50%。

第二，要提高新农合对各种大病的医疗保障机制，保持包括儿童白血病在内的22种重大疾病的安全机制，将保障机制扩大到新农合覆盖区域的一半以上，充分利用以疾病类型和疾病费用为主导的系统。我们还应该建立疾病应急救助的基本机制，协调基本医疗保障、城乡居民大病保险以及医疗救助。

第三，鼓励更多的商业保险公司经营新农合与大病保险的管理与服务。我们应该提高管理和服务，利用政府与市场，建立大病多级安全机制。

第四，加快推进新农合信息化建设，提高省域内即时报销服务，继续建设国家和省级信息平台，将信息化平台扩大到15个省，并都连接到国家信息平台。我们也应该推出跨省医疗费用的审核与报销试点项目。

第五，加强新农合精细化管理，推进支付方式改革，遏制医疗费用飞涨，进一步惠及农村居民。我们应该规范新农合基金使用和管理，确保其安全。

六、汉译英练习

Text 5

Commercial Medical Insurance

Commercial Medical Insurance is a component part of the health care system, participated by units and individuals on a voluntary base. The government encourages employers and individuals to participate in commercial medical insurance. Commercial Medical Insurance refers to profit earning medical insurance operated by companies. Consumers submit a certain amount to pay for insurance, and in the case of major diseases, they can get a certain amount of money for medical expenses from the insurance company.

Commercial Medical Insurance is a health insurance. Health insurance compensation includes not only the direct economic losses due to disease brought to people, but also the indirect economic loss caused by diseases. It gives economic compensation for child delivery, disability, and death.

The most obvious problem of current commercial medical insurance is its high price and low security level. Although the price for medical insurance is beyond the affordability of people, many insurance companies that operate this program are still making loses. This is caused mainly by two problems: one is adverse selection, namely the insured buy insurance when he knows that he is ill and hides from the insurance company his conditions in a variety of ways, therefore when he has bought his insurance, the insurance companies have to follow the terms of payment and pay for his medical expenses.

China's health care reform is aiming to establish a health care system that is commonly supported by the basic medical insurance, employers' supplementary insurance, and commercial medical insurance. Health care reform clarified that the employers pay 6% of the employees' total wages as pooled funds. When medical costs of the employees has surpassed more than 10% of the local average wage, then the pooled funds will start to pay for the employees, though the highest amount paid must be limited within four times of the average annual local wages.

Ⅰ. Where can you buy commercial medical insurance?

i. Buying It Online

With the development of the Internet, a number of online insurance service platform has been established. The consumers can find the basic content of insurance on the Internet, such as the amount of the premium, insurance coverage, timeliness and so on. Customers can easily fill in basic information and select insurance programs.

ii. Agent Service

Although a variety of insurance services are available in the market, traditional agent still has its advantages. They well understand their own insurance products, their own insurance companies actively provide them with financial planning training programs, as a result the agents can design more suitable insurance plans for the customers in accordance with their different occupations, ages, family structures and other factors. Another big advantage that an agent can offer is his service for insurance renewal, insurance claims and other customer service.

iii. Insurance Proxy Companies

If insurance agents can only sell the products of their company, they have the possibility to exaggerate their products and have non-objective introductions. The insurance proxy companies can recommend insurance plans of different insurance companies for the consumer to have comparison. They can objectively analyze various insurance plans and better satisfy the needs of the customers. The comparison of different insurance plans can provide a wider range of choices for the customer. This is also the biggest advantage of the insurance proxy company.

iv. Insurance Broker Companies

The insurance agent is one that represents the interests of the insurance company, while the broker is one that represents the interests of the insured. The brokers are still more objective than insurance agents or insurance proxy companies. They are more conducive for the insured to find the right insurance portfolio, and the customers can be less mislead by insurance agents or proxies.

v. The Bank Insurance

Usually the bank sells insurance of a relatively simple design, such as insurance in a way of consumer savings or of a participating pattern which is easy for the customer to understand. Those insurance products the terms of which need to be carefully understood are rarely seen at the bank counter, such as health insurance and life insurance. It is very convenient to buy insurance at the bank: the customer only needs to sign the insurance contract at the counter. The rate is usually lower.

Ⅱ. Features of Medical Insurance

i. Service Compensation

This is a bit different from cash compensation as imagined by many people. Customers must understand that when they buy the commercial medical insurance plan, they can enjoy the benefits brought by commercial medical insurance only when they fall ill and go to the hospital for medical treatment. Although the commercial medical insurance aims to give economic compensation to the insured, the compensation is presented to the insured in the form of medical service. That is to say, after you have bought a medical insurance plan, even if you are ill and stay in a hospital, what you are compensated is not cash compensation, medical services bought by the insurance. This is a point that a customer must be aware of, because it is directly related to how individual interests can be realized.

ii. Non-quota Compensation

This is another major feature of the commercial medical insurance. When they fall ill, the insured can enjoy the hospital treatment and medical services, and these services would not be affected by factors such as their economic status and social status. However, because of the difference of diseases and different levels of seriousness, the amount of money spent on each patient is different, so that the compensation paid by the insurance company is not the same. The insured must be very clear about this point: the amount of compensation is determined by the condition of the disease, rather than by the amount of insurance money they have paid. The greater an amount you pay the higher compensation you will obtain is not true in this context.

Ⅲ. Types of Insurance

With the reform of medical system, insurance companies are adapting their commercial medical insurance to the change. As a result, their insurance types are gradually multiplying. Then what are the major categories of commercial medical insurance? What do they insure? What don't they cover? What are the specific provisions for the insured? The following outlines several types of medical insurance.

i. General Medical Insurance

This medical insurance is an insurance that has one of the widest insurance liabilities in all medical insurances. It is responsible for paying the expenses of outpatient and hospitalization of the insured because of illness and accidental injury. General medical insurance are generally bought through group insurance, or as an additional responsibility of a long-term individual life insurance. It generally pays the medical insurance by way of compensation and prescribes the maximum compensation amount.

ii. Medical Insurance for Accidental Injury

This insurance takes the responsibility of medical expenses of the insured who suffers from an accidental injury, as an additional responsibility of the accident injury insurance. The insured amount can be the same as the basic insurance, or it can be different through additional agreement. It pays the medical insurance by way of compensation, therefore it prescribes that the insured amount is the prescribed limited amount, but also prescribes the duration of treatment.

iii. Medical Insurance for Hospitalization

This insurance takes the responsibility for medical expenses of hospitalization for the insured that fall ill or have an accidental injury. It has no responsibility for outpatient medical expenses of the insured. It can pay by way of compensation, or it can also pay by way of quota payment.

iv. Medical Insurance for Operation

The insurance is a single-item medical insurance. It takes the responsibility of paying for the medical expense of medical operation only; no matter it is outpatient operation or hospitalized operation. Medical insurance for operation can be bought singly, or bought as an additional insurance for accidental injury or life insurance. It pays the medical insurance for operation by way of compensation, prescribing only the cumulative maximum limited amount and paying the prescribed quota amount. That is, the insurance company pays only the prescribed quota in accordance with the operation categories.

Ⅳ. Insurance for Special Diseases

This insurance considers the specific diseases of the insured patient as an insurance accident. When the insured patient is diagnosed as suffering from certain diseases, the insurer pays the insurance in accordance with the agreed amount of payment, so as to satisfy the economic needs of the insured. An insurance policy for a special disease can cover only a specific disease, while it can also cover several specific diseases. It can be arranged separately, and it can also be bought as an additional insurance responsibility. It generally pays the insurance by way of quota payment. When the company pays the insured amount by way of one-time payment, its liability of insurance terminates.

Text 6

The Potential of 300 Billion Chinese Health Insurance Need to Be Tapped (Excerpts)

In order to promote the mutual cooperation and development, the 3rd Health Management and Health Insurance International Seminar, hosted by HMO and co-hosted by Ciming Health Checkup Management Group, was held on October 22nd, 2010 in Shanghai. Leaders from Health Executive Department, the Insurance Regulatory Department and CMDA (Chinese Medical Doctor Association) and experts in the insurance medicine from USA, Canada, Switzerland, Singapore and elsewhere met in Shanghai and exchanged experience they had in the medical insurance with China's elites in this field. Their advice and suggestions will promote the development of China's health insurance.

Great Potential and Promising Future Exists in China's Health Insurance

According to the data provided in the report by the foreign experts, the annual health insurance accounts for 25%-30% of the total premium in the western developed countries such as USA, Canada, Switzerland. The ratio in Singapore, which also locates in Asia just like China, has reached to 23%. Obviously, the health insurance has been the new force in the insurance products system in the developed countries. Back to China, the operational data in the insurance industry published by China Insurance Regulatory Commission shows that the premium income of China's health insurance in 2009 was about 5.74 million, which only accounted for about 5.15% of the then premium income of the annual original insurance, which is 11.137 million. The gap is 6 times compared with the developed countries in the west world. If the data reach the international level, it means that the health insurance will bring a large market with an annual output value of 300 billion. Its potential and the prospect cannot be estimated.

Back in 2002, the then Vice-Premier Wen Jiabao had commanded twice on the commercial health insurance. He hoped that the commercial health insurance should enjoy a rapid development with the incorporation of the social medical insurance. Around 2005, authorized by CIRC (China Insurance Regulatory Commission), PICC Health Insurance Company Ltd., Ping'an Insurance (Group) Company of China, Ltd. and other 3 professional health insurance companies started business. In the last 6 years, despite the 300 billion benefits, China's health insurance hesitated to move forward. The internal cause should be made in-depth exploration. With the reform of China's medical and health system going deeper and deeper, the important function that the commercial medical insurance plays in the medical reform has been paid attention by the government authorities. The health administrative sectors now authorize the Chinese Medical Doctor Association (CMDA) to conduct the commercial medical insurance to deepen the survey of medical reform service. The insurance medicine is the combination of medical treatment and insurance at the background of the current system which will bring a new opportunity.

The Lack of the Insurance Medicine System Is the Root Cause for the Development of China's Health Insurance

The experts from home and abroad attending the 3rd Health Management and Health Insurance International Seminar pointed out that China's health insurance is struggling at the moment. However, the market boasts a great potential and it will finally gain profits because the health insurance ranks the first in the insurance demand survey no matter for the official institution or for the public organization. Besides, many health insurance companies in the world have succeeded. In the western developed countries, endless cases prove that comprehensive insurance group could transfer to professional health insurance company, which points out the future trend. The biggest barrier for the profit pillar of insurance company is the lack of the insurance medicine system which specifically manifested in the insufficient cooperation between insurance and medical treatment, the lack of insurance doctor, the professional training, and the examination of the professional qualification, the promotion mechanism and the backward of the health insurance knowledge.

The combination of insurance and medicine has a history of about 200 years. The innovation of the insurance for major illness came from doctors instead of insurance company while the health management theory and the practices are first established by the insurance company instead of doctors. It fully proves that the medicine is the tool and spring of the insurance service innovation. The combination of insurance and medicine is beneficial to bring out the best in each other and promote the development of each other.

In this field, China is still at the stage of "referring to the foreign standard". A great gap exists in so many aspects. Many of the techniques used in the process of underwriting and claiming settlement in the insurance industry come from foreign countries. Some of the techniques don't bring expected operation benefits because of the inadaptation of China's national condition, which also make the development of China's health insurance lag behind in the long run. We have to focus and enhance the establishment and survey of China's insurance medicine to thoroughly change the situation.

Earlier this year, with the invitation of Siegfried Akermann, President of the International Insurance Medical Association, Hu Bo, Secretary-General of HMO, and Zhang Guofang, professor at the Insurance Institution at the Central University of Finance and Economics, attended the 23rd annual meeting of international insurance medicine held in Cape Town, South Africa. After the meeting, Mr. Hu pointed out several suggestions about the establishment and improvement of China's insurance medicine through the survey. His suggestions have attracted attention and gained confirm from the Health Executive Department and the Insurance Regulatory Department.

Cai Yu, Head of the Political Survey Office of the CIRC pointed out that the insurance industry cannot do without the support of the insurance medicine. He hoped that the professional association and the corporation enhance exchanges and communication and promote wide and efficient cooperation. Yang Jing, Standing Vice-Chairman of CMDA, said that more efforts should be made in the personnel training of the professional insurance doctor, the examination and registration of the qualification and the professional-title evaluation and promote, which will promote the smooth development of the health insurance in China.

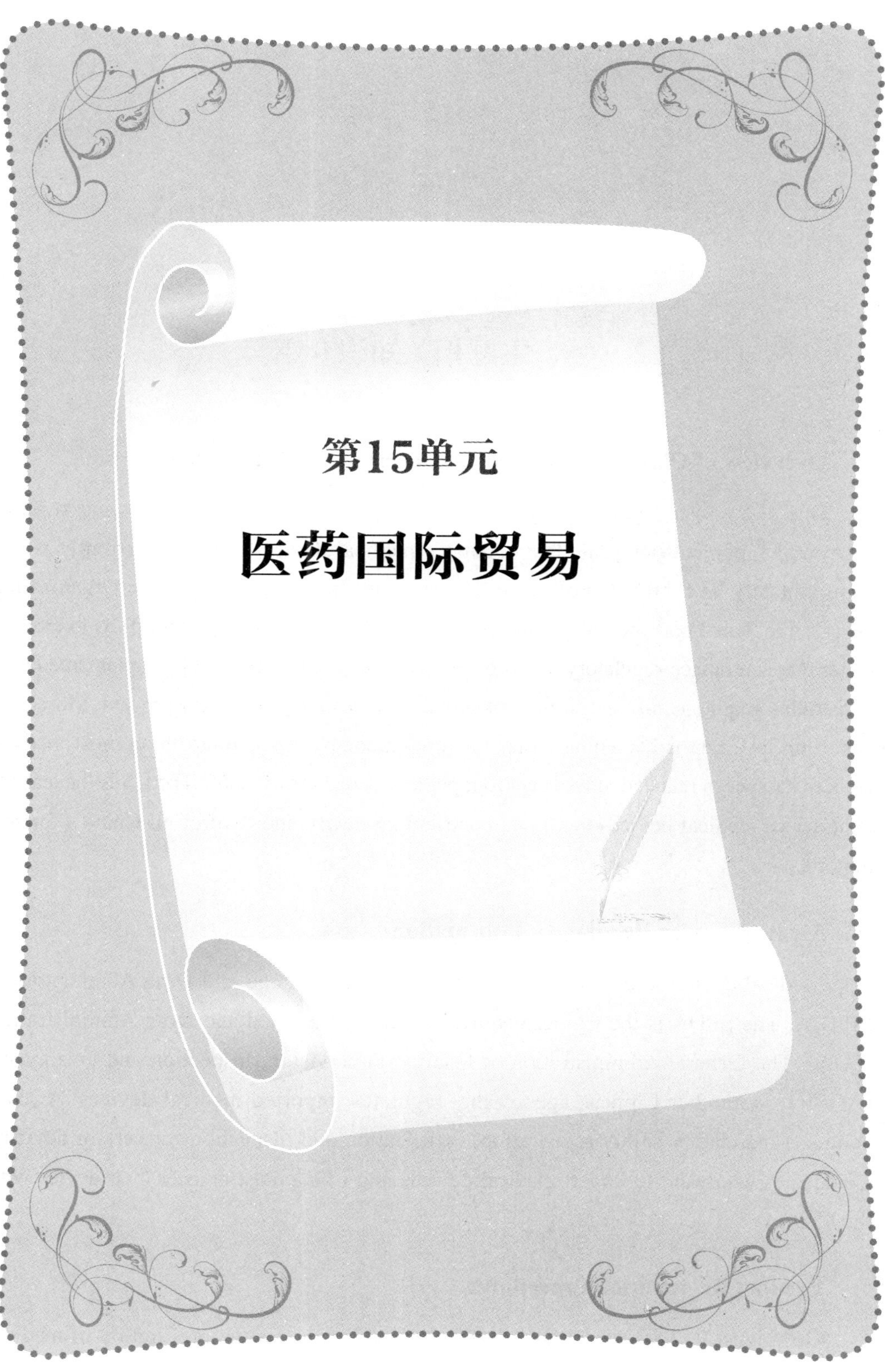

第15单元

医药国际贸易

一、主题相关知识介绍

Overview of China and Its Medical Device Market (Excerpts)

One of the fastest growing economies in the world today is China, growing at a rate of around 9 percent per year. The country's medical device market is currently worth approximately $3.5 billion. Following China's entry into the World Trade Organization (WTO), the State Food and Drug Administration (SFDA) is making greater efforts to create a better medical device regulatory environment. In August 2004, the SFDA implemented new registration requirements, simplifying the device application and review process. Moreover, exporting to China is becoming easier for foreign companies, and tariffs on most medical devices have been reduced to less than four percent as of January 2005. The US is the leading exporter of medical devices to China, contributing nearly one-third of all China's foreign imports.

Medical Device Regulatory Information

Medical devices are regulated in China by the State Food and Drug Administration (SFDA). The SFDA is the Chinese equivalent of the US Food and Drug Administration (FDA). The General Administration of Quality, Supervision, Inspection and Quarantine (AQSIQ) is another Chinese agency that regulates imported medical devices. AQSIQ conducts mandatory safety registration, certification and inspection for certain devices. Companies who want to import medical devices into China must register their device with the SFDA.

Product Registration Procedures

On August 9, 2004 the SFDA issued new regulations for the registration of medical devices in China. These new regulations have (to a certain extent) simplified the application and dossier review process for medical devices. Additionally, the Medical Device Clinical Trial Regulation, effective from April, 2004, has laid out more detailed requirements for clinical protocol, clinical hospitals and clinical reports in China.

Previously, a company prepared a dossier (with all required documents) and then applied to the SFDA for a specification validation (for approval of the specifications of the device to be imported). Once the specification validation was reviewed and approved, the company was then required to send samples to a testing center. A company would then file its dossier, with the approved specifications and the official testing report, to the SFDA. The SFDA would review the technical documents and judge whether to issue product approval.

The new regulations have combined the dossier preparation and specification application into one step. Companies no longer need to apply to the SFDA for specification validation. Instead, they may use their own specifications as a basis for a testing agency to provide testing. The company then includes these test results in its completed dossier and submits it to the SFDA. The SFDA sends this dossier to the Medical Device Evaluation Center (MDEC) to review the specifications, dossier, government certificate and clinical report, if needed. The MDEC sends their conclusion to the SFDA and if everything is acceptable, the SFDA will issue the product approval license. While these new regulations have somewhat streamlined the process, they have not significantly altered the timeframe for medical device registration in China.

However, there are now several situations that can lengthen the new registration process. First, if the MDEC requires a supplement dossier, companies must complete the supplement and re-submit it to the SFDA within 60 working days. Second, since the specification validation is not required before testing, the testing is completed based on the company's specifications. It is possible that the MDEC may request the company to revise its specifications and re-test, adding additional time and money to the registration process.

Product registration is valid for four years. In order to change manufacturing locations or add a new manufacturing location, a new product registration must be submitted. To change basic information, such as the manufacturer's name, product name, or name of the manufacturing location, etc., an amendment to the product registration can be submitted. Requests for renewal of product registration must be made 6 months before the initial registration expires. Along with renewal forms, a copy of the original registration must be submitted. Product quality follow-up reports must also be submitted.

The China Quality Certification Center requires that certain categories of medical devices obtain a CCC mark to ensure their safety. The CCC mark applies to several types of medical devices, including medical diagnostic x-ray equipment, haemodialysis equipment, hollow fiber dialysers, electrocardiographs and implantable cardiac pacemakers. Manufacturers can apply for the CCC mark directly to an Authorized Certification Body (ACB) or through a Chinese agent. Products requiring the CCC mark that are not properly marked may be held at the border by Chinese Customs and may be subject to other penalties.

Medical Device Regulation Updates

On July 8, 2004, the SFDA issued new regulations regarding inserts, labeling, and packaging for medical devices. This was the first regulation of this sort to exist in China. The new regulation contains detailed requirements for product inserts, labels and packaging. All medical devices exported to China must include this information in Chinese. Moreover, the inserts must be reviewed and approved by the SFDA during product registration. Following approval, the content of the insert cannot be changed. If any changes must be made, the insert must be resubmitted to the SFDA for approval again.

The SFDA released a second draft regulation for new diagnostic device registration procedures on July 29, 2004. The regulation only applies to diagnostic products categorized as a medical device, not those categorized as drugs. Registration requirements for some diagnostic devices are now similar to those for medical devices. The regulation requires three test batches of the diagnostic device for registration. However, the draft does not mention whether clinical trials will be required and this is normally determined on a case by case basis.

二、技巧指导：口译职业准则

本单元介绍职业口译员所应遵循的职业准则。由于职业准则是国家和行业的规范，因此这里直接转载国家的《翻译服务规范　第2部分：口译（试行）》和国际会议口译工作者协会的《会议口译员职业道德守则》。

Ⅰ. 口译服务国家标准

翻译服务规范　第2部分：口译（试行）

1. 目的

为了规范全国翻译服务企业协作网成员单位的现场口译服务质量，同时考虑到现场口译的特殊性，特制订本标准。本标准为推荐使用标准。

2. 适用范围

本标准仅适用于全国翻译企业协作网的各成员企业。

3. 定义

本标准所述的现场口译，仅指工程建设、技术交流、技术和工艺引进、工业设备引进等涉外工程项目建设从立项至结项全过程中的各类口译，属工程技术类口译范畴。

4. 现场口译服务质量是译员综合素质的体现，评判现场口译的服务质量，首先要确认译员的资质和素质。

4.1 译员资质

4.1.1 译员的资质按国家专业技术职务翻译系列评定标准，分为助理翻译、翻译、副译审、译审。

4.1.2 译员的资质，具有由各省、市、自治区外事部门或人事部门颁发的初级口译证书、中级口译证书、高级口译证书。

4.1.3 同声传译的资质具有国家有关部门颁发的同声传译证书或由各省、市、自治区外事部门或人事部门认可的同声传译资格。

4.1.4 经过长期现场口译实践具有4.1.1、4.1.2和4.1.3同等资质水平的译员。

4.1.5 译员的综合素质要求译员能够遵守一九九二年二月国务院发布的《涉外人员守则》十条，要求译员具有计算机、网络操作技能，要求译员有较深广的科技知识和文化知识。

4.2 现场口译分类及服务质量要求现场口译分为：施工现场翻译；商务和技术合同谈判翻译；随团出国翻译及其他翻译。

4.2.1 施工现场翻译服务质量要求。

（1）熟悉现场装置，在装置现场就位、机电仪安装、装置调试、开车和验收中，正确翻译并及时无误地向项目建设双方传达信息。

（2）正确翻译现场施工中项目建设双方的各类会谈纪要、备忘录、工作日志等有关工件资料。

（3）严格遵守现场安全施工的各项规定，工作认真负责、任劳任怨，积极主动。

4.2.2 商务和技术合同谈判翻译服务质量要求。

（1）熟悉项目建设的技术资料和文件，翻译正确、忠实、严谨、规范。

（2）正确校译合同及合同附件的中英文文本，译文忠实于原文原意。

（3）项目建设双方的会谈情况、双方合作意向以及合同内容要对外保密，不得泄露给第三方。

4.2.3 随团出国翻译服务质量要求。

（1）熟悉出访国的文化环境、风土人情和风俗习惯，熟悉出访的目的、背景，做好团长的参谋。

（2）遵守外事纪律，遵守保密守则，配合团长做好在国外的政治安全、交通安全，钱财物安全、护照安全。

（3）针对不同出访任务（考察、实习培训、设备采购、设计联络、技术交流等），做好出国前的（翻译）技术准备，在国外做到正确无误地翻译。

4.2.4 其他翻译服务质量要求

本标准所指的其他翻译服务是指与工程项目建设有关的技术交流翻译、培训讲座翻译、会议翻译等翻译服务，这些翻译服务质量要求参照4.2.2和4.2.3。

4.3 现场口译服务质量的分级

现场口译服务质量分为两级：合格和不合格。

（1）达到4.2本类服务质量要求的为合格。

（2）达不到4.2本类服务质量要求的为不合格。

4.4 合格译员的评判依据

合格译员的评判依据为五个方面：双语表达能力；工作态度和服务态度；翻译职业道德；纽带桥梁作用；用户对译员的评价和反映。

这五个方面是译员的基本素质要求，是评判各类合格译员的前提。

5. 关于现场口译对现场文书及文件笔译的质量要求（备忘录、现场工作日志、会议纪要等），参照TSS-102“工程技术类资料质量标准”。

6. 现场口译服务质量的评判，由全国翻译企业协作网（中国译协翻译服务工作委员会）专家组负责，通过译员在现场口译的音像带对用户访问做出评判。

7. 本标准由全国翻译企业协作网领导小组批准。

8. 本标准由全国翻译企业协作网领导小组解释。

Ⅱ. 会议口译员职业道德守则

国际会议口译员协会（AIIC）是专业会议口译人员的国际组织，以其入会资格之严苛著名，其会员身份是国际公认的合格会议口译人员的标志。因此，该协会制定的《职业道德守则》对于我国的口译人员有较高的参考价值。以下为会议口译员《职业道德守则》英汉对照全文，英文原文见国际会议口译员协会网站，中文译文由付蕾翻译，黄长奇审定。

AIIC: Code of Professional Ethics
会议口译员职业道德守则

Ⅰ. Purpose and Scope
一、目的和范围

Article 1

第1条

1. This Code of Professional Ethics (hereinafter called the "Code") lays down the standards of integrity, professionalism and confidentiality which all members of the Association shall be bound to respect in their work as conference interpreters.

1. 本《职业道德守则》（以下简称《守则》）规定了诚信、专业和保密的标准，所有会员均有义务在其作为会议口译员的工作中遵循这些标准。

2. Candidates shall also undertake to adhere to the provisions of this Code.

2. 候选会员（candidates）也应承诺遵守本守则的规定。

3. The Council, acting in accordance with the Regulation on Disciplinary Procedure, shall impose penalties for any breach of the rules of the profession as defined in this Code.

3. 按照《纪律程序条例》，理事会将对任何违反本守则所界定的职业规则的行为予以惩罚。

Ⅱ. Code of Honour
二、荣誉准则

Article 2

第2条

1. Members of the Association shall be bound by the strictest secrecy, which must be observed towards all persons and with regard to all information disclosed in the course of the practice of the profession at any gathering not open to the public.

1. 会员应受严格的保密准则约束。在任何不向公众开放的会议中，所有人员均需对口译过程中披露的所有信息严格保密。

2. Members shall refrain from deriving any personal gain whatsoever from confidential information they may have acquired in the exercise of their duties as conference interpreters.

2. 严禁会员利用会议口译员的职务之便，用可能获取的机密信息谋取任何私利。

Article 3

第3条

1. Members of the Association shall not accept any assignment for which they are not qualified. Acceptance of an assignment shall imply a moral undertaking on the member's part to work with all due professionalism.

1. 会员不得接受任何本人难以胜任的任务。接受任务则意味着会员在道义上承诺将以应有的专业水准工作。

2. Any member of the Association recruiting other conference interpreters, be they members of the Association or not, shall give the same undertaking.

2. 任何会员在招募其他会议口译员时，无论后者是否为本协会会员，都应给予客户同样的保证。

3. Members of the Association shall not accept more than one assignment for the same period of time.

3. 会员不得在同一时间里接受多项任务。

Article 4

第4条

1. Members of the Association shall not accept any job or situation which might detract from the dignity of the profession.

1. 会员不得接受任何可能有损本职业尊严的工作或职务。

2. They shall refrain from any act which might bring the profession into disrepute.

2. 会员应避免做出任何可能有损本职业声誉的行为。

Article 5

第5条

For any professional purpose, members may publicise the fact that they are conference interpreters and members of the Association, either as individuals or as part of any grouping or region to which they belong.

会员可以出于任何职业目的，宣传其为会议口译员和本协会会员这一事实，包括本协会个人会员身份和本协会任何下属机构或区域组织成员身份。

Article 6

第6条

1. It shall be the duty of members of the Association to afford their colleagues moral assistance and collegiality.

1. 会员有义务向同事提供道义援助和协作。

2. Members shall refrain from any utterance or action prejudicial to the interests of the

Association or its members. Any complaint arising out of the conduct of any other member or any disagreement regarding any decision taken by the Association shall be pursued and settled within the Association itself.

2. 会员应避免任何有损本协会或其会员利益的言语或行为。任何针对其他会员行为的申诉，或是对本协会所做出的任何决定有任何异议，应寻求在协会内部解决。

3. Any problem pertaining to the profession which arises between two or more members of the Association, including candidates, may be referred to the Council for arbitration, except for disputes of a commercial nature.

3. 任何两名或两名以上会员（包括候选会员），如产生任何与职业相关的争端，均可提交理事会仲裁，商业性质的争端除外。

Ⅲ. Working Conditions

三、工作条件

Article 7

第7条

With a view to ensuring the best quality interpretation, members of the Association:

为确保口译的最佳质量，协会会员：

1. shall endeavour always to secure satisfactory conditions of sound, visibility and comfort, having particular regard to the Professional Standards as adopted by the Association as well as any technical standards drawn up or approved by it;

1. 应根据本协会通过的《职业标准》以及由本协会制定或批准的任何技术标准，始终努力争取满意的声效、能见度和舒适度；

2. shall not, as a general rule, when interpreting simultaneously in a booth, work either alone or without the availability of a colleague to relieve them should the need arise;

2. 通常说来，在单独一人或在需要时没有同事可替换的情况下，不得在同传厢从事同传工作；

3. shall try to ensure that teams of conference interpreters are formed in such a way as to avoid the systematic use of relay;

3. 在组建会议口译团队时，应尽力避免经常使用接力；

4. shall not agree to undertake either simultaneous interpretation without a booth or whispered interpretation unless the circumstances are exceptional and the quality of interpretation work is not thereby impaired;

4. 不应同意从事耳语传译或在没有同传厢的条件下进行同声传译，除非情况特殊且口译工作的质量不会因此受到影响；

5. shall require a direct view of the speaker and the conference room. They will thus refuse to accept the use of television monitors instead of this direct view, except in the case of videoconferences;

5. 应要求可直接观察到发言者和会议室。因此，除非是视频会议，否则应拒绝接受使用电视屏幕代替直接观察的方式；

6. shall require that working documents and texts to be read out at the conference be sent to them in advance;

6. 应要求提前拿到将在会议上宣读的工作文件和演讲稿；

7. shall request a briefing session whenever appropriate;

7. 如果条件许可，应要求举办情况通报会；

8. shall not perform any other duties except that of conference interpreter at conferences for which they have been taken on as interpreters.

8. 在自己已被聘为会议口译员的会议上，不得从事会议口译之外的任何其他工作。

Article 8

第8条

Members of the Association shall neither accept nor, a fortiori, offer for themselves or for other conference interpreters recruited through them, be they members of the Association or not, any working conditions contrary to those laid down in this Code or in the Professional Standards.

对于任何违反本《守则》或《职业标准》规定的工作条件，协会会员均不得接受，更不得代表本人或本人招募的其他会议口译员（无论是否为协会会员）主动提出。

Ⅳ. Amendment Procedure

四、修订程序

Article 9

第9条

This Code may be modified by a decision of the Assembly taken with a two-thirds majority of votes cast, provided a legal opinion has been sought on the proposals.

相关提议在征求法律意见后，大会可在获得三分之二多数的投票后做出决定，对本《守则》予以修改。

关于职业原则，还可参考以下网站：

中国翻译协会：http://www.tac-online.org.cn

国际翻译家联盟（国际译联）（International Federation of Translators）：http://www.fit-ift.org

口译网：http://www.kouyi.org/thesis/499.html

三、词汇准备

Text 1

purchasing power parity (PPP) 购买力平价

per-capita GDP 人均国内生产总值

healthcare expenditure 医疗保健支出

World Health Organization (WHO) 世界卫生组织

intellectual property laws (IP) 知识产权法

research and development （R & D）研发

Ministry of Health (MOH) 卫生部

Bioinformatics Institute 生物信息学研究所

Genome Institute 基因组研究所

Institute of Bioengineering & Nanotechnology 生物工程与纳米技术研究所

Bioprocessing Technology Institute 生物工艺技术研究所

Institute of Medical Biology 医学生物学研究所

Institute of Molecular and Cell Biology 分子与细胞生物学研究所

Singapore Institute for Clinical Sciences 新加坡临床科学研究所

Bayer 拜耳公司

Roche 罗氏公司

Siena Biotech 锡耶纳生物技术公司

Novartis 诺华公司

Glaxo Smith Kline (GSK) 葛兰素史克

contract research organizations (CROs) 合同研究机构

A. Menarini Asia-Pacific 美纳里尼集团亚太公司（原Invida 英维达控股私人有限公司）

Eli Lilly 礼来公司

Takeda 武田药品工业株式会社
Merck 默克公司
Pfizer 辉瑞
Sanofi-Aventis and Abbot 赛诺菲-安万特和艾博特
Thermo Fisher Scientific（TFS） 赛默飞世尔科技
Tropical Diseases (NITD) 热带病
Amgen 安进

Text 2

outsourcing manufacturing 外包制造
government-approved trading companies 政府认可的贸易公司
specifications and required standards 规范和标准要求
price quote 报价
itemized quote 逐项报价
customs duties 关税
middleman 中间商

Text 3

AdvaMed 美国先进医疗技术协会
EucoMed 欧洲医疗器械行业协会
International Trade Administration （ITA） 国际贸易局（下属于美国商务部）
portfolio 职务，职责
National Export Initiative 国家出口计划
life expectancy 平均寿命
stroke 中风
breast cancer 乳腺癌
emerging market 新兴市场
profess 声称，公开表示
technical barriers to trade 技术性贸易壁垒
hamstring 削弱，使残废
US-China Joint Commission on Commerce and Trade's (JCCT) 美中商贸联合委员会
US-India High Technology Cooperation Group (HTCG) 美印高新技术合作组织
FDA (Food and Drug Administration) 食品和药物管理局
ANVISA (the Agencia Nacional Vigilancia de Sanitaria) 巴西国家卫生监督局

Text 4

Health, Welfare and Food (Health and Welfare) 香港食品卫生局
Permanent Secretary 常务秘书长
Hong Kong Trade Development Council 香港贸易发展局
Modernized Chinese Medicine International Association 现代化中医药国际协会
evidence-based Chinese medicine 循证中医药学
Hospital Authority 医院管理局
Hong Kong Chinese Materia Medica Standards 香港中药学标准

Text 5

国家基本药物制度 The National System for Essential Drugs
零差率销售 zero markup sales
国务院医改领导小组 Healthcare Reform Leading Group of the State Council
集中采购 centralized purchasing
统一配送 unified distribution
量价挂钩 linking quantity and price together
采购责任主体 liability subject for purchase
委托协议 consignment agreement
批量采购 bulk purchase
"双信封"招标方式 a "double envelop" method in biding
市场清退制度 elimination system

Text 6

医疗器械 medical device
年均复合增长率 compound annual growth rate
医药保健品行业 pharmaceutical and health products industry
医用敷料 medical dressings
耗材 consumables
环渤海湾 the rim of Bohai Bay
产业集群区 industrial clusters
一次性耗材 disposable consumables
按摩器 massage appliances
贴牌出口 OEM export
进出口垂直国际分工状态 vertical international division of labor in import and export

自主营销 independent marketing

四、摘要练习

请听下面英语语篇，第一篇用源语言复述此段主要信息逻辑点及层次，第二篇用译入语复述此段主要信息逻辑点及层次。注意信息点之间的逻辑联系。

Text 1

Singapore's Pharmaceutical Industry

Ames Gross

25 February 2014

Singapore, a small island nation in the South China Sea with a population of 5.5 million, has recently become a hot spot for sophisticated pharmaceutical research and manufacturing. In 2013, the country had an average purchasing power parity (PPP) per-capita GDP of over \$61,000, about \$10,000 more than in the US.

Healthcare expenditure in Singapore was over \$12 billion in 2013, representing 6% of GDP and approximately equal to healthcare spending in Thailand—which has a population 12 times as large. Total healthcare spending is expected to sky rocket to almost \$22.5 billion by 2018. Per-capita healthcare expenditure has increased almost 300% over the past decade to more than \$2,400 in 2013, second only to Japan in the Asian region. The country's healthcare system was ranked 6 worldwide by the World Health Organization (WHO).

Singapore also brings together a well-developed infrastructure and logistics network, strong intellectual property (IP) laws, a record of safety, a good regulatory environment, and active government support of the biomedical industry. For drug companies looking for an Asian country in which to manufacture pharmaceuticals, expand R & D, or sell their products, Singapore is a good choice.

Singapore's Pharmaceutical Market

The pharmaceutical market in Singapore is valued at almost \$1 billion, about one-fourth the size of the Philippine market—which has a population of over 100 million. Over the past two decades, Singapore has worked to create a solid foundation for the biomedical industry, with over 30 public-sector research institutes under the Ministry of Health (MOH) and the Agency for Science, Technology and Research (A*STAR). These include the Bioinformatics Institute, Genome Institute, Institute of Bioengineering & Nanotechnology, Bioprocessing Technology Institute, Institute of Medical Biology, Institute of Molecular and Cell Biology and the Singapore Institute for Clinical Sciences.

Singapore has also promoted public-private research institutes—such as with Bayer, Roche, Siena Biotech, Novartis, and GlaxoSmithKline (GSK)—as well as supporting the development of clinical contract research organizations (CROs). The government spent $2 billion investing in biomedical capabilities and infrastructure over the previous decade and earmarked more than $3 billion to support biomedical enterprises and research from 2011-2015.

There are a few domestic Singaporean pharmaceutical companies that are also successful in Singapore. For example, A. Menarini Asia-Pacific, formerly Invida, is a pharmaceutical company that was founded in 2005 in Singapore. In addition to its headquarters in Singapore, it has almost a dozen locations in other Asian countries, marketing branded pharmaceuticals, medical devices, and biotechnology to hospitals, pharmacies, and clinics. The company also has partnerships with a variety of multinational drug companies based in the US, EU and Japan.

Foreign Drug Companies in Singapore

More than 30 of the top global biomedical sciences firms—including Novartis, Eli Lilly, Takeda and GSK—have a R & D presence in Singapore. Of the top 10 biopharmaceutical companies, 7 manufacture some of their products in Singapore and 8 have regional headquarters in Singapore. GSK, Baxter and Roche all launched their first-in-Asia commercial production facilities in Singapore in 2009. Some companies, such as Merck, Pfizer, Sanofi-Aventis and Abbott, have chosen Singapore as their global manufacturing base. Within 5 years, Singapore will have 8 biologics production facilities—worth $2 billion.

Foreign biomedical companies spent approximately $500 million on R & D in Singapore last year, up from $40 million a decade ago. Nationally, public and private organizations spend almost $1.2 billion on biomedical R & D every year, with several thousand private- and public-sector researchers. In 2013, biomedical firms in Singapore manufactured products worth $25 billion, up from $5 billion in 2000.

For example, Thermo Fisher Scientific recently opened a new, 38,000 square foot production plant in Singapore. According to the company's Biosciences President, "Our new Singapore facility further strengthens our global presence, expands our manufacturing infrastructure and establishes local production capabilities to meet increased demand for biologic drug discovery and development in Asia."

Also, Novartis started building a new biologics production facility in February 2013, investing over $500 million. The plant should be operational by 2017. In Singapore, Novartis also has its Asia-Pacific head office, Institute for Tropical Diseases (NITD), a pharmaceutical manufacturing site and two production plants. Novartis is one of Singapore's top 3 biomedical investors, with almost $1 billion invested in pharmaceutical and healthcare products.

Recently, Amgen also began constructing its first Asian manufacturing facility in Singapore. The company plans to spend $200 million building the plant, which will be completed in 2015 and licensed in 2016. At the groundbreaking ceremony, Amgen's Executive Vice President of Operations said, "Singapore's rich talent pool and friendly business environment made it an ideal place to invest in a world-class manufacturing facility and to underscore our global expansion efforts."

复述要点提示（主要信息逻辑点及层次）

In 2013, Singapore's average PPP per-capita GDP was over $61,000, about $10,000 more than in the US; Healthcare expenditure was over $12 billion, is expected to rise to $22.5 billion by 2018. And its Per-capita spending in medicine has increased almost 300% in last 10 years to more than $2,400.

Singapore's healthcare system was ranked 6 worldwide by WHO. Supported by its excellent IP laws, very good infrastructure, logistic network, government support, and biomedical industry, it is excellent place for manufacture, selling and R & D in pharmaceuticals.

The pharmaceutical market in Singapore is valued at almost $1 billion.

Under its MOH and the Agency for Science, are over 30 public-sector research institutes, e.g.: Bioinformatics Institute, Genome Institute, Institute of Bioengineering & Nanotechnology, etc.

It also has many public-private research institutes, such as with Bayer, Roche, Siena Biotech, and many CROs. The government planned $3 billion to support biomedical enterprises and research from 2011-2015.

Successful domestic pharmaceutical companies include A. Menarini Asia-Pacific, which has wide business and connections in Asian countries, and partnerships with US, EU and

Japanese multinational drug companies.

Singapore has more than 30 world top biomedical science companies, they either have R&D or manufacture bases. These include Novartis, Eli Lilly, Takeda, GSK, Baxter, Roche, Merck, Pfizer, Sanofi-Aventis and Abbot, to name a few. In 2013, they spent $500 million while domestic firms spent $1.2 billion on R&D, and altogether they produce $25 billion products.

For example, Thermo Fisher Scientific recently opened a new, 38,000 square foot production plant in Singapore; Novartis has invested over $500 million for a new biologics production facility to operate in 2017. It has totally invested $1 billion in pharmaceutical and healthcare products. Also Amgen plans to spend $200 million build its first Asian facility which will be completed in 2015 and licensed in 2016.

Text 2

China's Medical Device Market 2005: Outsourcing of Medical Devices

As discussed in the beginning of this report, more US medical companies are now outsourcing manufacturing to China to reduce their costs. Chinese device manufacturers have made significant improvements in medical device technology and product quality. However, identifying the right factory in China can be a challenge.

Identifying Manufacturers of Your Product

Presently, one of the best places to begin searching for potential medical device manufacturers in China is on the Internet. In the past, Chinese manufacturers often used government-approved trading companies in order to export their products, so manufacturers typically did not have their own ability to sell their products overseas. However, as restrictions on import and export regulations have eased, Chinese manufacturers have begun doing their own direct sales and marketing, often via the Internet. Now, there is a wealth of information on the Internet for foreign companies interested in building relationships with manufacturers in China. Moreover, Chinese manufacturers are becoming more and more comfortable working and interacting with foreign companies and are accustomed to using English (albeit sometimes broken English) in many of their business dealings.

A good place to start your search is on a basic search engine. This will provide you with an initial list of manufacturers and is a relatively quick process. There are numerous websites that provide sizeable lists of manufacturers and often include contact information and a brief description of each manufacturer. However, this type of search should only be a starting point and should not be considered as a thorough investigation.

Once several potential manufacturers have been identified by the Internet search, each manufacturer's respective website should be examined. However, it is common for the Chinese version of the website to be much more detailed than the English version. In order to establish an accurate idea of the company, both websites should be viewed by a person fluent in both Chinese and English. Additionally, foreign companies should keep in mind that all the information on the Internet or an individual manufacturer's website may be misleading or inaccurate. It is vital for companies to take further measures in order to confirm the manufacturer's claims.

The Initial Contact

Once a list of Chinese manufacturers has been compiled, each of these manufacturers should be contacted directly. Many Chinese manufacturers today will have an English-speaking employee in their sales office. Nevertheless, it is always best for a foreign company to have a Chinese speaker available in order to make the communications go more smoothly. Initially, emails and phone calls should be used to establish trust and a good business relationship between the foreign and Chinese companies.

Trust is crucial to successful business in Asia, so this initial step should not be taken lightly. These emails and phone calls can also be used to answer initial questions and confirm the manufacturers' production capabilities. A foreign company should ensure that the manufacturer can produce their products to their specifications and required standards. Moreover, it is not unheard of for a Chinese company to claim that they are manufacturing a product, when, in fact, they are purchasing the product from another company and selling it for a higher price. Therefore, emails and phone calls are not 100 percent sufficient in deciding whether to pursue business with a company or manufacturer in China.

Determining the Price

After establishing a good business relationship and flow of communication with a manufacturer, the next step will be to obtain a price quote for your product. If you have a "standard" product, the price quote should be fairly straightforward. However, if your product has somewhat unique features or specifications, or if you are requesting a typical quantities, a general price quote may not be very useful. In this case, it may be necessary to ask the Chinese manufacturer for an itemized quote. Foreign companies should also keep in mind that Chinese manufacturers tend to use metric units and may not be familiar with inches or pounds. It is also important to ask the manufacturer how long they will honor their price quote. With a quickly growing economy, prices in China are often increasing, so a price quote may only be valid for a short period of time. Foreign companies must also add a number of other expenses into the overall costs of purchasing medical products from China. International and domestic shipping, customs duties and possible travel expenses need to also be included in the total cost of sourced products.

Trading Company vs. Factory

Even though Chinese manufacturers are increasingly exporting directly overseas, trading companies are still very common in China. Trading companies act as a "middleman," purchasing products from a Chinese manufacturer and selling the products to a foreign buyer.

Trading companies offer several advantages. First, these companies tend to have a wide variety of products available for purchase. A foreign company with numerous product lines may be able to use one trading company for most of their products, as opposed to a Chinese manufacturer that could only produce one or two lines. Second, trading companies can often purchase products for better prices since they already have well-established relationships (and may make larger purchases) with manufacturers in China. These prices, in some instances, may even be less than if a foreign company goes directly to a Chinese manufacturer. Third, it is usually easier dealing with a trading company since they tend to have more experience communicating with foreigners (many trading companies have English speakers) and more experience working with foreign companies. In general, trading companies offer short-term profits and business relationships with these companies can be established in less time.

Depending on a foreign company's objectives, trading companies are not always the best way to outsource. If a foreign company is looking to establish a long-term business relationship in China, direct contact with the Chinese manufacturer may be more beneficial. The foreign company can develop a long-standing relationship with a Chinese manufacturer, while also having more control over their product design and quality. By avoiding trading companies who may cut off your supply at any time, a direct relationship with a manufacturer will give the buyer a stronger sense of control and hopefully more leverage on prices as the relationship and volumes grow.

复述要点提示（主要信息逻辑点及层次）

1. 因为中国取消限制，企业自身可以自行向外销售或寻找市场，并且它们也逐渐习惯于与外国企业打交道。因此可以直接联系厂商。

2. 互联网是寻找中方企业的首选。先用基本搜索引擎搜索。互联网上有大量的生产厂家基本信息，并且提供联系方式。

3. 选定厂家之后，找厂家的互联网主页。主页中文版和英文版的介绍都要仔细看。但这还不够，还需与各制造商直接联系。

4. 与厂家接触时，虽然现在很多中国对外企业都雇有会说英文的雇员，但最好还是自带一个会说中文的翻译。

5. 在亚洲做生意，建立信任至关重要，要重视接触的第一步。用电子邮件和电话了解生产厂家的产能，确定厂家是否能按要求和标准生产产品。中方厂家称自己制造某一产品，但却从另一厂家购买并加价卖出，这种现象并不鲜见。因此要面谈。

6. 定价方面。如果您有“标准”产品，所报价格应当是相当直接的。但如果你的产品有某些独特的功能或规格，需逐项询问具体报价。由于经济发展及涨价问题，必须询问报价的时效。还需将国际运输、国内运输、关税以及可能的旅行费用计算在总成本之内。另外，需注意度量衡的问题，中企用公制。

7. 贸易公司与生产厂家有区别。贸易公司是中间商。与中间商做生意有几个好处：①有多种产品供选择。拥有各种生产线的外国厂家可以通过一个外贸公司销售大多数产品，而中企只能购买一两条生产线。②与中企关系成熟，他们拿到的价格可能比外国公司直接找生产厂家拿到的价格还低。③与外商打交道有经验，与中介做生意要容易且快捷一些。

8. 建立长久关系需直接与厂商接触。好处是关系可控，产品设计与质量可控，避免中介随时切断供货。随着关系发展和贸易量增加，会有更好的价格空间。

五、英译汉练习

Text 3

Remarks by Michael C. CamuÑez, US Assistant Secretary of Commerce at the 2012 International Medical Device Industry Compliance Conference

Stockholm, Sweden

10 May 2012

Thank you, Jeff, for that kind introduction. Good morning and thank you to AdvaMed[1] and EucoMed for hosting this event and for the invitation to be here with you today. As many of you know, this is the fifth consecutive year for this important compliance conference. What you may not know is that AdvaMed has been advancing issues of importance to the medical device industry since 1975—that's nearly 4 decades of advocacy. Until 2000, it was known as the Health Industry Manufacturers Association, but its core mission—to advance global health care by promoting a legal, regulatory and economic environment that promotes worldwide access to the benefits of medical technology—has remained unchanged. Your efforts are as important today as they have ever been. Let me also just add that the Department of Commerce has enjoyed a very strong working relationship over the years with AdvaMed and its leadership team, and I'd like to recognize and thank your President and CEO, Steve Ubl, your General Counsel, Chris White, and your Senior Vice President, Ralph Ives, for their leadership and partnership. I'd also like to acknowledge the important contributions made by EucoMed and its leadership team, including its Acting CEO Luciano Cattani.

When Steve and others first invited me to deliver the keynote address for this conference several months ago, I immediately expressed my interest in being here with you, and here's why: the medical technology industry is one of the most important drivers of growth and innovation in the world. In my capacity as Assistant Secretary of Commerce

---

1 AdvaMed: Advanced Medical Technology Association (美国先进医疗技术协会). AdvaMed advocates for a legal, regulatory and economic environment that advances global health care by assuring worldwide patient access to the benefits of medical technology. It promotes policies that foster the highest ethical standards, rapid product approvals, appropriate reimbursement, and access to international markets.

in the International Trade Administration, I have a global portfolio and responsibilities that require me to deal with virtually every industrial and services sector in the economy. Yet no sector has impressed me more than this one. Doing good for humanity while driving economic growth and prosperity is an uncommon combination—yet that's the hallmark of your industry. It's for that reason—this remarkable combination of human and commercial benefit—that the Department of Commerce is proud to partner with you. It's also why we have prioritized your sector under President Obama's National Export Initiative.

Your work begins with a commitment to unsurpassed quality in the delivery of patient care. And the impact of this commitment is remarkable: in the US, for example, between 1980 and 2000, advancements in medical technology contributed to, among other things, a three-year increase in life expectancy; a 50% reduction in deaths from heart disease; and a decrease in death from strokes of more than 30% and from breast cancer by 20%.

Beyond the life-saving benefits provided to countless patients, your industry also serves as an engine of employment and economic growth. According to industry figures, the medical device industry employs over 420,000 workers in the US, and that number is growing. Further, each of those 420-plus thousand workers generates an additional 4 jobs that are indirectly linked to this industry. Put differently, almost 2 million workers—including suppliers, manufacturers of component parts, service providers, and others—are now tied to the medical device sector in the US alone. And the US is not alone: the industry is experiencing significant growth in some of the world's most important emerging markets.

Despite the fact that so many economies profess their interest in attracting and supporting innovative industries like the medical technology sector, the reality is your companies continue to face substantial challenges that limit their competitiveness and impede their capacity to innovate. And in this twenty-first century, highly globalized, highly interconnected economy, these challenges most often take the form of technical barriers to trade—the so-called "behind the border" barriers that can hamstring an industry's growth and severely limit the benefits of free and open commerce. It's these challenges that the Department of Commerce's International Trade Administration (ITA) is most keenly focused on.

Many of our efforts on behalf of industry are raised through a wide range of bilateral engagements across the globe. In China, for example, our staff just returned from a meeting of the US-China Joint Commission on Commerce and Trade's (JCCT) Pharmaceutical and Medical Devices subgroup, which my department chairs. The meeting focused on issues of mutual interest to the two countries, including medical device safety standards and a pending Chinese regulation on the supervision of medical devices. In India, we regularly work with AdvaMed and others to resolve market access barriers through the US-India High Technology Cooperation Group (HTCG). And in Brazil, we have leveraged the US-Brazil Commercial Dialogue and other efforts to make progress on barriers relating to medical devices. For example, recently we helped launch the Information Exchange Forum, which saw Brazil's FDA equivalent, ANVISA, engage with the private sector in a public meeting for the first time. The discussions led to continued engagement between ANVISA and industry and to an MOU on data sharing between ANVISA and the US FDA. Just last year, I was pleased to join AdvaMed on a policy trip to Brazil that continued these efforts and resulted in significant progress on a number of important fronts, including an agreement between industry and the Brazilian government on a mutually beneficial action plan and the development of an industry-led alliance that includes three Brazil-based associations from the "Alliance of Brazilian Innovative Healthcare Industry."

These are, of course, just a few examples. As one of the most innovative industries in the world, you will no doubt continue to face market access barriers as you endeavor to introduce new products in new ways and push the innovation curve. Just know that the Department of Commerce is committed to working with and for you in an effort to help further the growth of your industry.

It is truly a pleasure and an honor for me to be here and to support you in your important work. If I am to leave you today with one message, it's this: government can't win this fight without your help, and we at the Department of Commerce look forward to continuing a long and successful partnership with AdvaMed and EucoMed and with each of your companies.

Thank you.

Text 4

Speech by PSHWF at HK International Medical and Health Care Fair

Sandra Lee, Permanent Secretary for Health, Welfare and Food

17 August 2006

Dr. Sun, Mr. Wong, Mr. Chan, Mr. Yeung, Mr. Kay,

Distinguished guests,

Ladies and gentlemen,

On behalf of the Hong Kong SAR Government, I extend a very warm welcome to you all. I would also like to thank the Hong Kong Trade Development Council and the Modernised Chinese Medicine International Association for inviting me to this conference and exhibition.The Government recognizes the important role of Chinese medicine in our healthcare system. Hong Kong is well placed in tapping the business potential for Chinese medicine given our expertise in marketing, trading, manufacturing, management, technology and standards setting. In the last few years, the Government has devoted much effort to facilitating the development of Chinese medicine in Hong Kong.

The Government's strategy is to develop a robust regulatory regime for Chinese medicine practitioners, traders and proprietary Chinese medicines, and to ensure a sufficient supply of practitioners through funding of relevant undergraduate courses. We believe that these elements are crucial to nurturing an enabling environment for the Chinese medicine industry to flourish.

At the same time, the Government is committed to promoting "evidence-based Chinese medicine" so that the data can be used for broader application. In this regard, we have set up six Chinese medicine clinics, and three more will be ready by the end of the year. We are planning more in future years. They are set up on a tripartite basis, between the Hospital Authority, NGOs and universities. One of the missions of these clinics is to participate in clinical research and assist in data collection. The Hospital Authority is also offering "evidence-based" clinical treatment using a combination of Chinese and Western Medicines in a few hospitals. Concurrently, our Department of Health is developing the Hong Kong Chinese Materia Medica Standards for 60 common herbal medicines. These standards will serve as a reference for the trade, benchmarks for quality and safety, and the basis for further research.

The Government's vision and direction for the development of Chinese medicine is clear. We will continue to strengthen the regulatory system and the infrastructure for this sector. Regulation is not meant to make things difficult for the trade. Rather it aims to protect public health and to set a common standard for the trade to follow. We hope that "registered in Hong Kong" will become a credible quality assurance for the Chinese medicine industry to develop their local and international markets. In a similar spirit, our intent of developing "evidence-based" Chinese medicine is to lay a solid foundation for the industry and academics to pursue further research and development.

I would also like to commend the private hospitals for their participation in the Fair to showcase the quality health and medical care services which Hong Kong offers. Together with the public sector, our private and public hospitals have earned for Hong Kong, an enviable reputation for high quality clinical standards and medical care.

The modernisation of Chinese medicine will not succeed without the active participation of the private sector. This event provides an important platform for this purpose. There will be ample opportunities for useful intellectual exchange and business collaborations. I am confident that you will have a lot to take home, be it insightful thoughts, valuable information or business opportunities. And I wish the conference success and all participants abundant health.

Thank you.

六、汉译英练习

Text 5

国务院医改办公室负责人就建立规范基本药物采购机制发布答记者问（节选）

问：国家基本药物制度实施已经一年多了，为什么要出台《采购机制》？

答：建立国家基本药物制度是惠及民生的重大制度创新，旨在保障群众基本用药。这项制度自去年启动实施以来，取得了明显进展和初步成效，截至目前，已有超过50%的政府办基层医疗卫生机构实施了基本药物制度，并实行零差率销售。但也出现了一些新情况、新问题，突出表现在基本药物集中招标采购不规范，药品价格虚高问题没有得到有效合理解决，一些地区部分药品出现了断供、缺货等情况，影响到基本药物制度的实施效果和群众的受益程度。按照国务院医改领导小组的指示精神，国务院医改办公室会同有关部门对基本药物招标采购的关键环节和存在的突出问题进行了深入分析，并积极借鉴国内外药品集中采购的成功经验，认真听取有关方面及国内外专家的意见和建议，提出了有针对性的措施，形成了《采购机制》初稿。经广泛征求有关部门、各地方意见，反复修改完善，形成《采购机制》送审稿，经国务院医改办公室全体会议讨论后，提交国务院医改领导小组全体会议审议通过，11月19日国务院办公厅正式印发了《采购机制》。

《采购机制》是国家基本药物制度的重要配套文件，必将有力地推进各地尽快建立规范的基本药物省级集中采购机制，构建起比较完善的基层基本药物供应保障体系，确保基本药物制度顺利实施。

问：此次《采购机制》出台的总体考虑是什么？有哪些创新性举措和亮点？

答：《采购机制》的总体思路是，实行以省（区、市）为单位的集中采购、统一配送；坚持政府主导与市场机制相结合，发挥集中批量采购优势，招标和采购结合，量价挂钩、签订合同，一次完成采购全过程，最大限度地降低采购成本，实现基本药物安全有效、品质良好、价格合理、供应及时，促进基本药物的生产和供应，使群众真正得到实惠。

《采购机制》针对各地存在的突出问题，围绕基本药物的质量、价格和供应三个核心要素，提出了一系列有针对性的创新措施，主要包括：一是明确采购责任主体，由省级卫生行政部门确定的采购机构作为采购主体负责基本药物采购，与政府办基层医疗卫生机构签订授权或委托协议，与药品供应商签订购销合同并负责合同执行。二是坚持量价挂钩，通过编制采购计划，明确采购数量（暂无法确定数量的采用单一货源承诺方式），实现一次完成采购全过程，签订购销合同，并严格付款时间。充分发挥批量采购的优势。三是质量优先，价格合理。坚持把质量放在首位，采取“双信封”招标方式，确保信誉高、质量好、供货能力强的企业参与竞争。同时，对基本药物市场实际购销价格进行全面调查，原则上集中采购价格不得高于市场实际购销价格，确保采购价格合理。四是严格诚信记录和信息公开制度，对违反合同、出现质量不达标、不按时供货等违规企业一律记录在案，并向社会公布，实行严格的市场清退制度，逾期不改的，两年内不得参与全国任何药品招标采购。通过网上采购平台，提高交易透明度，基本药物采购价格、数量和中标企业等要及时向社会公布，接受社会监督，从制度和机制上营造公开、公平和公正的采购环境。

Text 6

医疗器械贸易

医疗器械行业是当今世界发展最快、贸易往来最活跃的一个工业门类，随着科学技术的进一步发展，医疗器械逐步进入高科技工业企业行列。近年来，我国医疗器械出口贸易正步入一个新的高速增长期，2006～2010年，连续5年出口持续以2位数攀升，年均复合增长率达到20.94%，高于医药保健品行业平均增长水平。就出口主体而言，跨国巨头以我国为生产和加工基地辐射全球市场带动了高技术医院诊断与治疗设备的出口，国内众多民营企业则以中小型设备、医用敷料和耗材见长，成为该类产品出口的主力。

3 000多家外商投资企业带动了我国医疗器械出口增长，其出口总额已连续 5 年

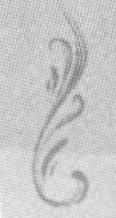

占据当年我医疗器械出口总额的“半壁江山”。据海关统计，2007～2011年外企出口额占比分别为58.51%、57.29%、59.01%、58.94%和52.59%，出口额年复合增长率为17.36%。随着国际医疗器械产业加速转移，国外先进技术和资本还将继续采用合资合作、技术输出等形式进入国内，部分依赖进口的仪器设备正逐步实现国产替代进口，使我国成为全球医疗器械重要的生产和研发基地。

民营企业出口呈快速增长趋势，年复合增长率为26.9%，远高于外企和国有企业增长水平，2007～2011年，民营企业出口额占比分别为28.12%、30.22%、30.26%、31.28%和37.3%，连年攀升，成为我医疗器械出口的主力军之一。

随着我国医疗器械产业的发展，珠江三角洲、长江三角洲及环渤海湾3个地区，依靠其地区工业技术、科学技术人才、临床医学基础及政策性优势，成为我国医疗器械三大产业集群区。据不完全统计，这三大区域医疗器械总产值和销量之和均占全国总量的80%以上。医疗器械出口布局也反映了这一特点，长三角和珠三角地区的出口额之和占全国出口总额的近70%。

一次性耗材、医用敷料和按摩器具等是我国出口的优势产品，属于技术含量相对较低的劳动力密集型产品，我国产品质量与国外同类产品相当但价格优势比较明显，因此国内企业在国际市场有明显的比较优势和竞争能力。据海关统计，民营企业该类产品出口占比达到43.31%，国有企业出口占比8.57%，以国内企业占主导。但我国企业出口有相当部分为贴牌出口，如一次性耗材以加工贸易出口占比为46.05%，保健康复用品加工贸易比重32.27%，国内企业仍须在打造自主品牌方面下苦功。

虽然经过多年发展，我国企业在部分领域出口逐年增加，在国际市场已占有相当份额，但必须看到国内企业素质还有待进一步提高。

当前，在进出口垂直国际分工状态下，医疗器械对外贸易输出低技术附加值产品、输入高技术附加值产品的状况仍不容乐观，品牌和自主营销渠道仍是制约国内企业真正“走出去”的主要障碍。提高企业素质，必须重视中小型高新技术企业的发展，从政府层面应加大政策扶持力度，促进企业素质提高和规模扩大，在鼓励医疗器械企业走出去扩大市场份额的同时，更要推动企业在国内市场占据有利空间，做大做强；在企业自身层面则有待于提高适应国际经营的管理水平、扩大产品销售范围，通过加强自主品牌建设、加大创新研发力度，提高企业竞争力。

资料来源：

Text 1 http://www.pacificbridgemedical.com/publications/singapores-pharmaceutical-industry-2014-update/

Text 2 http://www.pacificbridgemedical.com/publications/china-rsquo-s-medical-device-market-2005/

Text 3 http://trade.gov/press/speeches/2012/camunez-051012.asp

Text 4 http://www.fhb.gov.hk/en/press_and_publications/speech/shwf/2006/sp060817.htm

Text 5 http://www.moh.gov.cn/publicfiles/business/htmlfiles/mohbgt/s3577/201012/49985.htm

Text 6 http://www.cccmhpie.org.cn/Pub/1773/58229.shtml

参考答案

四、摘要练习

Text 1

新加坡医疗设备市场

埃姆斯·格罗斯

2014年2月25日

随着新加坡作为该地区医疗保健枢纽和优秀医疗保健中心的声誉日益加强，岛国的医疗设备市场将有望实现增长。

新加坡力争为其居民及国际医患市场提供一流的医疗保健服务体系，对尖端医疗设备需求较高。新加坡政府的目标是每年服务100万国外病患，贡献26亿新币（折合15.5亿美元）的附加值或1%的国内生产总值。

美国、日本、德国是新加坡的三大医疗设备供应商。大量的公司将区域总部设立于此，努力为其客户提供更加便捷、优质的服务。美国在此方面享有良好的声誉，因其先进的技术，高品质、先进、可靠的设备而得到行业的认可。

美国的公司在新加坡市场还算是新手，对出口新加坡颇有兴趣。他们可能会考虑指定一个当地的经销商来代理公司的产品和服务。由于岛国市场较小，大多数潜在的经销商都可能要求拥有产品的独家销售权。这样能保证他们将自身资源投入合适的终端用户的推销，并从销售所得中获得收益。同时，这也是美国出口商对当地市场承诺的体现。新加坡没有专门的代理协议法规，此类合同应基于双方都同意的条款和条件。

根据不同的医疗设备，美国公司需向经销商提供样品或对展示用商品给予特惠折扣。潜在的经销商将使用样品进行市场调研，确定产品收益。而展示用商品则被用于向潜在买家展示美国产品的技术。

美国医疗设备出口商应在公司市场的接触面、产品范围及其产品与美国公司产品的互补性等基础之上来评估经销商的适合程度。

Text 2

中国的医疗设备市场2005：医疗设备外包

正如本报告开始讨论的，目前越来越多的美国医疗公司正在中国寻求制造外包来降低成本。中国设备制造商已经在医疗设备技术和产品质量方面有明显改善。然而，想要在中国找到一家合适的工厂仍是一个挑战。

为产品寻找制造商

目前，在中国寻找潜在的医疗设备制造商最好的地方是互联网。过去，中国制造商经常使用政府认可的贸易公司来出口他们的产品，因此制造商通常自己没能力向海外销售产品。然而，随着进出口法规放宽限制，中国制造商已经开始通过互联网做自己的直接销售和市场营销。现在，对在中国与厂家建立关系感兴趣的外国公司可以在因特网上找到丰富的信息。此外，中国制造商在与外国公司一起工作和交往时越来越自如，并且在许多业务往来上已经习惯使用英语（尽管有时所说英语不连贯）。

基本的搜索引擎是您开始搜索的好地方。它将为您提供制造商名单，并且过程相对快捷。许多网站提供可观的制造商名单，通常包括联系信息与各厂家的简要说明。然而，这种类型的搜索应该只是一个起点，不是一个详尽的调查。

在互联网搜索发现了一些有可能与之建立关系的制造商之后，要仔细查看每个厂商的网站。通常，厂商网站的中文版要比英文版更详细，这是常见的。为了让自己对这些公司有一个准确的概念，要请一个能流利地说英语和汉语的人来审读中文和英文网站。此外，外国公司应记住，互联网上的所有信息或制造商网站上的信息可能会不准确并且会产生误导。外国公司应采取进一步的措施以确认制造商的要求，这一点很重要。

最初的接触

编制好中国制造商的名单后，要与各制造商直接联系。现在许多中国制造商的销售部都有一名讲英语的员工。然而，最好的方式仍然是外国公司自己有一名会说汉语的员工以使沟通更加顺利。一开始可通过电子邮件和电话来建立外国和中国公司之间的信任以及良好的业务关系。

信任是企业在亚洲成功的关键，所以这开始的一步不应掉以轻心。电子邮件和电话也可以用来回答最初的问题，并确认制造商的生产能力。外国公司应确保中国制造商能够按外国公司的产品规格和标准生产产品。此外，个别中国公司声称他们能够生产某种产品，但实际上他们从另一家公司购买该产品，然后再以更高的价格转卖，这样的事情也有发生。因此，在决定是否与中国公司或制造商进行业务往来之时，不能全靠电子邮件和电话。

决定价格

在与制造商建立了良好的业务关系和沟通流程后，下一步是获得产品报价。如果您有一个“标准”产品，所报价格应该是相当直接的。但如果您的产品有独特的功能或规格，或如果您要求的数量不合常规，一般报价方式可能不是很有用。在这种情况下，可能有必要向中国制造商询问分项报价。外国公司也应该记住，中国制造商倾向于使用公制单位，可能不熟悉英寸或磅。同样重要的是，应询问制造商他们报价的时效。中国经济增长快速，中国的价格也经常上扬，所以报价可能只在短时间内适用。外国企业在从中国购买医疗产品时，还必须增加一些其他的费用到整体成本之中。国际运输、国内运输、关税、可能的旅行费用也需要被纳入采购产品的总成本中。

贸易公司与和工厂的区别

尽管中国制造商越来越直接地出口海外，贸易公司在中国依然是很常见的。贸易公司是作为一个“中间人”从中国制造商处购买产品，并将该产品出售给外国买家。

贸易公司有以下一些优势。首先，这些企业往往有多种产品可供购买。一个拥有众多生产线的外国公司可以通过一家贸易公司来销售自己的大部分产品，相比之下，中国制造商只能生产一两条生产线。第二，贸易公司往往能够以更好的价格购买到产品，因为它们已经与中国的制造商建立起了成熟的关系（也可能大宗地购买）。在某些情况下，它们的价格甚至可能低于外国公司直接与中国制造商接洽的价格。第三，与贸易公司打交道通常要容易一些，因为它们在与外国人交流时往往更有经验（许多贸易公司都有英语为母语的人），与外国公司一起工作时也更有经验。一般来说，贸易公司提供短期利润，与这些公司建立业务关系，所用时间也较短。

贸易公司并不总是外包的最佳方式，这要以外国公司的目标为准。如果一家外国公司希望在中国建立长期的业务关系，与中国制造商的直接接触可能会更有益。外国公司可以与中国制造商发展长期合作关系，同时也可以控制自己产品的设计和质量。为了避免贸易公司在任何时间切断供货，与制造商直接联系会让买方有更强的控制感，并在关系发展、业务量增长之后对价格也可能进行控制。

五、英译汉练习

Text 3

美国商务部部长助理迈克尔C. 卡姆内兹在2012国际医疗设备行业规范会议上的讲话

瑞典斯德哥尔摩

2012年5月10日

杰夫，谢谢你热情的介绍。大家早上好，感谢美国先进医疗技术协会以及欧洲医疗器械行业协会主办此次活动，并邀请我参加。你们当中很多人都知道，今年是这一重要的规范会议连续举办的第五个年头。但你们可能有所不知，美国先进医疗技术协会自1975年起便致力于推动医疗设备行业重大事务的发展，已进行了近40年的宣传呼吁。直到2000年，其以医疗产业制造商协会而闻名，但核心任务并未改变，即通过建立合法、规范、经济的环境，形成有利于医疗技术发展的全球性准入，推动全球医疗卫生事业向前发展。你们今天的努力与他们曾经的付出同等重要。我还想指出，多年来，商务部都与先进医疗技术协会及其领导团队保持着紧密的工作伙伴关系。在此我想特别感谢你们的总裁兼首席执行官斯蒂夫、总顾问克里斯·怀特，以及高级副总裁拉尔夫·艾维斯，感谢他们卓越的领导力及合作精神。同时，对欧洲医疗器械行业协会及其领导，包括代理总裁卢西亚诺·卡达尼所做出的卓越贡献，我也在此一并致谢。

几个月前，斯蒂夫等人邀请我在此次大会上做主旨发言时，我便立即表达了希望到会的意愿，因为医疗技术行业是当今世界增长和创新最为重要的引擎之一。我作为商务部国际贸易局部长助理，职责涉及经济中几乎所有工业及服务业，但是医疗技术行业给我留下最深刻的印象。推动经济增长与繁荣的同时又有益于人类，这样少见的组合却是贵行业的特质。正是这种人类利益与商业利益的完美结合，让商务部以与你们合作而自豪。这也是为什么奥巴马总统国家出口计划将你们列为重点发展行业的原因。

你们的工作始于为病人提供质量一流的护理的承诺，而该承诺影响卓著。例如，在美国，1980年至2000年间医疗技术的进步使平均寿命延长了3年，心脏病死亡率下降50%，中风死亡率下降超过30%，乳腺癌死亡率下降20%。

除了为无数的病患带来拯救生命的福祉之外，贵行业同时也是就业与经济增长引擎。行业数据显示，医疗设备行业在美雇员超过42万人，且该数字呈上升趋势。另外，这42万多名雇员每人又衍生出4份与该行业间接相关的工作。换句话说，仅在美国就大约有200万工人——包括供应商、零件制造商、服务提供商等——从事医疗设备领域相关工作。不仅仅美国如此，在全球一些重要的新兴市场中，该行业也正经历着显著的增长。

尽管众多经济体都在吸引和支持医疗技术领域的创新行业方面表现出兴趣，但事实上，公司仍然面临着限制竞争力、阻碍创新的巨大挑战。置身于高度国际化、经济紧密相连的21世纪，这些挑战主要表现为技术性贸易壁垒，此类所谓的“境内”壁垒会阻碍一个行业的增长，极大地减少开放、自由贸易的益处，受到商务部国际贸易局的密切关注。

众多的行业代表性行动都是通过全球范围内种类繁多的双边交往来实现的。比如，就中国而言，我们的职员刚刚参加了由商务部主持的美中商贸联合委员会制药及医疗设备小组会议。会议集中讨论了关乎两国利益的议题，包括医疗设备安全标准和处于待审阶段的中国医疗设备监管条例。在印度，我们与先进医疗技术协会等组织开展定期合作，通过美印高新技术合作组织解决市场准入壁垒问题。在巴西，我们通过美巴商务对话及其他行动推进解决与医疗设备相关的壁垒问题。例如，近期，我们协助启动了信息交流论坛。此次论坛上，巴西的食品和药物管理局，即巴西国家卫生监督局，首次与私营部门公开会晤。论坛中所进行的讨论促进了国家卫生监督局与该产业的进一步交流接触，并促进巴西国家卫生监督局与美国食品和药物管理局签署数据共享备忘录。去年，我非常高兴能够与先进医疗技术协会共赴巴西政策之旅，并在一系列重大前沿事项上取得显著进展，其中就包括巴西政府与产业间签署的互利行动计划协议，建立起包括3家来自“巴西创新医疗保健行业联盟”的巴西本土协会的行业领头联盟。

当然，以上仅仅是一部分事例。作为全球最具创新力的行业之一，毫无疑问，你们在努力用新的方式引入新产品，延伸创新曲线的同时仍然会面临着市场准入壁垒问题。但是商务部承诺将与你们通力合作，为贵行业服务，努力促进贵行业的进一步发展。

我很高兴，也很荣幸今天能够来到这里，支持你们的工作。如果说我今天要给你们传达一个信息的话，那就是：没有你们的帮助，政府不可能赢得这场战斗，商务部希望与先进医疗技术协会和欧洲医疗器械行业协会及其下属公司保持长久、成功的伙伴关系。谢谢大家。

Text 4

香港食品卫生局常务秘书长李淑仪女士
在香港国际医疗及保健服务展上的讲话

2006年8月17日

尊敬的孙医生、王先生、陈先生、杨先生、凯伊先生、各位尊敬的来宾，女士们、先生们：

我谨代表香港特别行政区政府，向各位表示热烈的欢迎。同时，感谢香港贸易发展局和现代化中医药国际协会邀请我参加此次大会。香港政府十分认可中医药在卫生保健体系中的重要地位。我们在市场营销、贸易、制造、管理、技术以及标准定位等方面的专业知识让香港在挖掘中医药市场潜力方面处于有利地位。过去的几年中，政府始终致力于促进香港中医药事业的发展。

政府战略是建立强有力的针对中医药执业医师、贸易商及业主的管理机制，资助本科教学以保证有足够的执业医师。我们坚信，这些因素对于营造中医药行业繁荣发展的良好环境至关重要。同时，政府致力于提倡“循证中医药学”，让数据得到更广泛的应用。在此方面，我们已经建立起六家中医诊所，年末将新增三家，未来几年还将成立更多。诊所由医院管理局、非政府组织和高等院校三方共同设立，任务之一就是要参与临床研究，协助进行数据收集。医院管理局也在一些医院采用中西医结合的方式进行“循证”临床治疗。同时，卫生部针对60种常用中草药制定了香港中药学标准，供贸易、质量及安全基准参考，并为后续研究打下基础。

政府对中医药发展的蓝图和方向十分明晰。我们将会进一步加强监管体系，加快基础设施建设。监管的目的不是阻碍贸易，而是保护公共卫生，为贸易提供通用的准则。我们希望“香港注册”能够成为中医药行业在当地及国际市场的信誉和质量保障。本着同样的精神，发展循证中医药的目的是夯实该行业及中医药学界进一步研究和发展的基础。

对私立医院参加此次大会，展现香港卫生及医疗护理优质服务的行动，我表示十分赞赏。私立医院、公立医院携手公共部门，共同为香港赢得了令人羡慕的，拥有高临床标准和优质医疗护理服务的声誉。

没有私有领域的积极参与，就没有中医药的现代化。此次大会就是实现这一目标的重要平台，为知识交流和商业合作提供充足的机会。我深信大会上深刻的见解、宝贵的信息和商机会让诸位满载而归。预祝大会完满成功，诸位参会者身体安康。

谢谢大家。

六、汉译英练习

Text 5

Leaders from the Healthcare Reform Office of the State Council Take Questions from the Media on the Issue of Establishing the Purchasing Mechanism for Essential Drugs (Excerpt)

Q: The National System for Essential Drugs has been implemented for over a year, what are the reasons behind the issue of the Purchasing Mechanism?

A: The establishment of the National System for Essential Drugs, aiming at ensuring the basic drug use for the general public, is a major institutional innovation which benefits people's livelihood. Since it was put into effect last year, the system has achieved evident progress, and some initial effects can be seen in the process. To date, over 50% of the government supported grass root healthcare institutions have carried out the National System for Essential Drugs, practicing zero markup sales. Yet, there are some new problems popping up, highlighted by issues which haven't been addressed effectively and reasonably, like the irregular biding and purchasing of essential drugs, and drugs being overpriced. Some drugs are under supplied or stocked out in some region, which may affect the implementation of the National System for Essential Drugs and impact the benefit of the public. In accordance with the spirit and guidance of the Healthcare Reform Leading Group of the State Council, the Healthcare Reform Office of the State Council, together with other relevant department, will conduct deep analysis on the crucial links and prominent problems in the biding and purchasing of essential drugs, borrowing successful centralized purchasing experiences from both home and abroad, soliciting suggestions and opinions from both domestic and overseas experts in this field, so as to propose targeted measures, and draw the first draft of the Purchasing Mechanism. After soliciting opinions from relevant department and local governments, we have revised and improved the draft for several times, and finally produced an edition for the examination and approval of the State Council. Being discussed on the plenary meeting of the Healthcare Reform Office, and deliberated and approved by the plenary meeting of the State Council Healthcare Reform Leading Group, the Purchasing Mechanism has been printed and issued on November 19th by the General Office of the State Council.

Q: What are the overall considerations for the issue of the Purchasing Mechanism? Does it include any innovative measures and highlights?

A: The general thought of the Purchasing Mechanism is to conduct centralized purchasing and unified distribution at provincial (regional, municipal) scale. Combining the guidance of the government with the market mechanism, we should give scope to the advantages of centralized purchasing. Incorporating biding and purchasing, linking quantity and price together, signing contracts, making it a one-stop process, reducing the purchasing cost at the maximum scale, can help to make essential drugs safe and effective, and at the same time with higher quality, more reasonable price, and prompt supplement. Concurrently, they can promote the production and supplement of essential drugs, which brings concrete benefits to our people.

Focusing on those outstanding problems existing in various places, the Purchasing Mechanism has proposed a series of targeted innovative measures centered on quality, price and supplement, the three core elements of essential drugs, including: first, to clarify the liability subject for purchase. A purchasing institution appointed by the provincial health administration will take charge of the purchasing of essential drugs, signing authorization or consignment agreement with government supported grass root healthcare institutions, and sales and purchase contract with drug suppliers, and then fulfilling the contract. Second, adhere to the principles of combining quantity with price. Specify purchasing quantity by drawing up a purchasing plan which helps to make the whole purchasing process a one-stop one, sign the sales and purchase contract, and set a specific date for payment. It can give full play to the advantages of bulk purchase. Third, give priority to quality, and set a reasonable price. Persist in putting quality first, and adopt a "double envelop" method in biding, in order to allow those enterprises with good reputation, quality products and able supplement to participate in the competition. Meanwhile, carry out a thorough investigation on the actual price of essential drugs on the market. In principle, the price for centralized purchasing should be no higher than actual price on the market, so that we can ensure a reasonable purchasing price. Fourth, set up strict credibility record and information disclosure system. Enterprises who violate the rules, such as breach the contract, sell substandard products, or delay the supplement will be put on the record which will be disclosed to the society. We will carry out a strict elimination system. For those enterprises who do not correct their violations in two years, they cannot bid for any drug purchasing. To improve transparency by setting up an online purchasing platform; information like the purchasing price and quantity of essential drugs, and bid winners should be publicized on the internet, which can be supervised by the society, so that we can create an open, fair and just purchasing environment from an institutional perspective.

Text 6

Medical Device Trade

Medical device industry is an industry with the fastest growing speed, and the most active trade contacts in today's world. With the further development of science and technology, medical device industry has gradually become a high-tech one. In recent years, the export of medical equipments in China experiences rapid growth. From 2006 to 2010, medical equipments export enjoyed a double digit growth and 20.94% of compound annual growth rate for five consecutive years, which is higher than the average growth rate of the pharmaceutical and health products industry. In terms of the export subject, transnational tycoons establish production and processing bases in China which can radiate the global market and mobilize the export of high-tech diagnosis and treatment equipments. While private enterprises in China have strength in small and medium equipments, medical dressings and consumables, which makes them the mainstay in the export of the above products.

Over 3,000 foreign-funded enterprises mobilize the growth of China's medical apparatus export, taking half of the total export volume of medical devices for five years in a row. According to the statistics from the Customs, from 2007 to 2011, foreign enterprises shared 58.51%, 57.29%, 59.01%, 58.94% and 52.59% of the total export volume respectively, and their compound annual growth rate registered at 17.36%. As the international medical equipment industry speeding up it transfer, advanced technologies and capitals from abroad will continue to flow into China in the forms of joint cooperation and technology export. Domestic enterprises started to produce some apparatus that used to rely upon import, which enables our country to become an important production and R & D base for medical instruments in the world.

Private enterprises have seen a rapid growth in its export, with its compound annual growth rate registered at 26.9%, which towers over the growth rate of foreign and state owned enterprises. From the year 2007 to 2011, private enterprises took up 28.12%, 30.22%, 30.26%, 31.28% and 37.3% of the total export volume respectively, registering a successive rising, and becoming one of the main force in China's export of medical devices.

With the development of medical device industry, relying on its advanced industrial technologies, adequate scientific and technological talents, strong clinical medicine basis and advantageous policies, the Pearl River Delta, the Yangtze River Delta and the rim of Bohai Bay have become three industrial clusters for medical devices industry. According to the preliminary statistics, both the total output value and the total sales volume of the three regions account for over 80% of the national total. The export layout of medical equipments also reflects this feature, the sum of export volume in the Yangtze River Delta and the Pearl River Delta makes up 70% of the national total.

Disposable consumables, medical dressings and massage appliances are competitive products in China which require lower technologies and larger labor force. The quality of our products can rival those from abroad, while the price is more reasonable; therefore, domestic enterprises enjoy obvious comparative advantages and competitiveness. According to the statistics from the Customs, in terms of such products, private enterprises take up 43.31% of the export, while SOEs account for 8.57%, and domestic enterprises take the lead in this aspect. However, most of our domestic enterprises conduct OEM export. If disposable consumables are 46.05% of the export of the processed products, heath rehabilitation products are 32.27% of the processed products, vigorous efforts are needed in cultivating proprietary brands.

After many years of development, exports increase yearly in some of China's enterprises which have considerable market volume. However, there are still rooms for improvement for China's domestic enterprises.